2022

AF850187

ADVANCES IN MOLECULAR PATHOLOGY

EDITOR-IN-CHIEF

Gregory J. Tsongalis, PhD, HCLD

SECTION EDITORS

Ahmad N. Abou Tayoun, PhD, FACMG

Helen Fernandes, PhD

Andrea Ferreira-Gonzalez, PhD, HCLD(ABB), CC(ABB), FACC

Matthew Lebo, PhD, FACMG

Eric Y. Loo, MD

Ann M. Moyer, MD, PhD

ELSEVIER

Publishing Director, Medical Reference: Dolores Meloni
Editor: Taylor Hayes
Developmental Editor: Hannah Almira Lopez

Editorial Office:
Elsevier, Inc.
1600 John F. Kennedy Blvd,
Suite 1800
Philadelphia, PA 19103-2899

International Standard Serial Number: 2589-4080
International Standard Book Number: 13: 978-0-323-94039-9

ADVANCES IN MOLECULAR PATHOLOGY

CONTRIBUTORS

EDITOR

GREGORY J. TSONGALIS, PhD, HCLD
Professor, Department of Pathology and Laboratory Medicine, The Audrey and Theodore Geisel School of Medicine at Dartmouth, Hanover, New Hampshire, USA; Vice Chair for Research and Director, Laboratory for Clinical Genomics and Advanced Technology (CGAT), Department of Pathology and Laboratory Medicine, Dartmouth Hitchcock Medical Center, Lebanon, New Hampshire, USA

AUTHORS

NOURA S. ABUL-HUSN, MD, PhD
Institute for Genomic Health, Division of Genomic Medicine, Department of Medicine, Department of Genetics and Genomic Sciences, Icahn School of Medicine at Mount Sinai, New York, New York, USA

ERFAN AREF-ESHGHI, MD, PhD
Laboratory Genetics and Genomics Fellow, Division of Genomic Diagnostics, Children's Hospital of Philadelphia, Philadelphia, Pennsylvania, USA

RACHAEL E. BARNEY, BS
Clinical Genomics and Advanced Technology Laboratory, Department of Pathology and Laboratory Medicine, Geisel School of Medicine at Dartmouth, Dartmouth-Hitchcock Medical Center, Lebanon, New Hampshire, USA

ELIZABETH S. BARRIE, PhD
Assistant Professor, Department of Pathology, Virginia Commonwealth University Health System, Richmond, Virginia, USA

GREGORY J. BERRY, PhD
Associate Professor, Co-Director, Clinical Microbiology Service, Department of Pathology and Cell Biology, Columbia University Irving Medical Center, New York, New York, USA

JACOB BROWN, PharmD, MS
University of Minnesota College of Pharmacy, Duluth Department of Pharmacy Practice and Pharmaceutical Sciences, Duluth, Minnesota, USA

FANI CHATZOPOULOU, MSc, PhD
Laboratory of Pharmacology, School of Pharmacy, Aristotle University of Thessaloniki, Laboratory of Microbiology, School of Medicine, Aristotle University of Thessaloniki, Thessaloniki, Greece

ALLISON M. CUSHMAN-VOKOUN, MD, PhD, FCAP
University of Nebraska Medical Center, Omaha, Nebraska, USA

SOPHIE J. DEHARVENGT, PhD
Clinical Genomics and Advanced Technology Laboratory, Department of Pathology and Laboratory Medicine, Geisel School of Medicine at Dartmouth, Dartmouth-Hitchcock Medical Center, Lebanon, New Hampshire, USA

MARK G. EVANS, MD
Division of Pathology and Laboratory Medicine, The University of Texas MD Anderson Cancer Center, Houston, Texas, USA

HELEN FERNANDES, PhD
Professor of Pathology & Cell Biology, Department of Pathology and Cell biology, Laboratory of Personalized Genomic Medicine, New York, NY, USA

ANDREA FERREIRA-GONZALEZ, PhD, HCLD(ABB), CC(ABB), FACC
Professor and Chair, Molecular Diagnostics Division, Director, Molecular Diagnostics Laboratory Virginia Commonwealth University, Richmond, Virginia, USA

DANIEL A. GREEN, MD
Associate Professor, Co-Director, Clinical Microbiology Service, Department of Pathology and Cell Biology, Columbia University Irving Medical Center, New York, New York, USA

DAVID GREGORNIK, PharmD
Director, Pharmacogenomics Program, Children's Minnesota, Minneapolis, Minnesota, USA

SAFINA HAFEEZ, MD
University of Nebraska Medical Center, Omaha, Nebraska, USA

GUOHONG HUANG, PhD
Clinical Genomics and Advanced Technology Laboratory, Department of Pathology and Laboratory Medicine, Geisel School of Medicine at Dartmouth, Dartmouth-Hitchcock Medical Center, Lebanon, New Hampshire, USA

LOREN J. JOSEPH, MD
Assistant Professor, Department of Pathology, Harvard Medical School, Beth Israel Deaconess Medical Center, Boston, Massachusetts, USA

KRISTIN H. KARNER, MD
Associate Professor, Department of Pathology, ARUP Laboratories/University of Utah, Salt Lake City, Utah, USA

J. STEVEN LEEDER, PharmD, PhD
Professor of Pediatrics, Division of Clinical Pharmacology, Toxicology and Therapeutic Innovation, Department of Pediatrics, University of Missouri-Kansas City School of Medicine, Kansas City, Missouri, USA

JOEL A. LEFFERTS, PhD
Clinical Genomics and Advanced Technology Laboratory, Department of Pathology and Laboratory Medicine, Geisel School of Medicine at Dartmouth, Dartmouth-Hitchcock Medical Center, Lebanon, New Hampshire, USA

MARYLIN M. LI, MD
Professor of Pathology and Laboratory Medicine, Division of Genomic Diagnostics, Children's Hospital of Philadelphia, Philadelphia, Pennsylvania, USA

LANE MILLER, MD, MS
Center for Cancer and Blood Disorders, Children's Minnesota, Minneapolis, Minnesota, USA

GEORGE A. MYSTRIDIS, MSc, MBA
Laboratory of Pharmacology, School of Pharmacy, Aristotle University of Thessaloniki, Thessaloniki, Greece

DAMON OLSON, MD
Molecular Pathology Program, Children's Minnesota, Minneapolis, Minnesota, USA

COURTNEY PAETZNICK, PharmD
Pharmacogenomics Program, Children's Minnesota, Minneapolis, Minnesota, USA

GEORGE P. PATRINOS, PhD
Laboratory of Pharmacogenomics and Individualized Therapy, Department of Pharmacy, School of Health Sciences, University of Patras, Greece; Department of Genetics and Genomics, College of Medicine and Health Sciences, United Arab Emirates University, Zayed Center for Health Sciences, United Arab Emirates University, Al-Ain, Abu Dhabi, United Arab Emirates

LAURA B. RAMSEY, PhD
Associate Professor of Pediatrics, Divisions of Clinical Pharmacology and Research in Patient Services, Department of Pediatrics, Cincinnati Children's Hospital, University of Cincinnati College of Medicine, Cincinnati, Ohio, USA

SHIVAPRASAD H. SATHYANARAYANA, PhD
Clinical Genomics and Advanced Technology Laboratory, Department of Pathology and Laboratory Medicine, Geisel School of Medicine at Dartmouth, Dartmouth-Hitchcock Medical Center, Lebanon, New Hampshire, USA

PARTH S. SHAH, MD
Clinical Genomics and Advanced Technology Laboratory, Department of Pathology and Laboratory Medicine, Geisel School of Medicine at Dartmouth, Dartmouth-Hitchcock Medical Center, Lebanon, New Hampshire, USA

ANNA SHESTAKOVA, MD, PhD
Fellow, ARUP Laboratories/University of Utah, Salt Lake City, Utah, USA

EMILY R. SOPER, MS
Institute for Genomic Health, Division of Genomic Medicine, Department of Medicine, Icahn School of Medicine at Mount Sinai, New York, New York, USA

JASON A. SPROWL, PhD
Assistant Professor, Department of Pharmaceutical Sciences, School of Pharmacy and Pharmaceutical Sciences, University at Buffalo, State University of New York, Buffalo, New York, USA

CARLOS A. TORRES-CABALA, MD
Division of Pathology and Laboratory Medicine, The University of Texas MD Anderson Cancer Center, Houston, Texas, USA

IOANNIS S. VIZIRIANAKIS, PhD
Laboratory of Pharmacology, School of Pharmacy, Aristotle University of Thessaloniki, Thessaloniki, Greece; Department of Life and Health Sciences, University of Nicosia, Nicosia, Cyprus

JONATHAN B. WAGNER, DO
Associate Professor of Pediatrics, Division of Clinical Pharmacology, Toxicology and Therapeutic Innovation, Department of Pediatrics, University of Missouri-Kansas City School of Medicine, Ward Family Heart Center, Children's Mercy, Kansas City, Missouri, USA

MAXWELL D. WEIDMANN MD, PhD
Clinical Microbiology Fellow, Department of Pathology and Cell Biology, Columbia University Irving Medical Center, New York, New York, USA

FANN WU, MD, PhD
Associate Professor, Director of Molecular Diagnostics and Epidemiology in Clinical Microbiology Services, Department of Pathology and Cell Biology, Columbia University Irving Medical Center, New York, New York, USA

ADVANCES IN MOLECULAR PATHOLOGY

CONTENTS

VOLUME 5 • 2022

Hematopathology

Cutaneous T-cell lymphoma represents a genetically heterogeneous group of diseases thought to be derived from skin-homing lymphocytes. The genomic landscape of these conditions has been recently redefined to incorporate findings from cutting-edge molecular and cytogenetic testing. Recurrent genetic alterations that have been detected include those associated with chromatin modification, DNA repair, cell cycle control, JAK/STAT pathway activation, TCR/NFκB signaling, and MAPK pathway regulation. Many of these changes can be targeted by current/upcoming personalized therapies.

Accurate diagnosis of mature B-cell lymphomas is essential for adequate treatment. There is a morphologic and immunophenotypic overlap between high-grade B-cell lymphoma (HGBL) with *MYC* and *BCL2* and/or *BCL6* rearrangements, HGBL, not otherwise specified (NOS), and Burkitt-like lymphoma with 11q aberration. Therefore, cytogenetic and molecular testing are essential for an accurate diagnosis. HGBL with *MYC* and *BCL2* and/or *BCL6* rearrangements is defined by rearranged *MYC* and *BCL2* and/or *BCL6* genes, also known as double-hit and triple-hit lymphomas. Burkitt-like lymphoma with 11q is characterized by the absence of the rearrangement of the *MYC* gene and a peculiar aberration of 11q with proximal gain and terminal loss.

Peripheral T-cell lymphoma (PTCL) is a rare and heterogeneous group of mature T-cell malignancies. It is an aggressive form of the disease, which is frequently associated with a poor prognosis. It can be subdivided into four major categories based on the clinical presentation and location of the disease: nodal, extranodal, cutaneous, and leukemic. The diagnostic approach in PTCL requires multiple factors such as clinical presentation, morphology, immunophenotype, cytogenetics, and molecular genetic findings. The recent advances in gene expression profiling and next-generation sequencing technologies have opened up new insights into the pathogenesis and molecular genetic changes of different subtypes of PTCL. In this review article, we will focus on nodal PTCL.

Multiple Myeloma, *59*

By Loren J. Joseph

Multiple myeloma is a malignant clonal proliferation of plasma cells; it evolves through several stages of progressive pathology, marked by one or more of several specific cytogenetic abnormalities and subsequent accumulation of mutations in one or more of 80 driver genes, possibly in conjunction with alterations in stromal cells. Multiple lines of therapy have been developed, directed at different pathways. Each case bears a unique rearrangement of the IGH/L genes that permits sensitive detection of residual disease by next-generation sequencing. Overall survival has improved so dramatically that some experts have started using the "C(ure)" word.

Infectious Disease

Prevalence and Clinical Disease Severity of Respiratory Coinfections During the Coronavirus Disease 2019 Pandemic, *73*

By Maxwell D. Weidmann, Gregory J. Berry, Daniel A. Green, and Fann Wu

Respiratory tract infections represent a global health concern. More than 1 pathogenic organism in the respiratory tract has been widely recognized owing to the availability of molecular detection technologies. However, the association between the occurrence of multiple-pathogen infections and clinical disease severity remains unclear. Multiple infections fall into two broad categories: Coinfection occurs when a person is found to be infected by two or more micro-organisms, but which infection was established first cannot be clearly determined, while superinfection is an infection arising when one or more infections is already present. This review presents an overview of the prevalence and clinical disease severity of respiratory co-infections and superinfections and discusses possible mechanisms of the interactions between viral infections.

Applications of Long-Read Sequencing Technology in Clinical Genomics, *85*

By Shivaprasad H. Sathyanarayana, Sophie J. Deharvengt, Guohong Huang, Rachael E. Barney, Parth S. Shah, and Joel A. Lefferts

Next-generation sequencing (NGS) using traditional short-read sequencing (SRS) has transformed the field of clinical genetics and genomics research. Newer long-read sequencing (LRS) technologies have emerged more recently that are able to reveal specific types of genetic information that traditional SRS technologies may not be able to detect. Detection of structural variants and highly repetitive sequences, differentiating homologous genomic sequences, and establishing allele phasing are some benefits of LRS. This review article highlights the power of LRS technology in different clinical testing areas and addresses some of its current limitations and challenges.

Pharmacogenomics

SLCO1B1 Pharmacogenetics in Pediatrics, *109*

By Laura B. Ramsey, Jason A. Sprowl, J. Steven Leeder, and Jonathan B. Wagner

Organic polypeptide transporting polypetide 1B1 (OATP1B1), encoded by the *SLCO1B1* gene, is a major transporter involved in the hepatic uptake of several endogenous molecules and medications relevant to pediatrics. In children, the magnitude of effect of *SLCO1B1* allelic variation on systemic exposure of statins is similar to that observed in adults, but is associated within genotype variability (>10-fold) that exceeds reported variability in adults; sources of the intra-genotype variability appear to be drug-specific. For methotrexate, the influence of rare variants appears to be comparable to common variants. Taken together, existing pharmacogenetic-driven dosing guidelines based on adult experience may not be directly applicable to pediatric age groups and should be used with caution. Integration of *SLCO1B1* pharmacogenetics into clinical care will benefit from improved knowledge of non-genetic factors that contribute to inter-individual variability in drug disposition.

Implementation of a Clinical Pharmacogenomics Service in a Large Freestanding Pediatric Health System, *119*

By Courtney Paetznick, David Gregornik, Lane Miller, Damon Olson, and Jacob Brown

As a large, freestanding pediatric health system, Children's Minnesota is faced with unique challenges and opportunities with pharmacogenomics (PGx) implementation as compared with adult health systems. The PGx program was initially developed to meet a growing desire to incorporate PGx information into clinical decision-making, particularly in hematology/oncology and behavioral health, and to lead the clinical PGx implementation. Since the launch of the PGx program, new possibilities have emerged with contributions to PGx research and on going development of an in-house genotyping assay as ways to better serve our diverse pediatric population.

Artificial Intelligence/Machine Learning and Mechanistic Modeling Approaches as Translational Tools to Advance Personalized Medicine Decisions, *131*

By George A. Mystridis, Fani Chatzopoulou, George P. Patrinos, and Ioannis S. Vizirianakis

Nowadays, advancements in omics-based methodologies, data analysis, informatics, and bioinformatics, as well as nanotechnology have continuously led to a more digitized, robust, as well as information-based environment in biomedicine and health care. Precision in therapy will be ensured through the application of computerized platforms, as well as interdisciplinary integrated analysis and decision-making. In this review, artificial intelligence/machine learning approaches and mechanistic modeling methodologies will be discussed as translational tools aiming to advance personalized medicine decisions and patient care.

Solid tumors

This chapter will focus on a subtype of liquid biopsy that uses cell-free DNA as a blood-based biomarker to detect and monitor solid tumors. While this assay has clear advantages in terms of patient safety, improved turnaround time, and the ability to sample more frequently over time, the complexity lies in its application and interpretation.

Advances in Molecular Pathology 5 (2022) xv–xvi
ADVANCES IN MOLECULAR PATHOLOGY

Editorial

Monkeypox: Another Virus Gone Viral!

Monkeypox virus is a double-stranded DNA virus belonging to the *Orthopoxvirus* genus, which also includes variola (smallpox), vaccinia, and cowpox viruses. The virus can be transmitted to humans from animals and is therefore a zoonotic disease. In humans, Monkeypox transmission occurs from direct or indirect contact with the body fluids or infected lesions or via respiratory droplets. The symptoms in infected individuals are very similar to those seen in the past in smallpox patients, although it is clinically less severe.

The name monkeypox originates from the initial discovery of the virus in monkeys in 1958. A few years later, the disease was considered endemic in central and west African countries. Since then, sporadic cases, related to travel, were reported globally. In May 2022, outbreaks of the virus were reported in nonendemic countries. As of August 15, 2022, the Centers for Disease Control and Prevention (CDC) has reported over 38,000 confirmed cases in 387 countries worldwide, with the United States, Spain, Germany, and the United Kingdom having the largest number of reported cases (Fig. 1). The ensuing deaths prompted the World Health Organization (WHO) to declare Monkeypox virus a global health emergency.

There are two clades of monkeypox virus: West African clade and the Congo Basin (Central African) clade, that were recently renamed by the WHO as clade I and clade II, respectively. The differences in clinical presentation of the two known clades of the orthopoxvirus genome structure suggest that changes among a relatively small number of Open Reading Frames (ORFs) can be attributed to proteins that modulate viral pathogenesis or host response.[1,2] Sequencing studies suggest that the current outbreak is likely due to a virus from clade 1 (West African clade), which is often associated with milder disease and apparent human-to-human transmission.[3]

On May 17, 2022, the CDC developed, and the Food and Drug Administration cleared, the Non-variola Orthopoxvirus Real-time PCR Primer and Probe Set (nonvariola Orthopoxvirus assay) for testing through the Laboratory Response Network (LRN) member laboratories.[4] This polymerase chain reaction (PCR) diagnostic assay detects most commonly known human pathogenic Orthopoxviruses (eg, Vaccinia, Cowpox, and Monkeypox viruses) but not Variola virus, the causative agent of smallpox. The assay uses two sets of PCR primers and probes. One set of primers targets the Orthopoxvirus DNA polymerase gene (E9L; GenBank L22579). The second set amplifies the human RNase P gene as an internal control in monitoring specimen quality. Results of this assay are for the potential identification of nonvariola Orthopoxvirus DNA. Since the primers are not specific for monkeypox, positive results must be interpreted in conjunction with clinical presentation for the presumptive diagnosis and treatment of monkeypox. Confirmation of monkeypox is obtained from appropriate state or national public health authorities, including the CDC.

From the laboratory diagnostic perspective, rapid testing for the monkeypox virus did not ramp up fast enough to clamp down community spread of the virus. Testing for Orthopoxviruses beyond LRN members is just starting to establish itself, and screening sites are still trying to launch high-throughput testing. Furthermore, even though effective vaccines for monkeypox were available, the short supply and lack of organization affected access especially to high-risk individuals. The bottom line is we are still floundering at handling emerging pandemics. Mobilizing rapid testing and enhancing preventative measures to nip the problem in the bud continue to be daunting to health care. Emerging infections have gone viral over the past 3 years, and molecular testing methodologies can offer a clear path to identify and possibly control further infections.

Helen Fernandes, PhD
Department of Pathology and Cell biology
Columbia University Irving Medical Center
New York, NY 10032, USA

E-mail address: hf2340@cumc.columbia.edu

https://doi.org/10.1016/j.yamp.2022.08.003
2589-4080/22/

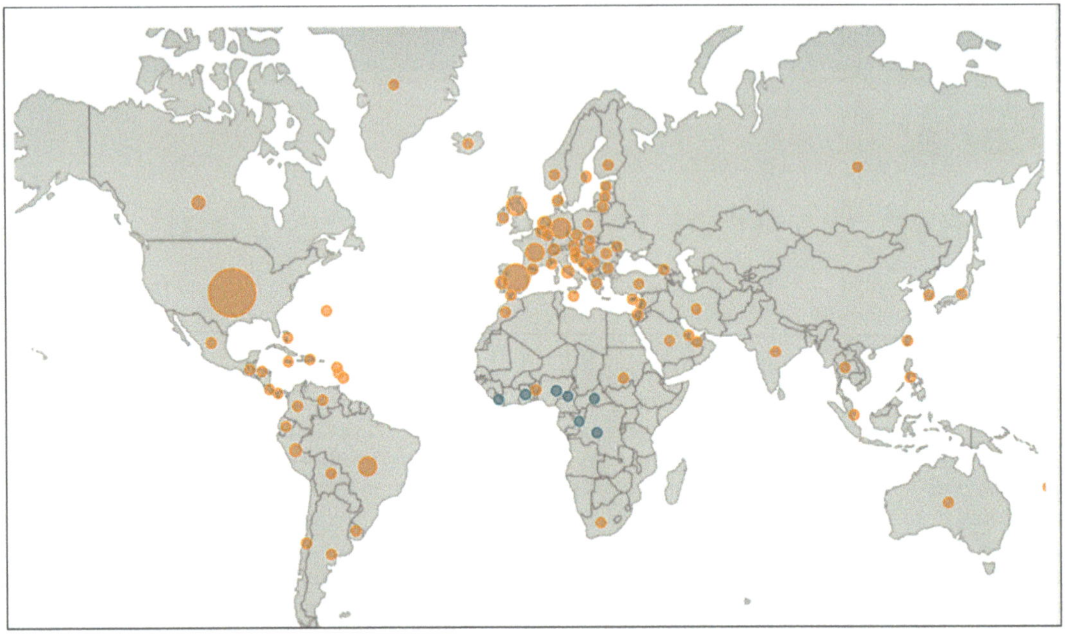

FIG. 1 Distribution of Monkeypox virus infections worldwide. (From 2022 Monkeypox Outbreak Global Map. Centers for Disease Control and Prevention. https://www.cdc.gov/poxvirus/monkeypox/response/2022/world-map.html. Published August 4, 2022.)

REFERENCES

1 2022 Monkeypox outbreak global map. Centers for Disease Control and Prevention. Available at: https://www.cdc.gov/poxvirus/monkeypox/response/2022/world-map.html. Accessed August 16, 2022.

2 Likos AM, Sammons SA, Olson VA, et al. A tale of two clades: monkeypox viruses. J Gen Virol 2005;86(Pt. 10): 2661–72.

3 Isidro J, Borges V, Pinto M, et al. Phylogenomic characterization and signs of microevolution in the 2022 multi-country outbreak of monkeypox virus. Nat Med 2022;28(8): 1569–72. https://doi.org/10.1038/s41591-022-01907-y.

4 Test procedure: non-variola orthopoxvirus generic real-time PCR test. Available at: https://www.cdc.gov/poxvirus/monkeypox/pdf/Non-variola-Orthopoxvirus-Generic-Real-Time-PCR-Test.pdf. Accessed August 16, 2022.

ADVANCES IN MOLECULAR PATHOLOGY

Preface

Molecular Pathology: Life Beyond the Pandemic

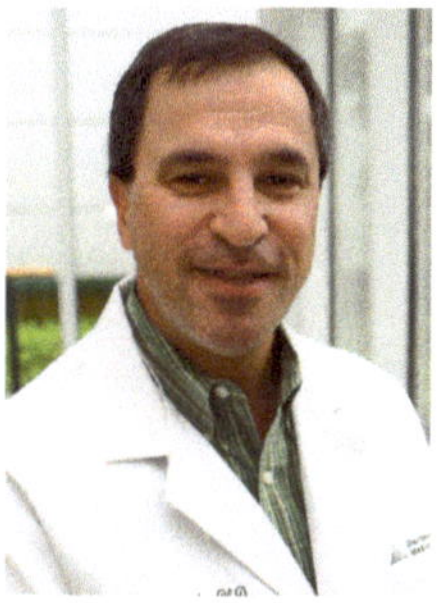

Gregory J. Tsongalis, PhD, HCLD
Editor-in-Chief

As most of our laboratories were called upon to provide some type of severe acute respiratory syndrome coronavirus 2 (SARS-CoV-2) testing during the pandemic, we also were charged with addressing major challenges in laboratory practices over the past 2.5 years. At the time of this writing, COVID-19 cases are back on the increase in the United States, and the BA.5 Omicron variant is now the dominant strain. Mortalities due to the virus, however, have significantly decreased. We are beginning to see relief in supply chain provisions, and instrument requests have subsided nationally. Staffing has become more permanent versus parttime or traveler-type technologists, and the polymerase chain reaction (PCR) has been forever engraved in the layperson's mind. It is hard to say if the SARS-CoV-2 will ever be abolished or if it will become another part of our "normalcy." What I am confident of is that molecular pathology efforts will once again be ramped up, and new and improved methods and clinical applications will rise from beneath the dark yet educational experiences of these past few years.

This fifth issue of *Advances in Molecular Pathology* embodies the fact that there is life in the laboratory beyond COVID-19 testing. We include articles that span the clinical applications of molecular technologies for genetic diseases, hematologic diseases, infectious diseases, pharmacogenomics, informatics, and solid tumors. I have opted not to include a "special" section on COVID-19, as we all must move past this and return to the R&D efforts of prepandemic times. This issue contains articles that discuss the latest clinical applications of molecular technologies from hereditary cancer syndromes through artificial intelligence applications in pharmacogenomics.

I am grateful to those friends and colleagues who once again agreed to becoming section editors and authors of the fantastic articles presented here.

Happy reading!

Gregory J. Tsongalis, PhD, HCLD
Department of Pathology and Laboratory Medicine
1 Medical Center Drive
Lebanon, NH 03756, USA

E-mail address: Gregory.j.tsongalis@hitchcock.org

https://doi.org/10.1016/j.yamp.2022.08.001
2589-4080/22/

Genetics

Advances in Molecular Pathology 5 (2022) 1–7
ADVANCES IN MOLECULAR PATHOLOGY

Polygenic Risk Scores in Clinical Care

Emily R. Soper, MS[a,b], Noura S. Abul-Husn, MD, PhD[a,b,c,*]
[a]Institute for Genomic Health, Icahn School of Medicine at Mount Sinai, One Gustave L. Levy Place, Box 1041, New York, NY 10029, USA; [b]Division of Genomic Medicine, Department of Medicine, Icahn School of Medicine at Mount Sinai, New York, NY, USA; [c]Department of Genetics and Genomic Sciences, Icahn School of Medicine at Mount Sinai, New York, NY, USA

KEYWORDS
• Polygenic risk score • Genomic medicine • Genomic risk • Common disease
• Genome-wide association study • Genetic risk

KEY POINTS
- Polygenic risk scores (PRS) combine risk from hundreds to millions of genetic variants in an individual to give an overall estimate of risk for a common disease.
- PRS can be generated from a saliva or blood sample using relatively inexpensive genotyping technologies.
- PRS may help to identify individuals at high risk of disease early on, potentially allowing for lifestyle modifications or clinical interventions to reduce disease risk.
- PRS may be combined with established clinical and other nongenetic risk factors to provide individualized risk assessments that guide clinical decision-making.
- Challenges remain to the clinical implementation of PRS, including a need for optimization in non-European ancestry populations, demonstration of clinical utility, and generation of evidence-based management guidelines.
- Despite the need for further research, PRS are increasingly available through direct-to-consumer testing and clinical testing, for example in hereditary cancer.

INTRODUCTION

In the last two decades, major investments have been made to generate large-scale genomic datasets and to perform genome-wide association studies (GWAS), in an effort to understand the genetic underpinnings of common diseases [1]. Today, large GWAS can include hundreds of thousands of individuals, and can explain large proportions of disease heritability [2]. These GWAS have uncovered the contributions of inherited variants to thousands of common diseases [3]. Importantly, GWAS have led to the understanding that the vast majority of common, adult-onset diseases are polygenic in nature, involving numerous common genetic variants (or risk alleles) that each contributes a small effect on disease risk. Although each of these variants in isolation is not informative for evaluating a patient's risk of disease, approaches to combine sets of variants from GWAS are increasingly being used to assess risk.

Polygenic risk scores (PRS) are a way of combining sets of genetic variants from GWAS, most commonly by calculating a weighted sum of the variants an individual carries. PRS can be generated from a saliva or blood sample using relatively inexpensive genotyping technologies. Compared with monogenic (single gene) disease risk, PRS have the potential to identify much larger proportions of the population at high risk for disease [4]. Despite concerns about the performance and clinical utility of PRS, many studies have shown that PRS can predict disease risk for an increasing number of common diseases. Here, we discuss how PRS are generated and validated, how they can be interpreted and used to guide clinical care, and ongoing

*Corresponding author, *E-mail address:* noura.abul-husn@mssm.edu

https://doi.org/10.1016/j.yamp.2022.07.001
2589-4080/22/

challenges and considerations for widespread implementation.

GENERATION, VALIDATION, AND EVALUATION OF POLYGENIC RISK SCORES

For most common diseases, which are multifactorial in nature, a single genetic variant is generally insufficient to inform disease risk. However, GWAS have uncovered thousands of risk variants linked to common diseases [1], and PRS are a way of aggregating and quantifying the effects of these to provide sufficient information to predict disease risk (Fig. 1) [4]. PRS development and validation are active areas of research. A common approach to generating a PRS is to calculate a weighted sum of the risk variants associated with a disease, based on current knowledge of these variants and their weights obtained from the largest or most informative GWAS [5]. The distribution of the PRS for a given disease in population samples is expected to be normal, and individuals at the extreme ends of the distribution may be at sufficiently increased (or decreased) risk of disease to warrant differential considerations for clinical care.

Once a PRS is developed, its performance must be validated in an independent sample with known case/control status for the disease. If the PRS is found to be predictive of disease, it can then be applied to individuals with unknown disease status. For each individual, the number of variants (0, 1, or 2) carried at each locus is summed, weighted by the effect size. The outcome is a single score quantifying the individual's risk for the disease, which is benchmarked against the population [5]. The validity of PRS can be evaluated by determining whether it can separate the population into categories with sufficiently distinct degrees of disease risk to guide decision-making, either alone or in combination with clinical risk factors [6].

There are several advanced methods to optimize variant selection and weight estimation for PRS calculation, including pruning and thresholding, penalized regression, and linkage disequilibrium prediction [7–9]. Many ongoing efforts aim to improve PRS calculation to yield the best predictive model for a given disease, which requires careful consideration of genetic architecture, sample size of discovery GWAS, thresholds for risk variant selection, linkage disequilibrium, and weight assignment for selected variants. An important consideration is that most GWAS to date have been conducted in European ancestry populations [10]. As a result, the predictive ability of PRS is attenuated in other population groups, particularly in those with African ancestry [11]. The predictive performance of PRS will improve with increasingly large sample sizes and the inclusion of ancestrally diverse populations in GWAS. Hence, the PRS estimated for an individual today is likely to change in the future.

Evaluation of the clinical utility of PRS in improving patient health is needed to support the widespread integration of PRS into clinical care. Mature PRS with potential to improve patient outcomes are already available for a few common diseases, such as coronary artery disease [12–15] and breast cancer [16–20]. For these and other diseases, individuals at the high end of the PRS distribution have been shown to have disease risk equivalent to that conferred by monogenic risk [4]. In addition, PRS can help further stratify disease risk when combined with monogenic risk information [21]. Based on this growing body of evidence, PRS-based stratification of disease risk should help to inform

FIG. 1 Generation, validation, and use of polygenic risk scores (PRS). To develop a PRS (*A* and *B*), summary statistics are first obtained from a genome-wide association study, from which risk variants are identified and weighted appropriately. The PRS must then be validated in an independent sample with known case/control status for comparison (*C*) before it can be used to calculate patient-specific risk to inform care (*D*). (A and B from Manhatton Plot GWAS study ALS, by Dr. Jan H. Veldink. https://commons.wikimedia.org/wiki/File:Manhatton_Plot_GWAS_study_ALS.png; under CC BY-SA 3.0)

surveillance and management strategies to mitigate risk, and improve patient outcomes. Although the clinical utility of single-gene testing for many monogenic conditions has been established, evidence for the clinical utility of PRS to reduce morbidity and mortality is lagging [22]. Clinical trials and other research studies to evaluate the clinical utility of PRS are underway.

TRANSLATING POLYGENIC RISK SCORES FROM RESEARCH INTO CLINICAL CARE

Several critical steps are involved in translating PRS from research into clinical care. First, as described above, are ongoing research efforts to optimize PRS performance through advances in statistical methods and the use of larger and more diverse study cohorts, and to show clinical utility. Evidence-based practices to integrate PRS into clinical care require standards for PRS reporting that facilitate reproducibility and generalizability [23]. The development of reporting standards is already underway. For example, the Clinical Genomics Resource consortium and the Polygenic Score Catalog published a joint statement to recommend reporting standards for PRS, which address components of analytical validity, clinical validity, clinical utility, and ethical considerations [24]. These standards aim to improve transparency in PRS development, acknowledge the limitations of these scores, and ultimately facilitate their translation into clinical care.

Once a PRS is considered suitable for clinical implementation, a clinical laboratory test is needed to generate and report PRS results from an individual patient's blood or saliva sample. This involves the development of an analytically and clinically valid testing pipeline to calculate, interpret, and report PRS results for an individual [25]. Finally, the PRS result must be framed in the context of the patient's full clinical picture to guide clinical decision-making. Neither PRS nor monogenic risk factors can be altered to change a patient's risk profile, unlike other nongenetic clinical or environmental risk factors (eg, reducing cholesterol levels to lower the risk of myocardial infarction). However, as one of many risk factors to consider for a common condition, PRS can be used to guide decision-making around risk management (eg, to better estimate the risk of developing coronary artery disease in an individual with a history of smoking, hypertension, and hypercholesterolemia [6]).

Ideally, PRS can be not just considered alongside but also combined with other risk factors to provide patients and their providers with a holistic risk estimate for a given disease. To date, this has been most commonly applied in the space of breast cancer and coronary artery disease, where integrated risk assessment models based on data from large research studies have been developed.

Breast cancer. The Breast and Ovarian Analysis of Disease Incidence and Carrier Estimation Algorithm (BOADICEA) model integrates a number of known risk factors to estimate the risk to develop breast cancer, including personal (lifestyle, hormonal, mammographic density) and family history [26,27]. It also incorporates monogenic and polygenic risk based on a 313-variant PRS [18]. Clinicians can apply this model via the CanRisk web tool (http://www.canrisk.org).

Coronary artery disease. The incorporation of PRS into some integrated risk models, such as the pooled cohorts equation [12], QRISK [12], and the Framingham risk score [15], shows promise in better predicting risk of coronary artery disease when combined with known family history and personal risk factors. This in turn may better identify who may benefit from risk-reducing therapies, with the goal of preventing disease [24].

REPORTING RISK FROM POLYGENIC RISK SCORES

Once a PRS has been developed and validated in the population(s) of interest, and a valid clinical assay is in place, clinical PRS results can be generated on an individual basis. One challenge is how to report this complex genetic information in a way that accurately describes risk and can be understood by both clinicians and patients. Importantly, PRS is not deterministic–even a patient with a high PRS will not definitively develop disease. It is critical to contextualize this risk information in such a way that it can be meaningfully translated into clinical care and decision-making.

As PRS have begun to make their way into the physician's office via clinical testing [28], direct-to-consumer tests [29], and clinical research initiatives [30], three common ways of presenting risk have emerged: percentile rank to place an individual's risk within the distribution of others in the population; a comparative risk, such as relative risk or odds ratio, to describe the magnitude of risk in relation to a reference population; and absolute risk denoting an estimated percentage risk to develop the associated disease within the lifetime or a specified length of time (Box 1) [31]. Each may provide different insights when incorporating PRS into clinical care.

A percentile rank provides a sense of where the patient stands relative to their peers, which may be

> **BOX 1**
> **Common methods of reporting polygenic risk.**
>
> - Percentile: Ranking an individual within the distribution of risk gives perspective on the proportion of individuals in a given population who have a higher and lower PRS than the patient.
> - Comparative risk: A comparative risk statistic, such as a relative risk or odds ratio, frames the individual's risk against that of the average risk in the population.
> - Absolute risk: The absolute risk can be reported as a percentage estimate of remaining risk over the lifetime or a specified period of time. PRS may be combined with clinical risk factors in a validated risk prediction model to hone absolute risk estimation.

motivating in making and adhering to lifestyle changes for those within the high-risk end of the distribution. It does not, however, provide insight into how likely the patient is to develop disease, as it does not account for the overall proportion of risk that is heritable. For conditions that are mainly driven by nongenetic factors, even someone at the highest end of PRS distribution may not be at high personal risk to develop disease.

A comparative risk statistic or absolute risk estimate speaks to the magnitude of risk. Where standard screening guidelines exist, these approaches to risk representation can help to clarify whether an individual crosses a risk threshold at which high-risk screening or preventive interventions would be typically considered (for example, consideration for the addition of annual surveillance magnetic resonance imaging for women with 20%–25% risk or higher for breast cancer [32]). Although absolute risk may be most readily conceptualized by patients and providers, accurate estimates will depend on the development of robust prediction models that adequately account for relevant risk factors and population differences.

In addition to a numeric risk statistic, PRS reports may include a more general description of risk (eg, "increased risk" or "typical risk" [29,33]). A PRS report may also include graphical representation of risk, such as an infographic pointing to an individual's placement along the normal distribution curve for percentile, a bar chart that represents the individual's risk relative to both the average population risk and an action threshold for a comparative risk, or a graph displaying risk over time, again typically displaying general population risk and a high-risk threshold.

Because of the challenges in portability of PRS across ancestry groups, PRS reports should include information about which population(s) the PRS is validated in, whether PRS is validated in the patient's specific ancestry group, and the degree of certainty regarding the risk statistic (eg, confidence intervals for an odds ratio).

CONSIDERATIONS IN COMMUNICATING POLYGENIC RISK SCORES

Although numerical values used to report risk based on PRS are typically quite specific, we emphasize that they are estimates, which by definition are imprecise. In addition, risk thresholds at which patients are advised to take medical action may be construed as dogma, when in fact many of these may be expert opinion-based rather than evidence-based [31]. The communication of this uncertainty to patients is key for contextualization and shared decision-making, and has not been shown to impact patient trust [34]. Genetic counselors receive specialized training in this type of risk communication and thus may facilitate patient understanding of complex genomic information. In addition to risk information, counseling around PRS could include a discussion of the following:

- The multifactorial nature of the common disease and an evaluation of other relevant risk factors in the individual
- Genetic and genomic risk information is not deterministic
- Although polygenic risk is inherited, it does not follow a straightforward inheritance pattern, and individuals from the same family may have a range of PRS
- PRS cannot be changed; however, other lifestyle and environmental risk factors can
- Research into the potential clinical utility of PRS in ongoing, which may lead to the future development of evidence-based clinical management guidelines
- Assessment of patient values and perceived personal utility of PRS to guide decision-making

POLYGENIC RISK SCORES TODAY AND IN THE FUTURE

PRS have the potential to enhance disease risk prediction, improve diagnosis of disease, predict disease progression, and tailor clinical decision making (Box 2) [6]. Because PRS can identify substantially larger

BOX 2
Potential benefits and limitations/challenges to current clinical use of polygenic risk scores.

Potential benefits (also see Fig. 2)

- Early diagnosis of existing disease leading to earlier treatment and improved outcomes
- Clarifying disease diagnosis to optimize appropriate treatment, for example, differentiating between type 1 versus type 2 diabetes [35]
- Identification of individuals with disease likely to benefit from a specific treatment option (precision medicine)
- Prompting beneficial health behavior modifications, for example, disclosure of PRS for coronary artery disease and increased sense of control and interest in health [36], lifestyle modifications [37], and uptake of statin therapy [14] in the MI-GENES study
- Clarifying risk in individuals with pathogenic variants in moderate penetrance genes (such as *CHEK2, ATM, PALB2,* and breast cancer risk), for example, clinical practice resource from the American College of Medical Genetics and Genomics recommends personalizing breast cancer risk assessment using a tool such as CanRisk, which may include PRS, in women who are positive for a *PALB2* pathogenic variant [38]
- Improving population health

Potential limitations/challenges

- Additional data on clinical utility and cost-effectiveness are needed
- Education about PRS for physicians and patients is needed
- No current standards exist for insurance coverage for PRS testing
- Insurance may not cover screening or risk-reducing interventions for individuals with high risk identified by PRS, as consensus guidelines have yet to be developed
- Portability of PRS across ancestry groups
    - Limited data in non-European ancestry populations creates the potential for exacerbation of health disparities due to poorer performance of PRS
    - Even with adequate data from diverse populations leading to better risk prediction in non-European ancestry populations, PRS has the potential to contribute to health disparities already in place [39]
- Concerns about privacy and genetic discrimination should be addressed, as with any genetic testing [39]

proportions of the population at high risk for disease than monogenic risk, PRS have greater potential for public health impact. Genetic information to calculate PRS for any number of conditions can be generated from a single, relatively inexpensive genetic test, and PRS reports are already available through certain clinical and direct-to-consumer tests. As such, clinicians can expect to engage with patients today about the current value of PRS-related information; for example, for individuals with clinical risk factors placing them near

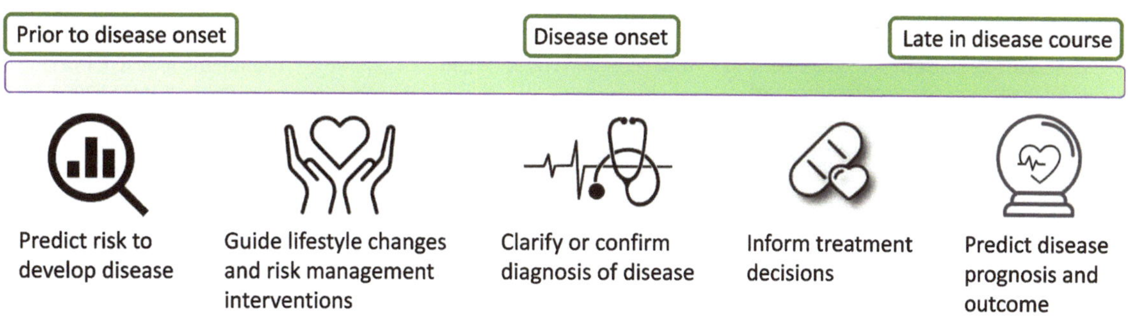

FIG. 2 Opportunities for the clinical use of polygenic risk scores (PRS) across the spectrum of disease course. Before the onset of a disease, even very early in life, PRS may help to predict risk and guide decisions around interventions for risk reduction and early detection. At disease onset, PRS may help to pinpoint or clarify a diagnosis and guide appropriate treatment. PRS may also be informative late in the course of disease by providing insight into prognosis and outcomes.

an action threshold, the addition of PRS may help with decision-making about an intervention (eg, initiating statin therapy to lower coronary artery disease risk) [6].

As with any emerging technology, PRS will take time to integrate appropriately and fully into patient care, and to establish clinical utility [22]. In essence, PRS represent a single point in a constellation of risk factors that apply to an individual patient, and should be framed in the context of the patient's full clinical picture. Understood in this way, PRS can be seen in the same way as other well-understood and widely used risk factors: another lens through which risk of common disease may be clarified.

CLINICS CARE POINTS

- Genome-wide association studies have led to the discovery of millions of genetic variants whose individual effect on common disease risk can be summed to create an overall polygenic risk score (PRS) with an appreciable impact on risk
- PRS must be validated separately in each population of interest
- Overall impact of PRS on total disease risk will depend on factors such as total heritability of disease, and the presence of other nongenetic and monogenic risk factors
- Different ways of reporting PRS are possible, such as a percentile rank or as a measure of risk magnitude, and counseling patients regarding the nature of risk will be key
- Clinical, direct-to-consumer, and clinical research reports may include PRS
- Validated risk models for breast cancer and coronary artery disease now allow for the incorporation of PRS into overall risk estimates in certain populations
- As PRS become more commonplace and clinical utility is clarified, clinicians should be prepared to consider them as one of many factors in assessing patients' risk for common diseases, and to appropriately counsel patients about their use

DISCLOSURE

NSA-H is a scientific advisory board member for Allelica. ERS has nothing to disclose.

ACKNOWLEDGEMENT

N.S.A.-H. is supported by the National Institutes of Health, National Human Genome Research Institute (NHGRI U01 HG011176) and National Heart, Lung, and Blood Institute (NHLBI R01 HL155356). N.S.A.-H. is an employee and equity holder of 23andMe; serves as a scientific advisory board member for Allelica; received personal fees from Genentech, Allelica, and 23andMe; received research funding from Akcea; and was previously employed by Regeneron Pharmaceuticals. E.R.S has nothing to disclose.

REFERENCES

[1] Visscher PM, Wray NR, Zhang Q, et al. 10 Years of GWAS Discovery: Biology, Function, and Translation. Am J Hum Genet 2017;101(1):5–22.

[2] Uffelmann E, Huang QQ, Munung NS, et al. Genome-wide association studies. Nat Rev Methods Primers 2021;1(1):1–21.

[3] Burdett T, Hastings E, Welter D. SPOT, EMBL-EBI, NHGRI. GWAS Catalog. Available at: https://www.ebi.ac.uk/gwas/. Accessed March 30, 2022.

[4] Khera AV, Chaffin M, Aragam KG, et al. Genome-wide polygenic scores for common diseases identify individuals with risk equivalent to monogenic mutations. Nat Genet 2018;50(9):1219–24.

[5] Chatterjee N, Shi J, García-Closas M. Developing and evaluating polygenic risk prediction models for stratified disease prevention. Nat Rev Genet 2016;17(7):392–406.

[6] Torkamani A, Wineinger NE, Topol EJ. The personal and clinical utility of polygenic risk scores. Nat Rev Genet 2018;19(9):581–90.

[7] Ge T, Chen CY, Ni Y, et al. Polygenic prediction via Bayesian regression and continuous shrinkage priors. Nat Commun 2019;10(1):1776. https://doi.org/10.1038/s41467-019-09718-5.

[8] Choi SW, O'Reilly PF. PRSice-2: Polygenic Risk Score software for biobank-scale data. Gigascience 2019;8(7). https://doi.org/10.1093/gigascience/giz082.

[9] Vilhjálmsson BJ, Yang J, Finucane HK, et al. Modeling Linkage Disequilibrium Increases Accuracy of Polygenic Risk Scores. Am J Hum Genet 2015;97(4):576–92. https://doi.org/10.1016/j.ajhg.2015.09.001.

[10] Fatumo S, Chikowore T, Choudhury A, et al. A roadmap to increase diversity in genomic studies. Nat Med 2022;28(2): 243–50. https://doi.org/10.1038/s41591-021-01672-4.

[11] Martin AR, Kanai M, Kamatani Y, et al. Publisher Correction: Clinical use of current polygenic risk scores may exacerbate health disparities. Nat Genet 2021;53(5): 763. https://doi.org/10.1038/s41588-021-00797-z.

[12] Elliott J, Bodinier B, Bond TA, et al. Predictive Accuracy of a Polygenic Risk Score–Enhanced Prediction Model vs a Clinical Risk Score for Coronary Artery Disease. JAMA 2020; 323(7):636. https://doi.org/10.1001/jama.2019.22241.

[13] Inouye M, Abraham G, Nelson CP, et al. Genomic Risk Prediction of Coronary Artery Disease in 480,000 Adults: Implications for Primary Prevention. J Am Coll Cardiol 2018; 72(16):1883–93. https://doi.org/10.1016/j.jacc.2018.07.079.

[14] Kullo IJ, Jouni H, Austin EE, et al. Incorporating a Genetic Risk Score Into Coronary Heart Disease Risk Estimates: Effect on Low-Density Lipoprotein Cholesterol Levels (the MI-GENES Clinical Trial). Circulation 2016;133(12):1181–8. https://doi.org/10.1161/CIRCULATIONAHA.115.020109.

[15] Abraham G, Havulinna AS, Bhalala OG, et al. Genomic prediction of coronary heart disease. Eur Heart J 2016;37(43): 3267–78. https://doi.org/10.1093/eurheartj/ehw450.

[16] Kapoor PM, Mavaddat N, Choudhury PP, et al. Combined Associations of a Polygenic Risk Score and Classical Risk Factors With Breast Cancer Risk. J Natl Cancer Inst 2021;113(3):329–37. https://doi.org/10.1093/jnci/djaa056.

[17] Kuchenbaecker KB, McGuffog L, Barrowdale D, et al. Evaluation of Polygenic Risk Scores for Breast and Ovarian Cancer Risk Prediction in BRCA1 and BRCA2 Mutation Carriers. J Natl Cancer Inst 2017;109(7). https://doi.org/10.1093/jnci/djw302.

[18] Mavaddat N, Michailidou K, Dennis J, et al. Polygenic Risk Scores for Prediction of Breast Cancer and Breast Cancer Subtypes. Am J Hum Genet 2019;104(1): 21–34. https://doi.org/10.1016/j.ajhg.2018.11.002.

[19] Zhang X, Rice M, Tworoger SS, et al. Addition of a polygenic risk score, mammographic density, and endogenous hormones to existing breast cancer risk prediction models: A nested case-control study. Plos Med 2018;15(9):e1002644. https://doi.org/10.1371/journal.pmed.1002644.

[20] Lakeman IMM, Hilbers FS, Rodríguez-Girondo M, et al. Addition of a 161-SNP polygenic risk score to family history-based risk prediction: impact on clinical management in non- breast cancer families. J Med Genet 2019; 56(9):581–9. https://doi.org/10.1136/jmedgenet-2019-106072.

[21] Fahed AC, Wang M, Homburger JR, et al. Polygenic background modifies penetrance of monogenic variants for tier 1 genomic conditions. Nat Commun 2020;11(1): 3635. https://doi.org/10.1038/s41467-020-17374-3.

[22] Kumuthini J, Zick B, Balasopoulou A, et al. The clinical utility of polygenic risk scores in genomic medicine practices: a systematic review. *Hum Genet* Published Online 2022. https://doi.org/10.1007/s00439-022-02452-x.

[23] Wand H, Knowles JW, Clarke SL. The need for polygenic score reporting standards in evidence-based practice: lipid genetics use case. Curr Opin Lipidol 2021;32(2):89–95. https://doi.org/10.1097/MOL.0000000000000733.

[24] Wand H, Lambert SA, Tamburro C, et al. Improving reporting standards for polygenic scores in risk prediction studies. Nature 2021;591(7849):211–9. https://doi.org/10.1038/s41586-021-03243-6.

[25] Hao L, Kraft P, Berriz GF, et al. Development of a clinical polygenic risk score assay and reporting workflow. Nat Med 2022. https://doi.org/10.1038/s41591-022-01767-6 Published online.

[26] Lee A, Mavaddat N, Wilcox AN, et al. BOADICEA: a comprehensive breast cancer risk prediction model incorporating genetic and nongenetic risk factors. Genet Med 2019;21(8): 1708–18. https://doi.org/10.1038/s41436-018-0406-9.

[27] Carver T, Hartley S, Lee A, et al. CanRisk Tool-A Web Interface for the Prediction of Breast and Ovarian Cancer Risk and the Likelihood of Carrying Genetic Pathogenic Variants. Cancer Epidemiol Biomarkers Prev 2021; 30(3):469–73. https://doi.org/10.1158/1055-9965.EPI-20-1319.

[28] RiskScore. Myriad MyRisk Published February 19, 2022. Available at: https://myriad.com/myrisk/riskscore/. Accessed March 31, 2022.

[29] How 23andMe predicted my likelihood of developing the "disease of kings." 23andMe Blog Published July 14, 2021. Available at: https://blog.23andme.com/health-traits/how-23andme-predicted-my-likelihood-of-developing-the-disease-of-kings/. Accessed March 22, 2022.

[30] welcome to eMerge > Collaborate. Available at: https://emerge-network.org/. Accessed April 17, 2022.

[31] Lewis ACF, Green RC, Vassy JL. Polygenic risk scores in the clinic: Translating risk into action. HGG Adv 2021;2(4): 100047. https://doi.org/10.1016/j.xhgg.2021.100047.

[32] ACS Breast Cancer Screening Guidelines. Available at: https://www.cancer.org/cancer/breast-cancer/screening-tests-and-early-detection/american-cancer-society-recommendations-for-the-early-detection-of-breast-cancer.html. Accessed May 5, 2022.

[33] Brockman DG, Petronio L, Dron JS, et al. Design and user experience testing of a polygenic score report: a qualitative study of prospective users. BMC Med Genomics 2021; 14(1):238. https://doi.org/10.1186/s12920-021-01056-0.

[34] van der Bles AM, van der Linden S, Freeman ALJ, et al. The effects of communicating uncertainty on public trust in facts and numbers. Proc Natl Acad Sci U S A 2020;117(14): 7672–83. https://doi.org/10.1073/pnas.1913678117.

[35] Polygenic Risk Score Task Force of the International Common Disease Alliance. Responsible use of polygenic risk scores in the clinic: potential benefits, risks and gaps. Nat Med 2021;27(11):1876–84. https://doi.org/10.1038/s41591-021-01549-6.

[36] Brown SAN, Jouni H, Marroush TS, et al. Effect of Disclosing Genetic Risk for Coronary Heart Disease on Information Seeking and Sharing: The MI-GENES Study (Myocardial Infarction Genes). Circ Cardiovasc Genet 2017;10(4). https://doi.org/10.1161/CIRCGENETICS.116.001613.

[37] Widén E, Junna N, Ruotsalainen S, et al. Communicating polygenic and nongenetic risk for atherosclerotic cardiovascular disease - An observational follow-up study. bioRxiv 2020. https://doi.org/10.1101/2020.09.18.20197137.

[38] Tischkowitz M, Balmaña J, Foulkes WD, et al. Management of individuals with germline variants in PALB2: a clinical practice resource of the American College of Medical Genetics and Genomics (ACMG). Genet Med 2021;23(8):1416–23.

[39] Lewis ACF, Green RC. Polygenic risk scores in the clinic: new perspectives needed on familiar ethical issues. Genome Med 2021;13(1):14.

Advances in Molecular Pathology 5 (2022) 9–27
ADVANCES IN MOLECULAR PATHOLOGY

Hereditary Cancer and Cancer Predisposition Syndromes

Erfan Aref-Eshghi, MD, PhD[1], Marylin M. Li, MD*
Division of Genomic Diagnostics, Department of Pathology and Laboratory Medicine, Children's Hospital of Philadelphia, Philadelphia, PA, USA

KEYWORDS
• Hereditary cancer • Cancer predisposition • Non-syndromic cancer • Polygenic cancer

KEY POINTS

- Cancer predisposition syndromes are frequently caused by a germline mutation in a tumor suppressor gene followed by a somatic loss of the functional allele.
- Genetic predisposition can be a feature of many other congenital syndromes with broad etiologies including chromosomal, imprinting, and single-gene defects.
- A new class of genes is emerging that cause non-syndromic cancers that do not always follow the traditional criteria for inherited malignancies.
- The involvement of hereditary factors in most cancers remains to be polygenic or multifactorial.
- The adaptation of genomic and transcriptomic testing in cancer is expected to expand our understanding of hereditary involvement in cancer.

INTRODUCTION

Despite being a genetic disease, most incidences of cancer are sporadic with no traceable family history. Occasionally, patients present with signs that raise the suspicion of an underlying hereditary involvement. These include an earlier age of onset, multiple primary tumors, bilateral involvement, rare malignancies, and a constellation of tumors specific to a recognizable syndrome. These so-called cancer predisposition syndromes have been most accountable for inherited malignancies, comprising approximately 10% of the cancer occurrences in the population. Although the list of these syndromes is growing, other classes of genetic predisposition to cancer are being recognized that do not fit the established criteria. Among these are genetic syndromes presenting cancer as a secondary phenotype, non syndromic genetic variants influencing tumor development, and polygenic contributions to cancer. This article discusses diverse genomic mechanisms and diagnostic testing advances in hereditary cancer.

CANCER PREDISPOSITION SYNDROMES IN CHILDREN AND ADULTS

Several hereditary syndromes are characterized by a predisposition to malignancy as the main/only clinical feature. These syndromes are often caused by inactivating mutations in tumor suppressor genes that encode proteins involved in restricting cell growth or regulating

[1] Present address. Abramson Research Center, Room 714J, 3615 Civic Center Boulevard., Philadelphia, PA, USA

*Corresponding author. Abramson Research Center, Room 716I, 3615 Civic Center Boulevard, Philadelphia, PA. *E-mail address:* Lim5@chop.edu

https://doi.org/10.1016/j.yamp.2022.07.002
2589-4080/22/

DNA repair. Less commonly, cancer predisposition syndromes are caused by activating mutations in oncogenes encoding receptor kinase or intracellular signaling proteins that promote growth. Most cancer-predisposing syndromes follow a dominant pattern of inheritance. Few syndromes have been described to result in cancer susceptibility in both dominant and recessive forms. In such cases, the biallelic mutation carriers show a more severe phenotype and tumor development during childhood [1]. The age of tumor development is otherwise variable in different syndromes. Retinoblastoma and *DICER1* tumor predisposition syndromes are among the examples of pediatric-onset conditions, whereas hereditary breast-ovarian cancer syndrome and hereditary polyposis and nonpolyposis colon cancer syndromes are the most characterized adult-onset hereditary cancers. Some other entities such as Li–Fraumeni syndrome can have varying ages of onset from pediatric to early adulthood. The tumor in these syndromes can be restricted to a single organ, or present as a broad range of malignancies. This section discusses a few of these syndromes to highlight the most recognized molecular basis of hereditary cancers as well as the diversity and variations in their phenotypic presentations. A comprehensive list of familial cancer syndromes is provided in Table 1.

Retinoblastoma

Retinoblastoma is the most common pediatric tumor of the embryonic neural retina, often occurring before 5 years of age [2]. Loss-of-function pathogenic variants in the *RB1* tumor suppressor gene are recognized as the genetic cause of retinoblastoma. The tumor development follows the "two-hit" model based on which two mutational events involving both alleles are necessary for tumor development. In line with this, the disease can be caused by two somatic mutations in each allele (unilateral disease), or by one germline mutation followed by a somatic aberration that renders the normal allele lost/inactive (often bilateral involvement). Germline carriers of pathogenic *RB1* variants develop retinoblastoma at an earlier age and are also at increased risk of developing other malignancies throughout their life, including sarcomas and melanoma [2]. The *RB1* gene product is a key substrate of the G1 cyclin-dependent kinases that phosphorylate the proteins required for the transition of a cell from G1 to S growth stages. Inactivation of RB1 is necessary for tumor development but other events including inactivation of the p53 pathway, chromosome instability, and epigenetic dysregulation of several cancer genes have also been proposed to be required for tumor progression [2]. In a small subset of tumors (~1%), no *RB1* variant is identified. Most of these are found to harbor amplification of the *MYCN* oncogene, highlighting the diverse mechanisms underlying retinoblastoma [3].

DICER1 tumor predisposition syndrome

The *DICER1* tumor predisposition syndrome is a relatively recently characterized syndrome presenting with dysontogenetic neoplasms in childhood. The most frequent tumor in this syndrome is pleuropulmonary blastoma, a rare pediatric lung cancer of embryonal origin [4]. Other tumors in this syndrome include nodular thyroid hyperplasia, papillary and follicular thyroid carcinoma, pituitary blastoma, cervical rhabdomyosarcoma, cystic nephroma, ovarian Sertoli–Leydig cell tumors, and Wilms tumor [5]. Pathogenic germline variants in *DICER1* have been identified in individuals affected by these tumors[4]. The gene encodes the ribonuclease Dicer, a helicase enzyme that cleaves the double-stranded pre-microRNA into microRNA, activating the RNA-induced silencing complex. The disease mechanism is proposed to follow the "two-hit" model, although with a variation. The germline mutations in *DICER1* are often loss-of-function variants resulting in protein reduction by half. Unlike retinoblastoma, the second hit is not a deactivating variant, possibly because a complete loss of *DICER1* is incompatible with cell survival. Instead, the second hit is a non-truncating somatic change in the RNase IIIb domain of the protein, knocking out the production of specific miRNAs [6].

An alternative mechanism for tumor development by *DICER1* is observed among carriers of germline missense mutations in the RNase IIIb domain in *de novo* mosaic status. These individuals present with global developmental delay, lung cysts, overgrowth, and Wilms tumor (GLOW syndrome), for whom the occurrence of the second hit for cancer development seems to be nonmandatory [7]. The phenotype is proposed to result from the activation of the PI3K/AKT/mTOR pathway [8]; as such, *DICER1* appears to act as an oncogene in these cases vs. a tumor suppressor gene in loss-of-function variant carriers. Patients with GLOW syndrome have a higher tumor burden and an earlier age of onset compared with germline loss-of-function variant carriers [9].

Li–Fraumeni syndrome

Li–Fraumeni syndrome is the most common cause of inherited pediatric cancers, resulting in more than 1% of all childhood malignancies [10]. This autosomal dominant cancer predisposition syndrome is caused by heterozygous mutations in the *TP53* gene

TABLE 1
Cancer predisposition syndromes with cancer as the main phenotype

Syndrome	Main Tumors Type or Site of Involvement	Onset	Genes
BAP1 tumor predisposition syndrome	Mesothelioma, atypical Spitz tumors, skin and uveal melanoma, and kidney cancer	Adulthood	*BAP1*
Birt–Hogg Dube syndrome	Renal tumors (hybrid oncocytic chromophobe, oncocytoma, chromophobe, and clear cell renal cell carcinoma)	Adulthood	*FLCN*
Carney complex	Myxoma, endocrine, and papillary thyroid	Childhood and adulthood	*PRKAR1A*
Constitutional mismatch repair deficiency syndrome (CMMRD or Turcot's syndrome)[a]	Hematologic malignancies, central nervous system tumors, colorectal tumors, and multiple intestinal polyps	Childhood	*MLH1, MSH2, MSH6,* and *PMS2*
Cowden syndrome	Hamartoma, glioma, prostate, and endometrial tumors	Childhood and adulthood	*PTEN*
Familial adenomatous polyposis (FAP)	Colorectal cancer	Adolescence and adulthood	*APC*
Familial breast cancer	Breast	Adulthood	*CHEK2*
Familial cylindromatosis; Familial trichoepithelioma; Brooke–Spiegler syndrome	Skin appendage tumors including cylindroma, trichoepithelioma, and spiradenoma	Adolescence and adulthood	*CYLD*
Familial malignant melanoma	Melanoma	Adulthood	*CDK4*
Familial paraganglioma	Paraganglioma and pheochromocytoma	Childhood and adulthood	*SDHA, SDHAF2, SDHB, SDHC,* and *SDHD*
Familial pleuropulmonary blastoma or *DICER1* syndrome	Pleuropulmonary blastoma	Childhood	*DICER1*
Familial retinoblastoma	Retinoblastoma, sarcoma, breast, and small cell lung carcinoma	Infancy and childhood	*RB1*
Gastric adenocarcinoma and proximal polyposis of the stomach	Gastric adenocarcinoma	Adulthood	*APC*
Hereditary breast and ovarian cancer	Breast, ovarian, and pancreas (*BRCA2* only)	Adulthood	*BRCA1* and *BRCA2*
Hereditary diffuse gastric cancer	Diffuse gastric cancer and lobular breast cancer	Adulthood	*CDH1*

(continued on next page)

TABLE 1
(continued)

Syndrome	Main Tumors Type or Site of Involvement	Onset	Genes
Hereditary leiomyomatosis and renal cell cancer	Leiomyomatosis and renal cancer	Adolescence and adulthood	*FH*
Juvenile polyposis syndrome	GI hamartomatous polyps and cancers (colorectal, esophageal, gastric, and pancreatic)	Childhood and adulthood	*BMPR1A* and *SMAD4*
Li–Fraumeni syndrome	Breast, sarcoma, adrenocortical carcinoma, glioma, and multiple other tumor types	Childhood and adulthood	*TP53*
Lynch syndrome (hereditary non-polyposis colorectal cancer)	Colorectal, endometrial, and ovarian tumors	Adulthood	*MSH2, MSH6, PMS1, MLH1, PMS2,* and *TGFBR2*
Melanoma-pancreatic cancer syndrome	Melanoma and pancreatic carcinoma	Adulthood	*CDKN2A*
Multiple endocrine neoplasia 1	Parathyroids, pancreatic islets, duodenal endocrine cells, and anterior pituitary	Childhood and adulthood	*MEN1*
Multiple endocrine neoplasia 2	medullary thyroid, papillary thyroid, and pheochromocytoma	Childhood and adulthood	*RET*
Multiple endocrine neoplasia 4	Pituitary and parathyroid	Adulthood	*CDKN1B*
MYH-associated polyposis[a]	Colon polyps, colorectal cancer, Duodenal polyps, and duodenal cancer	Adolescence and adulthood	*MUTYH (MYH)*
Nevoid basal cell carcinoma syndrome	Skin basal cell and medulloblastoma	Adolescence and adulthood	*PTCH1*
Peutz–Jeghers syndrome (PJS)	Jejunal hamartoma, ovarian, testicular, and pancreatic	Childhood and adulthood	*STK11*
POLE/POLD1-associated hereditary colorectal cancer	Colorectal cancer	Adulthood	*POLD1* and *POLE*
Von Hippel-Lindau syndrome	Renal cell cancer and hemangioma, pheochromocytoma	Childhood and adulthood	*VHL*

[a] Except for these syndromes, the inheritance pattern for all listed conditions is autosomal dominant.

and is characterized by a broad spectrum of tumors with onsets varying from childhood to late adulthood. The most recent studies estimate an average penetrance of 80% by age 70, which can be varied based on sex and mutation type [11]. Adrenal cortical carcinoma, choroid plexus carcinoma, rhabdomyosarcoma, medulloblastoma, and hypodiploid acute lymphoblastic leukemia (ALL) comprise the most common tumors in childhood [12]; although in early adulthood, breast cancer, osteosarcoma, soft tissue sarcomas, leukemia, astrocytoma/glioblastoma, colorectal and lung cancers become more prevalent. In late adulthood, the syndrome presents with pancreatic and prostate cancers [11].

The *TP53* gene encodes a transcription factor with binding sites specific to the promoters of many genes that promote DNA repair and tumor suppression. Most *TP53* mutations are missense changes in the DNA-binding domain, likely resulting in loss of function [13]; although, some are known to have dominant-negative effects [14]. In addition to germline predisposition to cancer, *TP53* is the most common somatically mutated gene in various tumors. These somatic mutations are found in over half of all tumors and involve the same hotspot as the germline variants [13].

Hereditary breast and ovarian cancers

Approximately 10% to 15% of breast and ovarian cancers occur in the context of inherited predisposition, most commonly due to germline pathogenic variants in *BRCA1* or *BRCA2* [15]. The penetrance for breast cancer development by age 80 is approximately 70% among the mutation carriers, which is varied depending on the variant position and type, modifying genetic polymorphisms, ethnicity, and environmental factors [16]. Most of the *BRCA1* breast tumors are basal-like, triple-negative (negative for estrogen receptor, progesterone receptor, and human epidermal growth factor receptor 2), although most *BRCA2* tumors express estrogen receptors [17]. Most of the disease-causing mutations in *BRCA1/2* are truncating variants [18]. The BRCA proteins are proposed to be involved in chromosome stability, homologous recombination (HR) DNA repair, DNA replication fork stabilization, and RNA-DNA hybrid processing during transcription [18]. Tumorigenesis is proposed to arise from the somatic loss of the wild-type allele, although recent studies have shown that the second hit is not always present in a subset of tumors [18,19]. Cells with loss of both *BRCA1/2* alleles are deficient in HR DNA repair and rely on the poly ADP-ribose polymerase (PARP) pathway for survival [18]. Inhibition of PARP results in selective death of these cells and is currently a therapeutic intervention for HR-deficient tumors [18]. Hereditary predisposition to breast or ovarian tumors also occurs in other cancer-predisposing conditions including Li–Fraumeni, Peutz–Jeghers, Cowden, and Lynch syndromes.

Hereditary polyposis and non-polyposis colorectal cancer syndromes

Hereditary cancer syndromes result in 5% to 10% of all colorectal tumors. These syndromes are caused by pathogenic variants in multiple genes and can be classified into polyposis, hamartomatous polyposis, and non-polyposis [20].

Familial adenomatous polyposis (FAP) is an autosomal dominant disorder presenting with hundreds of colorectal adenomas with a 100% risk of developing malignancy if left untreated [21]. Individuals with FAP are also at risk of developing extracolonic tumors including duodenal cancer, thyroid tumors, hepatoblastoma, and desmoid tumors. Sometimes FAP is accompanied by multiple benign extraintestinal lesions such as osteomas, fibromas, lipomas, and congenital hypertrophy of the retinal pigment epithelium. In these cases, the variant term "Gardner syndrome" is used to describe the condition [21]. A milder form of FAP with delayed onset, fewer polyps, and a lower chance of cancer transformation is known as attenuated FAP (AFAP) [21]. The genetic etiology in all these conditions is the *APC* gene, encoding a tumor suppressor protein with a functional role in the canonical Wnt signaling pathway and an involvement in DNA replication and chromosome segregation [22]. The mutation positions appear to correlate with the occurrence of AFAP and the presence of extracolonic features. Mutations in the extreme 5′ or 3′ of *APC* are proposed to result in AFAP [23]. A closely mimicking phenotype to AFAP is also described in individuals with biallelic germline mutations in the *MUTYH* (*MYH*) gene (*MYH*-associated polyposis), which can only be differentiated from AFAP through genetic testing [23].

Hamartomatous polyposis syndromes are rare autosomal dominant conditions that present with neoplastic gastrointestinal polyps. Peutz–Jeghers syndrome (PJS) is caused by loss-of-function mutations in *STK11* and presents with polyps, primarily in the small intestine, and melanotic macules on the lips, buccal mucosa, and fingertips [24]. The hamartomatous polyps in PJS can become very large and transform into adenomas and carcinomas [24]. Extraintestinal cancer may occur in the breast, uterus, and ovary of PJS patients [24]. Another syndrome in this category is *PTEN* hamartoma syndrome (also called Cowden syndrome), resulting from loss-of-function variants in *PTEN*. It presents with hyperplastic colon polyps, colonic adenomas, lipomas, and ganglioneuromas, as well as hamartomas of the hair follicle, and macrocephaly. The breast and thyroid are among the extracolonic organs at risk of cancer development [25]. Juvenile polyposis syndrome (JPS) presents with juvenile polyps in the colon. Half of JPS patients carry germline mutations in *SMAD4* or *BMPR1A* [20].

Hereditary non-polyposis CRC, also known as Lynch syndrome (LS), is the most common hereditary colorectal cancer syndrome. It results from heterozygous germline mutations in one of the mismatch repair (MMR) genes involved in post-replicative proofreading of DNA and genomic stability. The genes involved in LS are *MLH1*, *MSH2*, *MSH6*, and *PMS2* [26]. Germline deletion of the *EPCAM* gene is recognized as another etiology, leading to epigenetic silencing of *MSH2* in the downstream [26]. Loss of MMR activity results in microsatellite instability which is widely used as a screening marker for LS. The condition is characterized by neoplasia of the proximal colon with very few to no adenomas. The most frequent extracolonic tumor is endometrial cancer [26]. A variant of LS, Muir-Torre syndrome, is characterized by sebaceous and other skin tumors [26]. Biallelic germline mutations in MMR genes result in constitutional mismatch repair deficiency (CMMRD, also known as Turcot's syndrome), presenting with CRC, hematologic malignancies, neurofibromatosis-like presentations, brain tumor, and urinary tract malignancies at a very young age [27].

GENETIC SYNDROMES WITH CANCER PREDISPOSITION AS PART OF THE PHENOTYPE

Many genetic syndromes are initially diagnosed based on a spectrum of congenital anomalies but later in life predispose to cancer. The list includes various chromosomal anomalies, aneuploidies, single gene defects, and imprinting conditions, and each syndrome is associated with an increased risk of specific tumor/tumors (Table 2). The risk may arise from the underlying genetic defect or be secondary to the microenvironment of the syndrome. For instance, men with Klinefelter syndrome have a higher risk of developing breast cancer and a lower risk of developing prostate cancer. On the other hand, women with Turner syndrome, who also have a clone of cells with chromosome Y, have a high risk of gonadoblastoma but their chance of breast cancer is lower than the general population. These observations are proposed to be due to hormonal changes associated with imbalances of genetic material on sex chromosomes [28,29]. This section reviews some of the syndromes associated with cancer as one of the features of the underlying genetic defect.

Constitutional chromosomal abnormalities

Trisomy 21 (Down syndrome) is the most common chromosomal aneuploidy observed in human live births. Children with down syndrome have up to a 500-fold higher chance of developing a malignant form of acute myeloid leukemia (AML) with a megakaryoblastic phenotype (AMKL) [30]. Approximately 5% of individuals with trisomy 21 are born with a transient clonal megakaryocytosis syndrome, in 20% of which cases it transforms into AMKL. A characteristic of this malignancy is somatic mutations in *GATA1*, encoding a transcription factor regulating the normal development of multiple hematopoietic cell lineages [31]. These mutations occur in exon 2, inducing a premature stop codon and eliminating the transcriptional activation domain of the protein. It is proposed that the increased expression of chromosome 21 genes in fetal hematopoietic stem cells results in autonomous expansion of erythro-megakaryocytic progenitors, although the somatic *GATA1* mutations further disrupt megakaryoblastic differentiation. This will lead to a transient myeloproliferative disorder in newborn Down patients which later, with the acquisition of additional somatic changes, progresses into AMKL [32,33]. Down syndrome patients are also at increased risk of ALL, which has different cytogenetic and molecular characteristics from the ALL of the general pediatric population [34]. Among other constitutional chromosomal aneuploidies that predispose to cancer are mosaic trisomy 8 with an increased risk for myeloid neoplasms, and trisomy 18 with a higher chance of Wilms tumor and hepatoblastoma. Consistently, the acquired gain of chromosomes 8 and 18 are common findings in AML and Wilms tumor, respectively [35].

Chromosomal structural variants as well as microdeletion and microduplication syndromes are the next category of diseases that can predispose to cancer. The affected genomic regions may contain any of the known cancer-predisposing genes listed in Table 1. Deletion of these genes or disruption of their coding frame through these structural aberrations can result in haploinsufficiency and cancer predisposition when the involved gene is a tumor suppressor. Alternatively, they can disrupt the regulatory elements of a nearby gene, resulting in its abnormal expression [36]. Terminal deletion of *EPCAM*, upstream of *MSH2*, is an example of this phenomenon, resulting in Lynch syndrome.

In addition to unbalanced chromosomal aberrations, carriers of several balanced rearrangements may have an increased risk for specific malignancies [37]. For example, Emanuel syndrome is caused by the presence of a supernumerary derivative chromosome 22, inherited from a parent who carries a balanced reciprocal translocation between chromosomes 11 and 22. These asymptomatic carriers are known to have a higher chance of breast cancer [38]. Other examples are the carriers of the balanced

TABLE 2
Genetic syndromes with cancer as part of the phenotype

Syndrome	Main Clinical Features	Tumor Predispositions	Inheritance	Genes
Bone marrow failure syndromes				
Congenital amegakaryocytic thrombocytopenia	Bruises, organ dysfunction due to hemorrhagic events	AML and MDS	AR	*MPL*
Diamond–Blackfan anemia	Congenital abnormalities (craniofacial, upper limb, heart, and GU), growth deficiency, and macrocytic anemia	AML, MDS, and solid tumors including osteogenic sarcoma	AD and XL	*RPL/RPS* gene families, *GATA1*, and *TSR2*
Dyskeratosis congenita	Dysplastic nails, lacy reticular pigmentation of the upper chest and neck, oral leukoplakia, pulmonary fibrosis, and progressive BMF	AML, MDS, solid tumors (head/neck SCC, and anogenital cancer)	AD, AR, and XL	*ACD,CTC1,DKC1,NHP2, NOP10,PARN,RTEL1, TERC,TERT,TINF2*, and *WRAP53*
Schwachman-Diamond syndrome	Growth failure, hematologic abnormalities with cytopenia, and osteoporosis	AML and MDS	AR	*SBDS, EFL1, DNAJC21*, and *SRP54*
Severe congenital neutropenia	Neutropenia, osteopenia, and recurrent infections	AML and MDS	AD and AR	*ELANE* and *HAX1*
Bone marrow failure/chromosomal instability				
Fanconi Anemia	Congenital abnormalities, BMF, short stature, skin pigmentation, limb abnormalities, microcephaly, ophthalmic, and GU tract anomalies	AML, MDS, solid tumors (head & neck, GU tract, and skin)	AD, AR, and XL	*FANC-A, B, C, D1, D2, E, F, G, I, J, L, M, N, O, P, Q, R, S, T, U, V*, and *W*
Chromosomal instability syndromes				
Ataxia telangiectasia	Neurodegeneration, immunodeficiency, premature aging, and radiation sensitivity	Leukemia (T-ALL), lymphoma (B-cell), medulloblastoma, glioma, melanoma, and breast/ovarian cancer	AR	*ATM*
Bloom syndrome	Immunodeficiency and premature aging	Leukemia, lymphoma, and SCC	AR	*BLM*
		Oropharyngeal tumors	AD	*ATR*

(continued on next page)

TABLE 2
(continued)

Syndrome	Main Clinical Features	Tumor Predispositions	Inheritance	Genes
Familial cutaneous telangiectasia and cancer syndrome	Cutaneous telangiectasia, dental and nail anomalies, and patchy alopecia			
Mosaic variegated aneuploidy	IUGR, microcephaly, facial dysmorphism, ID, and seizures	RMS, Wilms tumor, and leukemia	AR	*BUB1B*, *TRIP13*, and *CEP57*
Nijmegen breakage syndrome	Progressive microcephaly, IUGR, short stature, recurrent sinopulmonary infections, and premature ovarian failure	T-cell and B-cell lymphomas, glioma, medulloblastoma, and RMS	AR	*NBN*
Rothmund Thomson syndrome type 2	Poikiloderma and congenital skeletal abnormalities	Osteosarcoma, skin basal cell carcinoma, and SCC	AR	*RECQL4*
Xeroderma pigmentosum	Photosensitivity and sunlight-induced ocular involvement	Sunlight-induced cutaneous neoplasms	AR	*DDB2*, *ERCC1-5*, *POLH*, *XPA*, and *XPC*
Cytogenetic abnormalities				
Chromosome 2p24.3 duplication involving *MYCN*	Psychomotor delay, facial anomalies and congenital heart defect	Wilms tumor	AD	*MYCN*
Down syndrome (Trisomy 21)	ID, brachycephaly, upslanting palpebral fissure, congenital heart, and multiorgan disease	AML with a megakaryoblastic phenotype and ALL		
Klinefelter syndrome	Tall stature, abnormal or absent puberty, small genitalia, and gynecomastia	Breast cancer		
rob(15;21) (q10;q10) and ring chromosomes involving chr21	Asymptomatic carrier	ALL with intrachromosomal amplification of chr21 (iAMP21)		
t(11;22) (q23;q11)	Asymptomatic carrier with risk of producing offspring with Emanuel syndrome	Breast cancer		
Translocations involving Chr3	Asymptomatic carrier	RCC		
Trisomy 18	Cleft palate, Clenched fists, rocker-bottom foot, and multiorgan defects	Wilms tumor and HBL		

Trisomy 8 (mosaic)	Facial features, ID, brain malformation, and multiorgan abnormalities	Myeloid neoplasms		
Turner syndrome with the presence of ChrY material	Short stature, delayed puberty, infertility, heart defects, and learning disabilities	Gonadoblastoma		
Imprinting disorders				
Beckwith–Wiedemann syndrome	Hemi-hyperplasia, exomphalos, macroglossia, macrosomia, and neonatal hypoglycemia	Wilms tumor, HBL, NBL, RMS, and adrenal carcinoma		*H19, CDKN1C, KCNQ1*, and *IGF2*
Kagami–Ogata syndrome	Skeletal abnormalities, dysmorphic facial features, growth retardation, and DD	HBL		*MEG3*
Metabolic disorders				
Argininosuccinate lyase deficiency	Neurocognitive defects, hepatitis, cirrhosis, trichorrhexis nodosa, and hypertension	Hepatocellular carcinoma	AR	*ASL*
Hemochromatosis	Iron overload-related symptoms, irregular heartbeat, cirrhosis, diabetes, skin hyperpigmentation, and arthritis	Hepatocellular carcinoma	AR	*HFE*
L-2-hydroxyglutaric aciduria	Developmental and growth deficiency, psychomotor regression, and seizures	Gliomatosis brain tumors	AR	*L2HGDH*
Tyrosinemia 1	Periodic neurologic crises with changes in mental status, abdominal pain, peripheral neuropathy, respiratory failure, renal tubular dysfunction, and acute intermittent porphyria	Hepatocellular carcinoma	AR	*FAH*
RASopathies				
Cardiofaciocutaneous syndrome	Cardiac abnormalities, distinctive craniofacial appearance, and cutaneous abnormalities	ALL and NHL	AD	*BRAF*
Costello syndrome		RMS, NBL, and bladder cancer	AD	*HRAS*

(*continued on next page*)

TABLE 2
(continued)

Syndrome	Main Clinical Features	Tumor Predispositions	Inheritance	Genes
	DD, ID, growth delay, short stature, coarse facial features, and multi-organ involvement			
Neurofibromatosis 1	Polyneuropathy, cutaneous lesions including café au lait patches, axillary & inguinal freckling, neurofibromas, and Lisch nodules	Glioma, RMS, malignant peripheral nerve tumor, JMML, breast cancer, and GI cancers	AD	*NF1*
Noonan syndrome	DD, characteristic facies, short stature, and congenital heart defect	JMML, NBL, ALL, glioma, RMS, AML, testicular cancer, and colorectal cancer	AD	*PTPN11, KRAS, SOS1, RAF1, RIT1, KRAS, GBL, SOS2, NRAS,* and *SHOC2*
Other single-gene disorders				
Cartilage-hair hypoplasia	Metaphyseal chondrodysplasia characterized by short-limbed short stature, and fine sparse hair	NHL and basal cell carcinoma	AR	*RMRP*
Denys–Drash syndrome, Frasier syndrome, Familial Wilms tumor	Progressive glomerulopathy and disorders of testicular development	Wilms tumor	AR	*WT1*
Neurofibromatosis 2	Neuropathy, vascular disease, and ocular features	Vestibular schwannomas, spinal tumors, and meningiomas	AD	*NF2*
Oligodontia-colorectal cancer syndrome	Oligodontia	Colorectal carcinoma	AR	*AXIN2*
Perlman syndrome	Overgrowth, hypotonia, DD, and facial dysmorphism	Wilms tumor	AR	*DIS3L2*
Rubinstein–Taybi syndrome	DD and distinctive facial features	HBL, NBL, RMS, CNS tumors, and carcinomas	AD	*CREBBP* and *EP300*
Schinzel–Giedion syndrome	Hypotonia, mild motor delays, ID, behavioral problems, refractive errors, and strabismus	Neuroepithelial tumors	AD	*SETBP1*
		Wilms tumor	XL	*GPC3*

Simpson–Golabi–Behmel syndrome	Pre/postnatal macrosomia, distinctive craniofacial features, and ID ± structural brain anomalies			
Sotos syndrome	DD, distinctive facial features, and overgrowth	NBL, ALL, AML, HBL, and SCT	AD	*NSD1*
Tuberous sclerosis complex	DD, ID, abnormalities of the skin, brain, kidney, heart, and lungs	Hamartoma, RCC, and tuberous sclerosis tuber	AR	*TSC1* and *TSC2*
Weaver syndrome	DD, distinctive facial features, and overgrowth	NBL and hematologic malignancies	AD	*EZH2* and *EED*
Werner syndrome	Premature aging	Osteosarcoma, meningioma, other tumor types	AR	*WRN*
WHIM syndrome	Immunologic dysregulations including neutropenia, and hypogammaglobulinemia	HPV and EBV-related malignancies, lymphoma, and skin cancer	AD	*CXCR4*
Wiskott–Aldrich syndrome	Thrombocytopenia with intermittent mucosal bleeding and recurrent infections	Lymphoma	XL	*WAS*

Abbreviations: AD, autosomal dominant; AML, acute myeloid leukemia; ALL, acute lymphoid leukemia; BMF, bone marrow failure; AR, autosomal recessive; DD, developmental delays; GI, gastrointestinal; GU, genitourinary; ID, intellectual disability; IUGR, intrauterine growth retardation; JMML, juvenile myelomonocytic leukemia; HBL, hepatoblastoma; MDS, myelodysplastic syndrome; NBL, neuroblastoma; NHL, non-Hodgkin lymphoma; RCC, renal cell carcinoma; RMS, rhabdomyosarcoma; SCC, squamous cell carcinoma; XL, X-linked.

Robertsonian translocation between chromosomes 15 and 21, and ring chromosomes involving chromosome 21, who have a significantly higher risk of developing ALL with intrachromosomal amplification of chromosome 21 (iAMP21). The instability of these chromosomal structures during mitosis is hypothesized to be the underlying mechanism for chromothripsis and iAMP21 [39].

Beckwith–Wiedemann syndrome

Beckwith–Wiedemann syndrome (BWS) is characterized by a spectrum of congenital anomalies including hemihyperplasia, exomphalos, macroglossia, macrosomia, and neonatal hypoglycemia. Approximately 8% of BWS cases develop cancer during childhood, including Wilms tumor, hepatoblastoma, neuroblastoma, rhabdomyosarcoma, and adrenal carcinoma. The disease is caused by an imprinting defect in chromosome 11p15 harboring two imprinting control (IC) regions. The involved genes include the paternally expressed *IGF2* and the maternally expressed *H19*, *CDKN1C*, and *KCNQ1*. In 50% to 60% of the cases, BWS results from the loss of methylation in IC2 on the maternal allele, leading to loss of *CDKN1C* and *KCNQ1* expressions. In 5% to 10% of sporadic cases and 40% of familial cases, maternally inherited pathogenic variants in *CDKN1C* induce a similar effect. In 5% of cases, a gain of methylation in IC1 on the maternal allele results in increased *IGF2* and decreased *H19* expressions. In 20% to 25% of cases, paternal uniparental disomy (UPD) results in all the above changes. The *CDKN1C* and *H19* genes are assumed to be tumor suppressors, whereas *IGF2* encodes a potent fetal growth factor. Patients with loss of IC2 methylation and those with *CDKN1C* mutations have the lowest risk for tumor development (3%–7%), whereas those with UPD and gain of methylation in IC1 have much higher risks (16% and 28%, respectively) [40].

RASopathies

"Rat sarcoma virus" (RAS) proteins belong to a family of GTPase molecules that regulate many signaling pathways involved in cell proliferation, growth, and differentiation. They are present in the cell in active and inactive forms, that is, guanosine triphosphate (GTP)- and diphosphate (GDP)-bound, respectively. Regulation of the RAS pathways is mediated through guanine nucleotide exchange factors (GEFs) that activate the RAS proteins, and the GTPase-activating proteins (GAPs) that switch them back to their inactive form. RASopathies are a group of autosomal dominant genetic syndromes that result from increased RAS signaling due to mutations in different components of the RAS pathway and its regulators. They include neurofibromatosis type 1, Noonan, Costello, Legius, cardiofaciocutaneous, capillary malformation-arteriovenous, and autosomal dominant intellectual disability type 5 syndromes. They share many clinical features including cardiac malformations, craniofacial dysmorphia, learning difficulties, and an increased risk of cancer [41].

Neurofibromatosis type 1 arises from loss-of-function mutations in *NF1*, encoding the GAP protein neurofibromin which has an inhibitory effect on the NRAS and HRAS proteins. Loss of the NF1 protein results in overactivation of the RAS pathway and thus *NF1* is considered a tumor suppressor gene. The clinical presentations include hyperpigmented macules (café-au-lait spots), inguinal/axillary freckling, iris hamartomas, optic gliomas, peripheral nerve sheath tumors (neurofibromas), and osseous lesions. In addition to neurofibromas, the patients have increased incidences of central nervous system (CNS) tumors, as well as breast and gastrointestinal cancer [42]. Of note, neurofibromatosis 2 is caused by loss-of-function mutations in *NF2*, which encodes another tumor suppressor protein known as merlin or schwannomin. This protein does not belong to the RAS family. The disease is also distinct from neurofibromatosis 1 and represents a different spectrum of tumors including schwannomas, meningiomas, and ependymomas [43].

Activating mutations in *PTPN11*, *SOS1*, *RAF1*, *RIT1*, *KRAS*, *NRAS*, *CBL*, *LZTR1*, and *BRAF* can result in Noonan or a Noonan-like syndrome. *PTPN11* is the most mutated gene, encoding a tyrosine phosphatase in the RAS-MAPK pathway. These mutations impair the protein's ability to switch to the inactive form, resulting in increased RAS signaling. Noonan syndrome is associated with an increased risk of malignancy, including CNS tumors, neuroblastoma, ALL, rhabdomyosarcoma, as well as myeloproliferative disorders. Activating mutations in *HRAS* cause Costello syndrome that has a higher risk of malignancy development compared with Noonan syndrome. Rhabdomyosarcoma, neuroblastoma, and bladder cancers are the most common malignancies in this syndrome. A similar range of malignancies can be observed in cardiofaciocutaneous syndrome, caused by mutations in *BRAF*, *MAP2K1*, *MAP2K2*, and *KRAS* [41,44].

Bone marrow failure and chromosomal instability syndromes

Inherited bone marrow failure (BMF) syndromes are a group of heterogeneous disorders characterized by insufficient production of one or more blood cell lineages, congenital anomalies, and a predisposition to both solid and hematological malignancies. Inherited BMF syndromes are caused by defects in genes involved in various housekeeping pathways and are predominantly inherited in an autosomal recessive fashion. The most common inherited BMF syndromes include Fanconi anemia (DNA repair issue), dyskeratosis congenita (telomerase maintenance disorder), Schwachman-Diamond syndrome (ribosome maturation defect), Diamond-Blackfan anemia (ribosomal biogenesis defect), and severe congenital neutropenia (protein folding/trafficking defect). In addition to cancer predisposition and BMF, these syndromes may also present with various other features such as short stature, skin pigmentation lesions, skeletal abnormalities, and defects in extremities [45].

A classic example of BMF is Fanconi anemia (FA) caused by mutations in over 20 genes involved in a complex network involved in DNA damage repair. The genes are grouped based on the order of activation in the pathway as upstream genes (*FANCA, B, C, E, F, G, L, M,* and *T*), ID complex (*FANCD2* and *I*), and downstream genes (*FANCD1, J, N, O, P, Q, R, S, U, V,* and *W*). Individuals with FA have a high chance of developing various malignancies including myelodysplastic syndrome (MDS), AML, and squamous cell carcinomas [46]. The risk level depends on the underlying genetic defect, such that biallelic mutations in the downstream genes *BRCA2/FANCD1* and *FANCN/PALB2* are associated with the highest risk with up to 97% chance of developing cancer by age 5 [47]. Of note, the heterozygous asymptomatic carriers of pathogenic variants in some of the FA genes, for example, *BRCA2*, are also at increased risk of developing cancer. Cytogenetically, cells of FA patients show hypersensitivity to agents that cause DNA inter-strand crosslinks, resulting in a significant increase in chromosomal breaks and radial figures, a characteristic diagnostic finding [48]. In this regard, FA overlaps with chromosomal instability syndromes and is also classified as one.

Chromosomal instability syndromes are characterized by an increased frequency of chromosomal breaks and rearrangements and a higher risk of cancer due to DNA repair deficiency. Some of the most common disorders in this group are FA, Nijmegen breakage, ataxia-telangiectasia, and Bloom syndromes. They represent overplaying clinical features including immunodeficiency, light-sensitive skin lesions, ataxia, and increased predisposition to various solid and hematopoietic tumors [49]. Further details on these syndromes are provided in Table 2.

GERMLINE MUTATION CONTRIBUTIONS TO NON-SYNDROMIC CANCER PREDISPOSITION

Evidence is accumulating to support the presence of high penetrant germline mutations in up to ~20% of individuals who develop cancer without a syndromic involvement [19,50–53]. Most of these cases do not meet the criteria based on clinical/family history to be eligible for germline genetic testing [50,52]. The most well-recognized examples include genes predisposing to hematological malignancies, such as *RUNX1, ANKRD26, ETV6, CEBPA,* and *DDX41*. Although somatic changes in many of these genes are long known in hematological malignancies, their germline involvements have only been recently recognized [54]. Individuals with loss-of-function or dominant-negative mutations in these genes have a susceptibility to developing various forms of myeloid and lymphoid neoplasms. These patients do not have additional features, although carriers of pathogenic variants in *RUNX1, ANKRD26,* and *ETV6* can have mild to moderate thrombocytopenia [54].

The *ETV6* gene is a transcription factor containing a DNA binding domain known as "erythroblast transformation specific (ETS)". This domain recognizes a specific DNA sequence present in many gene promoters and acts as a transcriptional repressor. Most of the reported mutations in *ETV6* affect the nuclear localization of the protein through a dominant-negative effect. Reduced presence in the nucleus decreases the inhibitory effect of ETV6 on many genes involved in hematopoiesis, leading to abnormal erythroid/megakaryocytic differentiation [55]. This results in an autosomal dominant disorder among the mutation carriers with mild to moderate thrombocytopenia and predisposition to hematological malignancies. They can develop both myeloid (MDS/AML) and lymphoid (ALL) malignancies, although ALL occurrence is twice as common. Solid tumors have rarely been documented in these patients. The penetrance of malignancies is incomplete, and the lifetime risk of malignancy is yet to be determined [56]. Germline mutations in *RUNX1* and *ANKRD26* result in autosomal dominant phenocopies but with a preferential predisposition to MDS/AML [57,58].

Most patients with non-syndromic tumors and a germline etiology do not undergo germline genetic testing and the cause of their tumors remains unknown. The growing use of paired tumor-normal paired sequencing is providing an opportunity for the discovery of novel cancer-predisposing genes. Examples include the identification of germline mutations in DNA damage repair genes in metastatic prostate cancer [59], *CHEK2* in renal cell carcinoma [60], and novel non-MMR DNA repair genes in urothelial cancers [61]. A list of genes associated with non-syndromic cancer predisposition is provided in Table 3.

POLYGENIC HEREDITARY CONTRIBUTION TO CANCER

For most cancer incidences, there is no underlying cancer predisposition syndrome or an identifiable genetic etiology. Most tumors are thought to begin with somatic mutations that occur by chance or due to environmental exposures. Yet, genomic variants influence the process of cancer development including mutation selection and carcinogenic transformation [90]. This involvement can account for the polygenic/multifactorial susceptibility to cancer. As polygenic contribution to disease is traditionally estimated by twin studies, efforts have been made to compare the concordance of cancer among monozygotic and dizygotic twins. Such studies have estimated a moderate heritability of 33% for common cancers, with some malignancies, such as melanoma, yielding the highest heritability (58%) [91]. The estimates are higher when the onset of cancer is earlier. This has been shown for hematological malignancies, where a heritability of 55% is measured for those with the onset of cancer before 40 years of age but only 20% to 25% for those older than 55 [92].

The genetic susceptibility to common cancers is thought to result from the cumulative and interactive contribution of many genetic variants, each harboring a small effect. Although most of the genetic variants underlying cancer heritability are still not discovered, genome-wide association studies have identified many cancer-associated single-nucleotide polymorphisms (SNPs) that cumulatively explain 10% to 30% of the cancer heritability [93]. These SNPs can be combined to generate a cumulative risk level for cancer, known as a polygenic risk score (PRS) [94]. Individuals within the top 20% of the PRS distribution may constitute up to 30% of the population incidences of cancer [94]. These scores may also modify the risk of monogenic cancer predisposition syndromes such as the risk of ovarian and breast cancer development among *BRCA1/2* mutation carriers [95]. Combining the clinical, demographic, and lifestyle factors with PRS may provide a more holistic cancer risk [96].

The potential utility of PRS would be in population screening programs, guiding therapeutic interventions, refining familial cancer risk, and determining diagnostic/prognostic outcomes [96]. At the time being, this technology is yet to provide a competitive performance to the current cancer screening programs and is not ready for use in the clinical setting [97].

GENOMIC TESTING IN HEREDITARY CANCER

Identification of individuals at risk for inherited cancer susceptibility is dependent upon characterizing the clinically relevant cancer-predisposing genes, understanding their mechanism, and determining appropriate indications for genetic testing. Resources including Clinical Genome Resource (ClinGen) working groups are actively curating the genes associated with cancer predisposition [98]. Clinical practice guidelines in oncology for genetic testing of hereditary cancer are also being published by organizations including National Comprehensive Cancer Network (NCCN) [15]. Although the bulk of the guidelines and curated gene lists are yet exclusively available for historically established cancer genes such as *BRCA1/2*, *TP53*, and MMR genes, large panels containing hundreds of cancer-predisposing genes are increasingly being used for screening and diagnosis.

The most popular approach for hereditary cancer testing uses multi-gene next-generation sequencing (NGS) panels. This approach provides relatively good leverage for simultaneous sequencing and copy number assessment in most of the recognized genes in hereditary cancer. However, certain challenges remain, which require additional experiments. As an example, sequencing genomic regions of low complexity, for example, genes with pseudogenes and repetitive elements, requires long-range PCR amplification before NGS or long-read sequencing. Several other conditions require additional specific designs in the panels, such as detection of microsatellite instability in Lynch syndrome, or measurement of telomere length in dyskeratosis congenita.

Additional testing to complement the NGS findings includes RNA analysis, which can assist with the classification of noncoding variants and refinement of structural genetic changes with breakpoints in the noncoding regions [99]. Another area of testing that is gaining popularity includes paired tumor-normal testing that enables differentiation of somatic vs. germline variants contributing to the tumor development or progression [100]. Detection of germline variants in patients with no apparent family history will have clinical implications for the prevention and risk management of subsequent malignancies in survivors [101].

TABLE 3
Genes with germline mutations that predispose to non-syndromic cancer

Gene	Tumors	Reference
ALK	Neuroblastoma	Mossé YP et al. [62] 2008
ANKRD26	MDS/AML	Klco JM [54] 2021
AR	Breast/prostate cancer	Koochekpour S [63] 2010
CDC73	Parathyroid adenoma and ossifying jaw fibroma	Shattuck TM, et al. [64] 2003
CEBPA	AML	Smith et al. [65] 2004
DDX41	MDS/AML	Polprasert C et al. [66] 2015
EGFR	Non-small-cell lung cancer	Ikeda K et al. [67] 2008
ERBB3	Non-small-cell lung cancer	McInerney-Leo AM et al. [68] 2021
ETV6	ALL	Feurstein S, [56] 2017
FAT1	Pancreatic cancer	Abe K et al. [69] 2021
FEN1	Breast cancer	Chung L et al. [70] 2015
HNF1A	Hepatic adenoma and hepatocellular carcinoma	Willson JS et al. [71] 2013
KDR	Melanoma	Silva IP et al. [72] 2016
KIT	Gastrointestinal stromal tumor (GIST) and epithelioma	Nishida T, et al. [73] 1998
LMO1	Neuroblastoma	Wang K, et al. [74] 2011
LZTR1	Glioblastoma and schwannoma	Piotrowski A, et al. [75] 2014
MAX	Pheochromocytoma	Comino-Méndez I, et al. [76] 2011
PALB2	Breast cancer	Rahman N, et al. [77] 2007
PDGFRA	Gastrointestinal stromal tumors	Chompret A, et al. [78] 2004
PHOX2B	Neuroblastoma	Trochet D et al. [79] 2004
POLQ	Breast cancer	Brandalize AP et al. [80] 2014
PRF1	Leukemia and lymphoma	Clementi R et al. [81] 2002
RAD51 C	Ovarian cancer	Yang X et al. [82] 2020
RECQL	Breast cancer	Bowden AR [83] 2019
RUNX1	MDS/AML	Klco JM [54] 2021
SMARCA4	Rhabdoid tumor	Schneppenheim R et al. [84] 2010
SMARCB1	Malignant rhabdoid tumors	Swensen JJ et al. [85] 2009
SMARCE1	Meningioma	Smith MJ et al. [86], 2013
SPOP	Prostate cancer	Zuhlke KA et al. [87], 2014
SUFU	Medulloblastoma	Aavikko M et al. [88]2012
TERT	Melanoma	Horn S et al. [89] 2013

With the advancement of technology and decrease in sequencing cost, genome-wide testing strategies including exome, genome, and transcriptome sequencing are expected to become the tier one diagnostic approach for cancer predisposition.

CONCLUDING REMARKS

The field of hereditary cancer has grown from a few pediatric-onset Mendelian syndromes to include many sporadic cancer incidences. As such, many tumors are being recognized to have a hereditary background.

With the growing use of genomic approaches in gene discovery and clinical testing, it is expected that a greater number of cancer incidences can be explained by germline variation. This will increase germline testing in cancer patients, which will be followed by demands for the development of clinical surveillance guidelines. We expect that early etiologic diagnosis and appropriate surveillance will improve the survival and quality of life for pediatric and adult populations with hereditary cancer.

DISCLOSURE

This work is partially supported by the Department of Pathology and Laboratory Medicine (EAE and MML), Center for Childhood Cancer Research, Children's Hospital of Philadelphia (MML); and NIH Grant U2CHL138346 (MML).

REFERENCES

[1] Rahman N. Realizing the promise of cancer predisposition genes. Nature 2014;505(7483):302–8. https://doi.org/10.1038/nature12981.

[2] Rodriguez-Galindo C, Orbach DB, VanderVeen D. Retinoblastoma. Pediatr Clin North Am 2015;62(1):201–23.

[3] Schwermer M, Hiber M, Dreesmann S, et al. Comprehensive characterization of RB1 mutant and MYCN amplified retinoblastoma cell lines. Exp Cell Res 2019;375(2):92–9. https://doi.org/10.1016/j.yexcr.2018.12.018.

[4] Hill DA, Ivanovich J, Priest JR, et al. DICER1 mutations in familial pleuropulmonary blastoma. Science 2009;325(5943):965. https://doi.org/10.1126/science.1174334.

[5] Abbo O, Pinnagoda K, Brouchet L, et al. Wilms tumor, pleuropulmonary blastoma, and DICER1: case report and literature review. World J Surg Oncol 2018;16(1):164. https://doi.org/10.1186/s12957-018-1469-4.

[6] González IA, Stewart DR, Schultz KAP, et al. DICER1 tumor predisposition syndrome: an evolving story initiated with the pleuropulmonary blastoma. Mod Pathol 2022;35(1):4–22. https://doi.org/10.1038/s41379-021-00905-8.

[7] Klein S, Lee H, Ghahremani S, et al. Expanding the phenotype of mutations in DICER1: mosaic missense mutations in the RNase IIIb domain of DICER1 cause GLOW syndrome. J Med Genet 2014;51(5):294–302. https://doi.org/10.1136/jmedgenet-2013-101943.

[8] Klein SD, Martinez-Agosto JA. Hotspot Mutations in DICER1 Causing GLOW Syndrome-Associated Macrocephaly via Modulation of Specific microRNA Populations Result in the Activation of PI3K/ATK/mTOR Signaling. Microrna 2020;9(1):70–80.

[9] de Kock L, Wang YC, Revil T, et al. High-sensitivity sequencing reveals multi-organ somatic mosaicism causing DICER1 syndrome. J Med Genet 2016;53(1):43–52. https://doi.org/10.1136/jmedgenet-2015-103428.

[10] Gröbner SN, Worst BC, Weischenfeldt J, et al. The landscape of genomic alterations across childhood cancers. Nature 2018;555(7696):321–7. https://doi.org/10.1038/nature25480.

[11] Amadou A, Achatz MIW, Hainaut P. Revisiting tumor patterns and penetrance in germline TP53 mutation carriers: temporal phases of Li-Fraumeni syndrome. Curr Opin Oncol 2018;30(1):23–9. https://doi.org/10.1097/CCO.0000000000000423.

[12] Winter G, Kirschner-Schwabe R, Groeneveld-Krentz S, et al. Clinical and genetic characteristics of children with acute lymphoblastic leukemia and Li-Fraumeni syndrome. Leukemia 2021;35(5):1475–9. https://doi.org/10.1038/s41375-021-01163-y.

[13] Olivier M, Hollstein M, Hainaut P. TP53 mutations in human cancers: origins, consequences, and clinical use. Cold Spring Harb Perspect Biol 2010;2(1):a001008. https://doi.org/10.1101/cshperspect.a001008.

[14] Willis A, Jung EJ, Wakefield T, et al. Mutant p53 exerts a dominant negative effect by preventing wild-type p53 from binding to the promoter of its target genes. Oncogene 2004;23(13):2330–8. https://doi.org/10.1038/sj.onc.1207396.

[15] Samadder NJ, Giridhar KV, Baffy N, et al. Hereditary Cancer Syndromes-A Primer on Diagnosis and Management: Part 1: Breast-Ovarian Cancer Syndromes. Mayo Clin Proc 2019;94(6):1084–98. https://doi.org/10.1016/j.mayocp.2019.02.017.

[16] Kuchenbaecker KB, Hopper JL, Barnes DR, et al. Risks of Breast, Ovarian, and Contralateral Breast Cancer for BRCA1 and BRCA2 Mutation Carriers. JAMA 2017;317(23):2402–16. https://doi.org/10.1001/jama.2017.7112.

[17] Mavaddat N, Barrowdale D, Andrulis IL, et al. Pathology of breast and ovarian cancers among BRCA1 and BRCA2 mutation carriers: results from the Consortium of Investigators of Modifiers of BRCA1/2 (CIMBA). Cancer Epidemiol Biomarkers Prev 2012;21(1):134–47. https://doi.org/10.1158/1055-9965.EPI-11-0775.

[18] Venkitaraman AR. How do mutations affecting the breast cancer genes BRCA1 and BRCA2 cause cancer susceptibility? DNA Repair (Amst) 2019;81:102668. https://doi.org/10.1016/j.dnarep.2019.102668.

[19] Huang KL, Mashl RJ, Wu Y, et al. Pathogenic Germline Variants in 10,389 Adult Cancers. Cell 2018;173(2):355–70.e14.

[20] Samadder NJ, Baffy N, Giridhar KV, et al. Hereditary Cancer Syndromes-A Primer on Diagnosis and Management, Part 2: Gastrointestinal Cancer Syndromes. Mayo Clin Proc 2019;94(6):1099–116. https://doi.org/10.1016/j.mayocp.2019.01.042.

[21] Dinarvand P, Davaro EP, Doan JV, et al. Familial Adenomatous Polyposis Syndrome: An Update and Review of

Extraintestinal Manifestations. Arch Pathol Lab Med 2019; 143(11):1382–98. https://doi.org/10.5858/arpa.2018-0570-RA.
[22] Hankey W, Frankel WL, Groden J. Functions of the APC tumor suppressor protein dependent and independent of canonical WNT signaling: implications for therapeutic targeting. Cancer Metastasis Rev 2018;37(1):159–72. https://doi.org/10.1007/s10555-017-9725-6.
[23] Leoz ML, Carballal S, Moreira L, et al. The genetic basis of familial adenomatous polyposis and its implications for clinical practice and risk management. Appl Clin Genet 2015;8:95–107. https://doi.org/10.2147/TACG.S51484.
[24] Sandru F, Petca A, Dumitrascu MC, et al. Peutz-Jeghers syndrome: Skin manifestations and endocrine anomalies (Review). Exp Ther Med 2021;22(6):1387. https://doi.org/10.3892/etm.2021.10823.
[25] Pilarski R. PTEN Hamartoma Tumor Syndrome: A Clinical Overview. Cancers (Basel) 2019;11(6):844. https://doi.org/10.3390/cancers11060844.
[26] Sinicrope FA. Lynch Syndrome-Associated Colorectal Cancer. N Engl J Med 2018;379(8):764–73. https://doi.org/10.1056/NEJMcp1714533.
[27] Wimmer K, Kratz CP, Vasen HF, et al. Diagnostic criteria for constitutional mismatch repair deficiency syndrome: suggestions of the European consortium 'care for CMMRD' (C4CMMRD). J Med Genet 2014;51(6):355–65. https://doi.org/10.1136/jmedgenet-2014-102284.
[28] Swerdlow AJ, Schoemaker MJ, Higgins CD, et al. Cancer incidence and mortality in men with Klinefelter syndrome: a cohort study. J Natl Cancer Inst 2005; 97(16):1204–10. https://doi.org/10.1093/jnci/dji240.
[29] Kwon A, Hyun SE, Jung MK, et al. Risk of Gonadoblastoma Development in Patients with Turner Syndrome with Cryptic Y Chromosome. Mater Horm Cancer 2017;8(3):166–73. https://doi.org/10.1007/s12672-017-0291-8.
[30] Hitzler JK, Zipursky A. Origins of leukaemia in children with Down syndrome. Nat Rev Cancer 2005,5(1): 11–20. https://doi.org/10.1038/nrc1525.
[31] Wechsler J, Greene M, McDevitt MA, et al. Acquired mutations in GATA1 in the megakaryoblastic leukemia of Down syndrome. Nat Genet 2002;32(1):148–52. https://doi.org/10.1038/ng955.
[32] Chou ST, Opalinska JB, Yao Y, et al. Trisomy 21 enhances human fetal erythro-megakaryocytic development. Blood 2008;112(12):4503–6. https://doi.org/10.1182/blood-2008-05-157859.
[33] Gruber TA, Downing JR. The biology of pediatric acute megakaryoblastic leukemia. Blood 2015;126(8):943–9. https://doi.org/10.1182/blood-2015-05-567859.
[34] Kubota Y, Uryu K, Ito T, et al. Integrated genetic and epigenetic analysis revealed heterogeneity of acute lymphoblastic leukemia in Down syndrome. Cancer Sci 2019;110(10):3358–67. https://doi.org/10.1111/cas.14160.
[35] Ganmore I, Smooha G, Izraeli S. Constitutional aneuploidy and cancer predisposition. Hum Mol Genet 2009;18(R1):R84–93. https://doi.org/10.1093/hmg/ddp084.
[36] Pócza T, Grolmusz VK, Papp J, et al. Germline Structural Variations in Cancer Predisposition Genes. Front Genet 2021;12:634217. https://doi.org/10.3389/fgene.2021.634217.
[37] Panani AD. Is there an association with constitutional structural chromosomal abnormalities and hematologic neoplastic process? A short review. Ann Hematol 2009;88(4):293–9. https://doi.org/10.1007/s00277-008-0672-8.
[38] Schoemaker MJ, Jones ME, Higgins CD, et al. Mortality and cancer incidence in carriers of constitutional t(11; 22)(q23;q11) translocations: A prospective study. Int J Cancer 2019;145(6):1493–8. https://doi.org/10.1002/ijc.32031.
[39] Harrison CJ, Schwab C. Constitutional abnormalities of chromosome 21 predispose to iAMP21-acute lymphoblastic leukaemia. Eur J Med Genet 2016;59(3): 162–5. https://doi.org/10.1016/j.ejmg.2016.01.006.
[40] Wang KH, Kupa J, Duffy KA, et al. Diagnosis and Management of Beckwith-Wiedemann Syndrome. Front Pediatr 2020;7:562. https://doi.org/10.3389/fped.2019.00562.
[41] Dunnett-Kane V, Burkitt-Wright E, Blackhall FH, et al. Germline and sporadic cancers driven by the RAS pathway: parallels and contrasts. Ann Oncol 2020; 31(7):873–83. https://doi.org/10.1016/j.annonc.2020.03.291.
[42] Wilson BN, John AM, Handler MZ, et al. Neurofibromatosis type 1: New developments in genetics and treatment. J Am Acad Dermatol 2021;84(6):1667–76. https://doi.org/10.1016/j.jaad.2020.07.105.
[43] Coy S, Rashid R, Stemmer-Rachamimov A, et al. An update on the CNS manifestations of neurofibromatosis type 2. Acta Neuropathol 2020;139(4):643–65. https://doi.org/10.1007/s00401-019-02029-5.
[44] Tajan M, Paccoud R, Branka S, et al. The RASopathy Family: Consequences of Germline Activation of the RAS/MAPK Pathway. Endocr Rev 2018;39(5): 676–700. https://doi.org/10.1210/er.2017-00232.
[45] Wilson DB, Link DC, Mason PJ, et al. Inherited bone marrow failure syndromes in adolescents and young adults. Ann Med 2014;46(6):353–63. https://doi.org/10.3109/07853890.2014.915579.
[46] Fiesco-Roa MO, Giri N, McReynolds LJ, et al. Genotype-phenotype associations in Fanconi anemia: A literature review. Blood Rev 2019;37:100589. https://doi.org/10.1016/j.blre.2019.100589.
[47] Triemstra J, Pham A, Rhodes L, et al. A Review of Fanconi Anemia for the Practicing Pediatrician. Pediatr Ann 2015;44(10):444–5.
[48] Moreno OM, Paredes AC, Suarez-Obando F, et al. An update on Fanconi anemia: Clinical, cytogenetic and

molecular approaches (Review). Biomed Rep 2021; 15(3):74. https://doi.org/10.3892/br.2021.1450.

[49] Taylor AMR, Rothblum-Oviatt C, Ellis NA, et al. Chromosome instability syndromes. Nat Rev Dis Primers 2019;5(1):64. https://doi.org/10.1038/s41572-019-0113-0.

[50] Zhang J, Walsh MF, Wu G, et al. Germline Mutations in Predisposition Genes in Pediatric Cancer. N Engl J Med 2015;373(24):2336–46. https://doi.org/10.1056/NEJMoa1508054.

[51] Schrader KA, Cheng DT, Joseph V, et al. Germline Variants in Targeted Tumor Sequencing Using Matched Normal DNA. JAMA Oncol 2016;2(1):104–11. https://doi.org/10.1001/jamaoncol.2015.5208.

[52] Mandelker D, Zhang L, Kemel Y, et al. Mutation Detection in Patients With Advanced Cancer by Universal Sequencing of Cancer-Related Genes in Tumor and Normal DNA vs Guideline-Based Germline Testing. JAMA 2017;318(9):825–35. https://doi.org/10.1001/jama.2017.11137.

[53] Lowery MA, Wong W, Jordan EJ, et al. Prospective Evaluation of Germline Alterations in Patients With Exocrine Pancreatic Neoplasms. J Natl Cancer Inst 2018;110(10):1067–74.

[54] Klco JM, Mullighan CG. Advances in germline predisposition to acute leukaemias and myeloid neoplasms. Nat Rev Cancer 2021;21(2):122–37. https://doi.org/10.1038/s41568-020-00315-z.

[55] Feurstein S, Godley LA. Germline ETV6 mutations and predisposition to hematological malignancies. Int J Hematol 2017;106(2):189–95. https://doi.org/10.1007/s12185-017-2259-4.

[56] Di Paola J, Porter CC. ETV6-related thrombocytopenia and leukemia predisposition. Blood 2019;134(8):663–7. https://doi.org/10.1182/blood.2019852418.

[57] Noris P, Favier R, Alessi MC, et al. ANKRD26-related thrombocytopenia and myeloid malignancies. Blood 2013;122:1987, −1989.

[58] Simon L, Spinella JF, Yao CY, et al. High frequency of germline RUNX1 mutations in patients with RUNX1-mutated AML. Blood 2020;135(21):1882–6. https://doi.org/10.1182/blood.2019003357.

[59] Abida W, Armenia J, Gopalan A, et al. Prospective Genomic Profiling of Prostate Cancer Across Disease States Reveals Germline and Somatic Alterations That May Affect Clinical Decision Making. JCO Precis Oncol 2017;2017:00029. https://doi.org/10.1200/PO.17.00029, PO.17.

[60] Carlo MI, Mukherjee S, Mandelker D, et al. Prevalence of Germline Mutations in Cancer Susceptibility Genes in Patients with Advanced Renal Cell Carcinoma. JAMA Oncol 2018;4(9):1228–35. https://doi.org/10.1001/jamaoncol.2018.1986.

[61] Carlo MI, Ravichandran V, Srinavasan P, et al. Cancer Susceptibility Mutations in Patients with Urothelial Malignancies. J Clin Oncol 2020;38(5):406–14. https://doi.org/10.1200/JCO.19.01395.

[62] Mossé YP, Laudenslager M, Longo L, et al. Identification of ALK as a major familial neuroblastoma predisposition gene. Nature 2008;455(7215):930–5. https://doi.org/10.1038/nature07261.

[63] Koochekpour S. Androgen receptor signaling and mutations in prostate cancer. Asian J Androl 2010;12(5):639–57. https://doi.org/10.1038/aja.2010.89.

[64] Shattuck TM, Välimäki S, Obara T, et al. Somatic and germ-line mutations of the HRPT2 gene in sporadic parathyroid carcinoma. N Engl J Med 2003;349(18):1722–9. https://doi.org/10.1056/NEJMoa031237.

[65] Smith ML, Cavenagh JD, Lister TA, et al. Mutation of CEBPA in familial acute myeloid leukemia. N Engl J Med 2004;351(23):2403–7. https://doi.org/10.1056/NEJMoa041331.

[66] Polprasert C, Schulze I, Sekeres MA, et al. Inherited and Somatic Defects in DDX41 in Myeloid Neoplasms. Cancer Cell 2015;27(5):658–70. https://doi.org/10.1016/j.ccell.2015.03.017.

[67] Ikeda K, Nomori H, Mori T, et al. Novel germline mutation: EGFR V843I in patient with multiple lung adenocarcinomas and family members with lung cancer. Ann Thorac Surg 2008;85(4):1430–2. https://doi.org/10.1016/j.athoracsur.2007.10.012.

[68] McInerney-Leo AM, Chew HY, Inglis PL, et al. Germline ERBB3 mutation in familial non-small-cell lung carcinoma: expanding ErbB's role in oncogenesis. Hum Mol Genet 2021;30(24):2393–401. https://doi.org/10.1093/hmg/ddab172.

[69] Abe K, Kitago M, Kitagawa Y, et al. Hereditary pancreatic cancer. Int J Clin Oncol 2021;26(10):1784–92. https://doi.org/10.1007/s10147-021-02015-6.

[70] Chung L, Onyango D, Guo Z, et al. The FEN1 E359K germline mutation disrupts the FEN1-WRN interaction and FEN1 GEN activity, causing aneuploidy-associated cancers. Oncogene 2015;34(7):902–11. https://doi.org/10.1038/onc.2014.19.

[71] Willson JS, Godwin TD, Wiggins GA, et al. Primary hepatocellular neoplasms in a MODY3 family with a novel HNF1A germline mutation. J Hepatol 2013;59(4):904–7. https://doi.org/10.1016/j.jhep.2013.05.024.

[72] Silva IP, Salhi A, Giles KM, et al. Identification of a Novel Pathogenic Germline KDR Variant in Melanoma. Clin Cancer Res 2016;22(10):2377–85. https://doi.org/10.1158/1078-0432.CCR-15-1811.

[73] Nishida T, Hirota S, Taniguchi M, et al. Familial gastrointestinal stromal tumours with germline mutation of the KIT gene. Nat Genet 1998;19(4):323–4. https://doi.org/10.1038/1209.

[74] Wang K, Diskin SJ, Zhang H, et al. Integrative genomics identifies LMO1 as a neuroblastoma oncogene. Nature 2011;469(7329):216–20. https://doi.org/10.1038/nature09609.

[75] Piotrowski A, Xie J, Liu YF, et al. Germline loss-of-function mutations in LZTR1 predispose to an inherited disorder of multiple schwannomas. Nat Genet 2014; 46(2):182–7. https://doi.org/10.1038/ng.2855.

[76] Comino-Méndez I, Gracia-Aznárez FJ, Schiavi F, et al. Exome sequencing identifies MAX mutations as a cause of hereditary pheochromocytoma. Nat Genet 2011; 43(7):663–7.

[77] Rahman N, Seal S, Thompson D, et al. PALB2, which encodes a BRCA2-interacting protein, is a breast cancer susceptibility gene. Nat Genet 2007;39(2):165–7. https://doi.org/10.1038/ng1959.

[78] Chompret A, Kannengiesser C, Barrois M, et al. PDGFRA germline mutation in a family with multiple cases of gastrointestinal stromal tumor. Gastroenterology 2004;126(1):318–21. https://doi.org/10.1053/j.gastro.2003.10.079.

[79] Trochet D, Bourdeaut F, Janoueix-Lerosey I, et al. Germline mutations of the paired-like homeobox 2B (PHOX2B) gene in neuroblastoma. Am J Hum Genet 2004;74(4):761–4. https://doi.org/10.1086/383253.

[80] Brandalize AP, Schüler-Faccini L, Hoffmann JS, et al. A DNA repair variant in POLQ (c.-1060A > G) is associated to hereditary breast cancer patients: a case-control study. BMC Cancer 2014;14:850. https://doi.org/10.1186/1471-2407-14-850.

[81] Clementi R, Emmi L, Maccario R, et al. Adult onset and atypical presentation of hemophagocytic lymphohistiocytosis in siblings carrying PRF1 mutations. Blood 2002;100(6):2266–7. https://doi.org/10.1182/blood-2002-04-1030.

[82] Yang X, Song H, Leslie G, et al. Ovarian and Breast Cancer Risks Associated With Pathogenic Variants in RAD51C and RAD51D. J Natl Cancer Inst 2020;112(12):1242–50. https://doi.org/10.1093/jnci/djaa030.

[83] Bowden AR, Tischkowitz M. Clinical implications of germline mutations in breast cancer genes: RECQL. Breast Cancer Res Treat 2019;174(3):553–60. https://doi.org/10.1007/s10549-018-05096-6.

[84] Schneppenheim R, Frühwald MC, Gesk S, et al. Germline nonsense mutation and somatic inactivation of SMARCA4/BRG1 in a family with rhabdoid tumor predisposition syndrome. Am J Hum Genet 2010;86(2): 279–84. https://doi.org/10.1016/j.ajhg.2010.01.013.

[85] Swensen JJ, Keyser J, Coffin CM, et al. Familial occurrence of schwannomas and malignant rhabdoid tumour associated with a duplication in SMARCB1. J Med Genet 2009;46(1):68–72. https://doi.org/10.1136/jmg.2008.060152.

[86] Smith MJ, O'Sullivan J, Bhaskar SS, et al. Loss-of-function mutations in SMARCE1 cause an inherited disorder of multiple spinal meningiomas. Nat Genet 2013; 45(3):295–8. https://doi.org/10.1038/ng.2552.

[87] Zuhlke KA, Johnson AM, Tomlins SA, et al. Identification of a novel germline SPOP mutation in a family with hereditary prostate cancer. Prostate 2014;74(9): 983–90. https://doi.org/10.1002/pros.22818.

[88] Aavikko M, Li SP, Saarinen S, et al. Loss of SUFU function in familial multiple meningioma. Am J Hum Genet 2012;91(3):520–6. https://doi.org/10.1016/j.ajhg.2012.07.015.

[89] Horn S, Figl A, Rachakonda PS, et al. TERT promoter mutations in familial and sporadic melanoma. Science 2013;339(6122):959–61. https://doi.org/10.1126/science.1230062.

[90] Hyndman IJ. Review: the Contribution of both Nature and Nurture to Carcinogenesis and Progression in Solid Tumours. Cancer Microenviron 2016;9(1):63–9. https://doi.org/10.1007/s12307-016-0183-4.

[91] Mucci LA, Hjelmborg JB, Harris JR, et al. Familial Risk and Heritability of Cancer Among Twins in Nordic Countries. JAMA 2016;315(1):68–76. https://doi.org/10.1001/jama.2015.17703.

[92] Clemmensen SB, Harris JR. Mengel-From J, et al. Familial Risk and Heritability of Hematologic Malignancies in the Nordic Twin Study of Cancer. Cancers (Basel) 2021;13(12):3023. https://doi.org/10.3390/cancers13123023.

[93] Fanfani V, Citi L, Harris AL, et al. The Landscape of the Heritable Cancer Genome. Cancer Res 2021;81(10):2588–99. https://doi.org/10.1158/0008-5472.CAN-20-3348.

[94] Kachuri L, Graff RE, Smith-Byrne K, et al. Pan-cancer analysis demonstrates that integrating polygenic risk scores with modifiable risk factors improves risk prediction. Nat Commun 2020;11(1):6084. https://doi.org/10.1038/s41467-020-19600-4.

[95] Kuchenbaecker KB, McGuffog L, Barrowdale D, et al. Evaluation of Polygenic Risk Scores for Breast and Ovarian Cancer Risk Prediction in BRCA1 and BRCA2 Mutation Carriers. J Natl Cancer Inst 2017;109(7): djw302. https://doi.org/10.1093/jnci/djw302.

[96] Yanes T, McInerney-Leo AM, Law MH, et al. The emerging field of polygenic risk scores and perspective for use in clinical care. Hum Mol Genet 2020;29(R2): R165–76. https://doi.org/10.1093/hmg/ddaa136.

[97] Sud A, Turnbull C, Houlston R. Will polygenic risk scores for cancer ever be clinically useful? NPJ Precis Oncol 2021;5(1):40. https://doi.org/10.1038/s41698-021-00176-1.

[98] Ritter DI, Rao S, Kulkarni S, et al. A case for expert curation: an overview of cancer curation in the Clinical Genome Resource (ClinGen). Cold Spring Harb Mol Case Stud 2019;5(5):a004739. https://doi.org/10.1101/mcs.a004739.

[99] Xu F, Aref-Eshghi E, Wu J, et al. A Novel TP53 Tandem Duplication in a Child with Li-Fraumeni Syndrome. Cold Spring Harb Mol Case Stud 2022;a006181. https://doi.org/10.1101/mcs.a006181.

[100] Mandelker D, Zhang L. The emerging significance of secondary germline testing in cancer genomics. J Pathol 2018;244(5):610–5. https://doi.org/10.1002/path.5031.

[101] Cullinan N, Schiller I, Di Giuseppe G, et al. Utility of a Cancer Predisposition Screening Tool for Predicting Subsequent Malignant Neoplasms in Childhood Cancer Survivors. J Clin Oncol 2021;39(29):3207–16.

Hematopathology

Advances in Molecular Pathology 5 (2022) 29–40
ADVANCES IN MOLECULAR PATHOLOGY

Expanding the Molecular Landscape of Cutaneous T-Cell Lymphoma

Mark G. Evans, MD*, **Carlos A. Torres-Cabala, MD**
Division of Pathology and Laboratory Medicine, The University of Texas MD Anderson Cancer Center, 6565 MD Anderson Boulevard, Unit 1053, Houston, TX 77030, USA

KEYWORDS
• Cutaneous T-cell lymphoma • Mycosis fungoides • Next-generation sequencing • JAK/STAT pathway activation • MAPK pathway regulation • NFκB pathway signaling

KEY POINTS

- Cutaneous T-cell lymphoma (CTCL) consists of a heterogeneous collection of subtypes, each associated with a unique clinical presentation, histologic features, molecular/cytogenetic findings, and overall outcomes.
- Recent studies have incorporated state-of-the-art technologies, including whole-exome/genome sequencing and RNA-sequencing, to detect genetic abnormalities in CTCL that were previously unknown.
- Many of the genomic alterations described in CTCL serve as current or potential drug targets.

INTRODUCTION

Cutaneous T-cell lymphoma (CTCL) consists of a heterogeneous collection of lymphoproliferative disorders composed of malignant skin-homing T cells. Early diagnostic criteria have been frequently revised, culminating in the 2018 World Health Organization-European Organization for Research and Treatment of Cancer (WHO-EORTC) classification system, which has incorporated gene expression data into the description of CTCL subtypes [1]. Diagnosis of these diseases still relies on the integration of clinical, histopathological, and molecular findings [2]. In only the past 20 years has the molecular genetic profile of these diseases truly begun to be explored. Starting with cytogenetic and array-based methodologies, studies since 2012 have introduced next-generation sequencing (NGS) techniques to enrich our understanding of the biology of CTCL. Moreover, this research has identified potential gene targets for therapies that provide new hope for patients with CTCL.

The goal of this review is to outline recent genetic findings discovered in the various CTCL subtypes (Fig. 1). We shall exclude from our discussions those diseases that frequently occur within extracutaneous sites, including adult T-cell leukemia/lymphoma, lymphomas with T follicular helper phenotype, extranodal NK/T-cell lymphoma, nasal type, and peripheral T-cell lymphoma, not otherwise specified. Ultimately, we intend to capture the current understanding of the molecular landscape of T-cell lymphomas localized to the skin.

CLASSICAL SUBTYPES OF CUTANEOUS T-CELL LYMPHOMA: MYCOSIS FUNGOIDES AND SÉZARY SYNDROME

Mycosis fungoides (MF) represents the most common form of CTCL, accounting for approximately 50% of cases [3]. It presents as erythematous patches or plaques that represent early clinical stages of disease and are associated with a favorable 10-year survival of 88%.

*Corresponding author, *E-mail address:* MGEvans@mdanderson.org

https://doi.org/10.1016/j.yamp.2022.05.001
2589-4080/22/

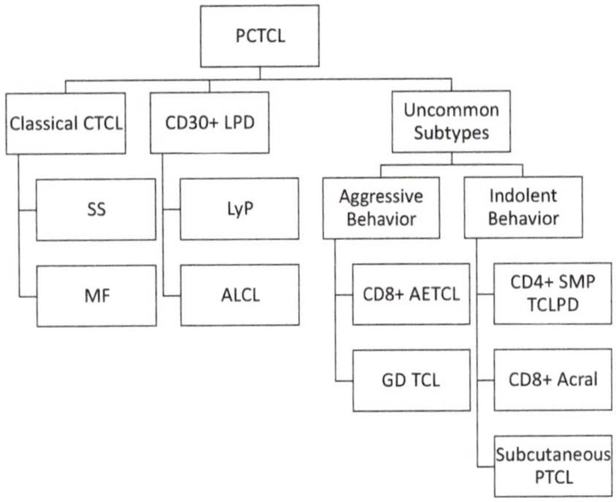

FIG. 1 CTCL subtypes. The subtypes of CTCL included in the revised WHO-EORTC 2018 classification system [1]. The most common (classic) types of CTCL are MF and SS. The CD30-positive T-cell lymphoproliferative disorders comprise a spectrum of diseases that include lymphomatoid papulosis and primary cutaneous anaplastic large cell lymphoma. The uncommon types may be divided in two subgroups: the usually aggressive cytotoxic T-cell lymphomas such as primary cutaneous CD8-positive aggressive epidermotropic cytotoxic T-cell lymphoma (Berti's lymphoma) and primary cutaneous gamma delta T-cell lymphoma; the more indolent entities including subcutaneous panniculitis-like T-cell lymphoma, primary cutaneous acral CD8-positive T-cell lymphoma, and primary cutaneous CD4-positive small/medium pleomorphic T-cell lymphoproliferative disorder. ALCL, anaplastic large cell lymphoma; CD30+ LPD, CD30-positive T-cell lymphoproliferative disorders; CD4+ SMP TCLPD, primary cutaneous CD4-positive small/medium pleomorphic T-cell lymphoproliferative disorder; CD8+ Acral, primary cutaneous acral CD8-positive T-cell lymphoma (provisional entity); CD8+ AETCL, primary cutaneous CD8-positive aggressive epidermotropic cytotoxic T-cell lymphoma (provisional entity); GD TCL, gamma delta T-cell lymphoma; LyP, lymphomatoid papulosis; MF, mycosis fungoides; PCTCL, primary cutaneous T-cell lymphoma; SS, Sézary syndrome; Subcutaneous PTCL, subcutaneous panniculitis-like T-cell lymphoma.

Microscopically, these lesions feature epidermotropism of atypical small-to-medium-sized lymphocytes (Fig. 2A, B). Within the epidermis, the atypical cells form Pautrier microabscesses in proximity to antigen-presenting cells and can often be seen tagging the dermal–epidermal junction. Typically, there is little spongiosis or accompanying plasma cells or eosinophils. Increasing tumor burden within the dermis manifests clinically as deeply infiltrating plaques or tumors (Fig. 2C, D). These lesions may indicate progression to late-stage disease and has been associated with a 42% of 10-year survival [4]. In patients who develop visceral organ or lymph node involvement by the atypical lymphocytes, only 20% are alive at ten years.

In contrast, Sézary syndrome (SS) is a leukemic subtype of CTCL that is characterized by large body-surface-area erythroderma and lymphadenopathy (Fig. 2E). Moreover, at least 1000 circulating tumor cells (Sézary cells) are appreciated per cubic milliliter of peripheral blood [4]. These lymphocytes demonstrate irregular, cerebriform nuclear contours, condensed nuclear chromatin, indistinct nucleoli, and variable amounts of non-granular cytoplasm (Fig. 2F). Afflicted patients often develop brittle nails, eye ectropion, and scaling of the hands and feet. Their erythrodermic skin is pruritic and develops superimposed bacterial infections that cause considerable morbidity and mortality—10-year survival is less than 30% [4,5].

Until 2002, the genetic basis of MF and SS was unexplored. Instead, most early molecular studies had emphasized the importance of T-cell receptor (TCR) gene rearrangement in the development of CTCL. Current methodologies detect rearrangements of TCR genes (alpha, beta, gamma, and delta) created during recombination of V/J or V/D/J segments that are unique to the monoclonal neoplastic cells. Unfortunately, some non-neoplastic conditions can demonstrate clonal TCR rearrangement patterns, and clinical–pathological correlation is required for confirming the presence of CTCL [6]. Interestingly, only 3.7% of pathologists rely on TCR gene rearrangement studies to properly identify cases [7]. Instead, molecular studies provide supplemental information to the major morphologic and immunohistochemical findings essential for diagnosis.

TCR gene rearrangement analysis is of great utility in early-stage disease, as a limited number of atypical lymphocytes may be difficult to identify histologically or to distinguish from a benign dermatosis that lacks a clonal recombination [8,9]. One of the commonly used techniques involves polymerase chain reaction (PCR)-based assays that demonstrate a variable sensitivity of 44% to 90% in these scenarios [10–12]. This range has been attributed to specimen disease burden, interobserver variability, methodology, primers used, and the specific PCR products [13]. The limitations are seemingly overcome by the use of high-throughput NGS, which demonstrates 85% sensitivity compared with the 44% sensitivity documented with PCR [14].

Assessment of TCR gene rearrangement has important implications beyond the diagnosis of CTCL, as it has recently been used in monitoring for minimal

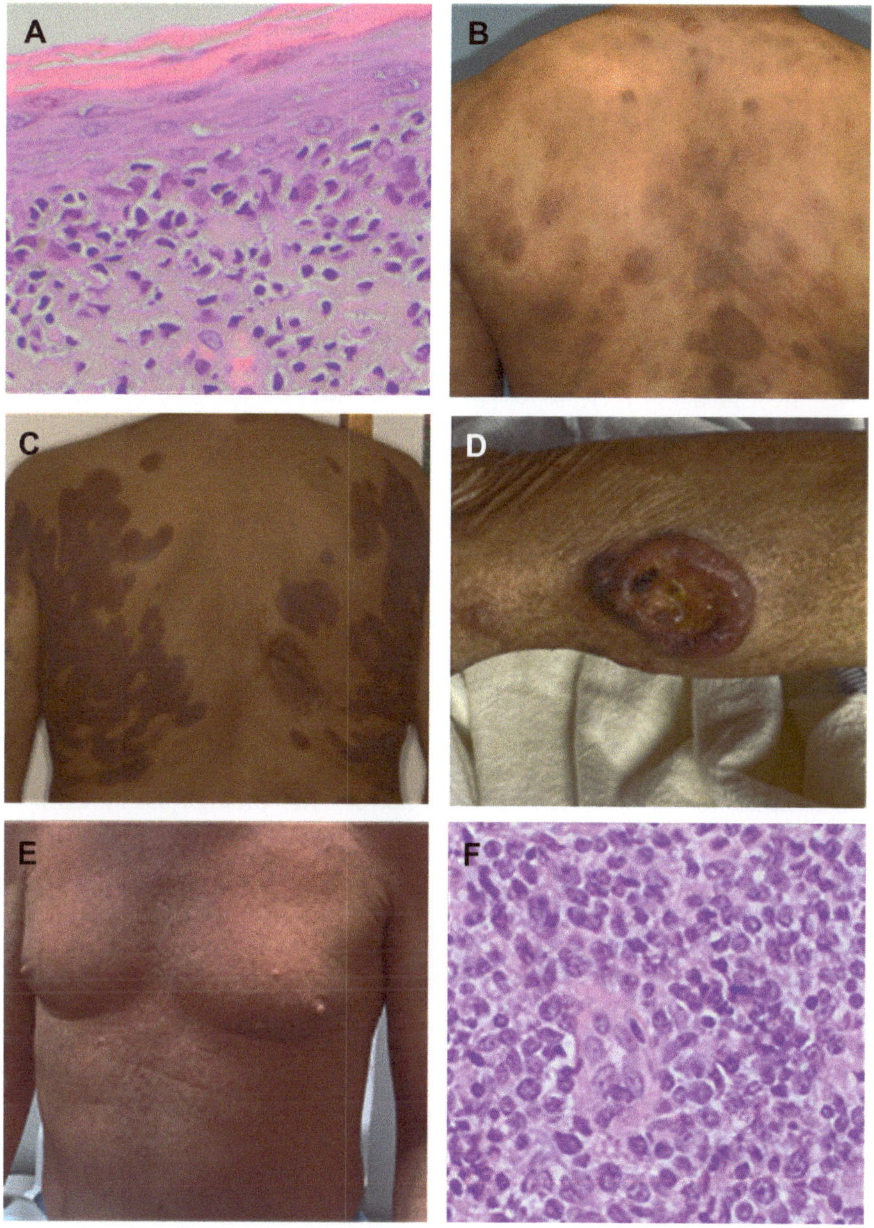

FIG. 2 Presentations of classical CTCL. Hematoxylin and eosin staining of a patch-stage MF lesion demonstrates epidermotropism by atypical lymphocytes (**A**, 20x magnification). Clinically, MF can present as skin patches (**B**), plaques (**C**), and tumors (**D**). In contrast, SS manifests as diffuse cutaneous erythroderma (**E**). Histologically, the skin in SS is densely infiltrated by small to medium-sized lymphocytes with irregular nuclear contours, conspicuous nucleoli, and variable amounts of cytoplasm (**F**, 40x magnification).

residual disease (MRD). Specimens obtained subsequently during a treatment course are compared with the initial, diagnostic specimens to ascertain whether recurring monoclonal TCR gene rearrangements are present. Compared with conventional flow cytometric techniques for assessing leukemic disease, PCR-based molecular studies provide superior sensitivity and specificity [15]. Another research provided proof of concept that NGS monitoring of CTCL was possible during the less than 2 years of follow-up [16]. A larger survey of 200 MF patients also implied the prognostic significance of MRD analysis such that no survival difference was observed, regardless of test positivity or negativity, over a 4-year time span [17].

Recently, NGS has given rise to the concept of tumor clone frequency (TCF). Although the identification of a monoclonal TCR gene rearrangement has little prognostic significance [17,18], quantitating the extent of neoplastic infiltration according to TCF directly correlates with progression-free/overall survival in MF. In particular, clone frequencies greater than 25% serve as strong indicators of poor prognosis [19]. Ultimately, detecting low-level disease by PCR or NGS has important therapeutic implications, particularly when attempting to determine whether a new cutaneous finding represents disease recurrence in patients with a history of CTCL, or when the degree of disease burden warrants more aggressive treatment.

NGS, in conjunction with cytogenetic and array-based studies, has revealed more than the presence of TCR gene rearrangements in cases of MF and SS (Table 1). Comprehensive whole-exome/genome and RNA-sequencing has ultimately provided gene expression profiling that redefines our knowledge of these diseases. Research as early as 2002 identified frequent copy number alterations–deletions of *CDKN2A* were observed in both MF and SS, with other cases of SS demonstrating loss of *RB1* or gain of *MYC* [21,22]. Interestingly, most of the subsequent 12 NGS-based analyses tested samples from patients with SS, or a combination of specimens with SS and MF, and only one focused exclusively on MF. Thus, the medical literature provides a greater wealth of information regarding the molecular biology of SS compared with MF [20,23–33].

Overall, the NGS-based testing demonstrated somatic gene alteration rates in SS that were comparable to those observed in solid tumors [24]. In addition, gene abnormalities resulted most frequently from copy number alterations, as opposed to single nucleotide variations. In addition to changes in the cell cycle control (*CDKN2A* and *RB1*), recurrent abnormalities have been demonstrated in genes related to apoptosis (ie, *FAS*, TNFRSF10 A), DNA damage repair (*TP53* and *ATM*), MAPK pathway (ie, *MAPK1, KRAS, BRAF*), and chromatin modification (ie, *ARID1A, DNMT3A, KMT2C*) [20,30,34]. Another study postulated that the loss of tumor suppressor gene copies resulted in significant genomic instability by altering the function of DNA-cutting enzymes [20]. Copy number alterations are particularly relevant for the genes on chromosomes 8, 10, and 17, which are completely or partially lost in many cases of MF/SS [35]. When single nucleotide changes occur, several genes, including *RHOA, TP53,* and *DNMT3A*, are frequently altered [20]. Recent studies have indicated that *TP53*-altered MF demonstrates poor survival and may require stratification into clinical trials with intense chemotherapy [36]. Curiously, nearly 40% to 75% of single nucleotide abnormalities observed in MF/SS result from the C > T substitution [24,31]. This phenomenon is commonly associated with the mutational signature of ultraviolet light exposure (disrupting NpCpG sites) or of aging (affecting NpCpC areas). Whether light or aging is important for the pathogenesis of CTCL remains unknown.

Molecular analyses ultimately implicate disrupted T-cell signaling in the pathogenesis of MF and SS. Upregulation frequently occurs with the fusion of genes encoding the co-stimulatory molecules CTLA4 and CD28; use of the anti-CTLA4 therapy, ipilimumab, has therefore shown some clinical benefit [25]. Moreover, genes giving rise to TCR-related proteins (ie, *PLCG1*) are frequently altered, in addition to TCR transcription repressors like *ZEB1* [20,24,31]. This gene, in particular, has been associated with overproduction of Th2 cytokines. Recent emphasis has been placed on determining whether MF cases manifest a Th1 or Th2 immunophenotype. The presence of increased Th2 cytokines, including IL4, IL5, IL13, IL15, , IL16, IL17 A, IL17 F, IL22, IL23, and IL25, has been associated with tumor development and poor prognosis [37]. The presence of *ZEB1* point abnormalities or deletions may ultimately prove important for identifying patients with high-risk disease that could benefit from more aggressive therapies.

Changes in genes involved in thymic T-cell development, such as *TOX*, have also been described in cases of late-stage MF and SS. Increased *TOX* expression has proven helpful in distinguishing lymphoma from benign dermatoses, and when observed, portends a worse prognosis that warrants intensified therapy [38–40]. Likewise, disruptions to apoptosis caused by overexpression of *CD158k/KIR3DL2* demonstrate similarly poor prognosis in SS and in advanced-stage of MF [41]. Additionally, dysregulation of the NFκB signaling pathway has been implicated. Point alterations of *TNFRSF1B, CARD11*, or amino acid substitutions in the C-terminus of NFκB lead to constitutive activation and impaired expression of growth factors such as TNFα, IL-2, IL-6, TGFβ, IFNβ, which potentiates lymphomagenesis [24,28,42]. Finally, activation of the JAK/STAT pathway by changes in including *STAT3,*

TABLE 1
Genomic Alterations in Classical CTCL

Biological Function	Affected Genes
DNA repair	*ATM, TP53*
Epigenetic regulators/ chromatin modifications	*DNMT3A, ARIDIA, CTCF*
Cytokine/cell signaling	*ZEBI, PRKCQ, RHOA, PLCG1, CD28, STAT5B, IRF4, TNFA1P3, NFKB2, BRAF*
Cell cycle regulation	*CDKN2A, FAS*

Summary of findings from comprehensive whole-genome/exome sequencing and RNA-sequencing performed by Choi et al. [20]. The genes listed in the table were found to demonstrate copy number changes and/or single nucleotide variations in the referenced study.

STAT5B, *JAK1*, and *JAK3*, was observed in some cases of MF, which could serve as targets for therapy [20,30,31,43]. The immunohistochemical expression of pSTAT3 has been associated with advanced stage of MF and may represent a marker of progression [44].

Given the considerable genetic heterogeneity of MF/SS suggested by the various NGS, cytogenetic, and array-based studies, some experts advocate for gene expression profiling to aid in accurate diagnosis. One publication presented a 17-gene panel that demonstrated good specificity for distinguishing MF/SS from benign dermatoses [45]. By examining genes such as *CCR4*, *STAT5A*, IL2RA, and *TOX*, the authors were also able to predict disease progression in a cohort of patients. Other studies have instead proposed sequencing four (*Twist1*, *PLS3*, *NKp46*, and *CD158k/KIR3DL2*) and five (*CD1D*, *TRAIL*, *GATA3*, *STAT4*, and *PLS3*) genes [46,47]. These limited gene panels were capable of diagnosing 91% and 100% of cases of SS, respectively. Whether the use of gene expression profiling for identifying MF or SS becomes widespread remains uncertain, especially when pathologists were previously comfortable toward their assessment based on histologic and immunohistochemical findings alone.

Most recently, the molecular landscape of MF and SS has emphasized the importance of microRNAs (miRNA). CTCL can now be reliably distinguished from benign dermatoses based on the expression of three miRNAs: miR-205, miR-203, and miR-155 [48]. Moreover, these molecules may serve as important markers for MRD during patient monitoring. From a prognostic standpoint, analyzing three separate miRNAs (miR-338-3p, miR-148-3p, and miR-106b-5p) can stratify patients into high-risk and low-risk cohorts [49]. Unfortunately, the therapeutic implications of miRNAs have yet to be established. However, as our understanding of the diverse copy number alterations, single nucleotide variations, and miR profiles grows, we move closer to harnessing this knowledge to identify new drug targets that will benefit countless patients suffering from MF and SS.

CD30-POSITIVE T-CELL LYMPHOPROLIFERATIVE DISORDERS

The primary cutaneous CD30-positive T-cell lymphoproliferative disorders represent the second most prevalent manifestations of CTCL, accounting for 25% of cases [2]. They include lymphomatoid papulosis (LyP) and primary cutaneous anaplastic large cell lymphoma (C-ALCL), which represent opposing ends of clinical and histologic spectrum. LyP presents as clusters of papules or nodules on typically the torso or extremities that occur at various stages of development, but are ultimately self-healing and eventually recurrent [50]. In contrast, anaplastic large cell lymphoma (ALCL) generally occurs as a single ulcerated nodule or tumor, and unlike LyP, multiple lesions are observed in only 20% of cases [51]. These solitary lesions require localized surgical intervention or radiotherapy, and are associated with an encouraging 90% of 10-year overall survival [50].

Histologically, LyP represents infiltration of the epidermis and dermis, sometimes appearing wedge-shaped, by atypical lymphocytes of various sizes. The most recent WHO-EORTC classification system has designated five histologic subtypes (A–E) that are beyond the scope of this review [1]. Each of the subtypes is associated with similar favorable prognosis, and many patients experience resolution of disease with limited topical therapy or even without treatment. Conversely, the skin lesions of C-ALCL consist of diffuse sheets of large pleomorphic lymphocytes with irregular, sometimes horseshoe-shaped nuclei and prominent nucleoli. These so-called "hallmark cells" are helpful in distinguishing this disease from the LyP subtypes characterized by large-sized lymphocytes [51]. Although CD30 expression is usually detected in a large number of the tumor cells in both C-ALCL and LyP, this finding is not specific and other CTCL, like MF with large cell transformation, may also show expression of CD30.

Cytogenetic studies investigating cases of LyP have uncovered no specific genetic alterations. However, molecular testing has demonstrated frequent overexpression of *SATB1* [52]. In less than 10% of cases, translocations involving chromosome 6p25.3 have been detected, resulting in the *DUSP22::IRF4* rearrangement [53]. This alteration is hypothesized to produce uncontrolled TCR signaling by means of downregulated DUSP22. The prognostic significance of *DUSP22:IRF4* is unknown, but its presence has prompted the creation of a separate clinical-histological subtype by the WHO-EORTC system [1]. In particular, these lesions are notable for extensive epidermotropism composed of small-to-medium lymphocytes and the presence of larger atypical cells in the dermis, all demonstrating variable CD30-positivity [51].

Similar to LyP, *DUSP22:IRF4* translocations are detected in 25% of C-ALCL cases [54]. Additional studies have demonstrated frequent gains of chromosome 7q31 and losses of 13q34 and 6q16-21 [55,56]. Also, the *NPM1::TYK2* fusion has been observed in rare cases of both LyP and C-ALCL, leading to upregulation of STAT5 signaling [57]. However, the molecular findings observed in C-ALCL are not identical to those identified in systemic ALCL (Fig. 3). C-ALCL rarely demonstrates rearrangements of *ALK* that typify ALK-positive systemic ALCL. The few described cases ALK-positive C-ALCL have produced highly variable clinical outcomes that warrant additional investigation. Some patients presented with indolent, slow-growing lesions, whereas others were afflicted by rapidly progressive tumors that were responsible for shortened survival [58,59]. From a treatment standpoint, poor prognosis is also observed in C-ALCL when *TP63* rearrangements are detected [60,61]. Such cases would therefore benefit from intensive systemic therapies.

UNCOMMON SUBTYPES OF CUTANEOUS T-CELL LYMPHOMA

Indolent Subtypes: Primary Cutaneous CD4-Positive Small/Medium Pleomorphic T-Cell Lymphoproliferative Disorder and Primary Cutaneous Acral CD8-Positive T-Cell Lymphoma

Primary cutaneous T-cell CD4-positive small/medium pleomorphic T-cell lymphoproliferative disorder accounts for only 2% of cutaneous lymphomas [2]. Patients generally present with a single erythematous nodule on the neck, upper torso, or face [62,63]. Histology of this lesion is composed of a dense dermal infiltrate of small to medium-sized T cells that demonstrate surface CD4-positivity, follicular T helper phenotype, and no expression of cytotoxic proteins by immunohistochemistry. Only rare larger cells may be appreciated.

Another indolent cutaneous lymphoma representing less than 1% of CTCL cases is primary cutaneous acral CD8-positive T-cell lymphoma, which has been recognized by the WHO as a provisional disease entity. It appears as solitary erythematous nodules or papules on the ear, nose, or sole of the foot [63]. The lesions consist of monotonous infiltrates of medium-sized atypical lymphocytes into the dermis with minimal epidermotropism. Immunohistochemical stains reveal that the cells are CD3/CD8-positive T cells that co-express TIA1. Although the presence of dot-like Golgi TIA1 staining could raise concern for another more aggressive subtype of CD8-positive CTCL, other cytotoxic makers are typically negative, indicating a non-activated cytotoxic phenotype, and the Ki67 proliferation index is typically low.

Molecular testing of cases of primary cutaneous CD4-positive small/medium T-cell pleomorphic lymphoproliferative disorder and primary cutaneous acral CD8-positive T-cell lymphoma reveal monoclonal TCR gene rearrangements [64]. Unfortunately, no other genetic alterations specific to these diseases have been identified [65]. However, of note, the prognosis for both conditions is excellent, and patients typically experience complete remissions with the use of surgical intervention, radiation therapy, or intralesional steroids [63].

Subcutaneous Subtype: Subcutaneous Panniculitis-like T-Cell Lymphoma

Representing less than 1% of CTCL cases, subcutaneous panniculitis-like T-cell lymphoma manifests as multiple plaques or nodules localized to the subcutaneous tissues of the extremities or trunk [66]. Histology of pleomorphic lymphocytes of varying size are seen infiltrating fat lobules, often sparing the septa, with associated apoptotic activity and fat necrosis. The cells are typically CD8-positive alpha beta T lymphocytes that co-express with the cytotoxic proteins TIA1, granzyme B, and perforin, identified by immunohistochemistry. Patients present with systemic symptoms in approximately 50% of the cases, and hemophagocytic syndrome develops in 15–20% overall [67]. Although survival rates of 80% have been documented at 5 years, this figure drops precipitously if hemophagocytosis occurs [68].

The earliest studies investigating the molecular basis of subcutaneous panniculitis-like T-cell lymphoma uncovered numerous chromosomal gains and losses, as well as changes in the neural tumor suppressor *NAV3* that upregulate IL-23R protein expression [69]. More recent research has detected germline abnormalities in

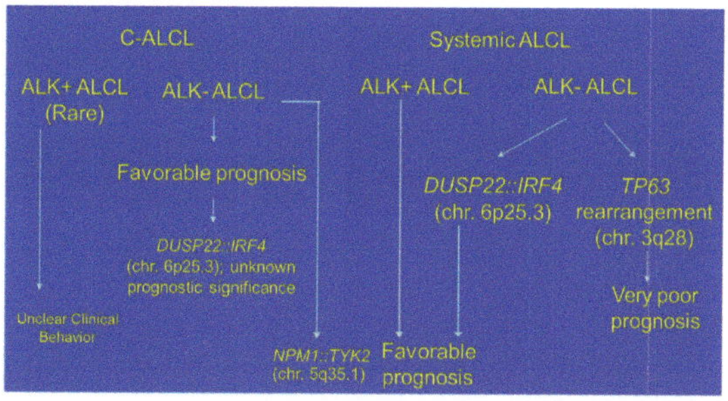

FIG. 3 Major genomic alterations in C-ALCL and systemic ALCL. The diagram outlines the common chromosomal translocations specific to ALK-negative C-ALCL (ie, *NPM1::TYK2*), shared between ALK-negative C-ALCL and ALK-negative systemic ALCL (*DUSP22::IRF4*), and those observed in ALK-negative systemic ALCL (*TP63* rearrangements), as well as the associated prognostic significance. Not represented in the figure are rare case reports of ALK-negative C-ALCL harboring *TP63* rearrangements, which have demonstrated exceptionally poor prognosis [60,61].

HAVCR2, which encodes TIM-3, a protein found on the surface of T cells that maintains immune system activity [70]. Specifically, altered TIM-3 potentiates production of inflammatory cytokines, which has been postulated as contributing to the development of hemophagocytic syndrome in some patients. In the future, assessing TIM-3 expression, even by immunohistochemical staining, may prove fruitful in predicting outcomes and the development of hemophagocytosis in subcutaneous panniculitis-like T-cell lymphoma.

Aggressive Subtypes: Primary Cutaneous Gamma Delta T-Cell Lymphoma and Primary Cutaneous CD8-Positive Aggressive Epidermotropic Cytotoxic T-Cell Lymphoma

Primary cutaneous gamma delta T-cell lymphoma, accounting for 1% of CTLC cases, occurs as a proliferation of activated gamma delta T lymphocytes that are usually negative for CD4/ CD8 and express cytotoxic proteins has been identified by immunohistochemistry [71]. The tumor cells may be limited to the epidermis, dermis, or subcutaneous tissue typically of the extremities, manifesting clinically as patches, plaques, or deeper tumors with variable surface necrosis or ulceration. Hemophagocytosis, B symptoms, and dissemination to extranodal areas, such as mucosal sites, are particularly common and contribute to the overall poor survival of 31 months was demonstrated in one large study [72].

The genetic profile of gamma delta T-cell lymphoma was unknown until a study using comprehensive whole-genome/exome sequencing and RNA-sequencing on 29 cases was published in 2020 [73]. The authors demonstrated by NGS that the cellular origin of the neoplastic lymphocytes depended on the skin compartment to which they were localized. This research confirmed the reported distinct clinical–pathological features between the indolent predominantly epidermotropic variant of gamma delta T-cell lymphoma and the aggressive dermal/subcutaneous gamma delta T-cell lymphoma [74]. Cells occurring in the epidermis and superficial dermis were generally derived from Vδ1 cells, whereas Vδ2 cells gave rise to disease within the subcutaneous fat. This research also demonstrated a heterogeneous collection of single nucleotide alterations and copy number variations in numerous genes of the MYC, MAPK, JAK/STAT, and chromatin modification pathways. Many of these genes, particularly involving JAK/STAT signaling, were hypothesized by the authors as important target for therapies, such as using JAK1/2 inhibitor ruxolitinib. Although the findings suggest exciting new avenues for treatment, whether the medications actually have proven clinical benefit warrants additional study.

Similar to the lethal presentation of primary cutaneous gamma delta T-cell lymphoma, primary cutaneous CD8-positive aggressive epidermotropic cytotoxic T-cell lymphoma manifests as a generalized skin eruption of ulcerated nodules or tumors observed in less than 1% of patients with CTCL [63] and is another provisional disease entity recognized by the WHO. The lesions consist of small-medium or medium-large pleomorphic CD8-positive T cells that co-expresscytotoxic markers. The neoplastic lymphomas demonstrate marked epidermotropism and produce surface breakdown and blister formation; they frequently infiltrate deeper into the skin, resulting in adnexal destruction and angioinvasion. In keeping with the concerning histologic appearance, the median survival rate is only 12 to 15 months [75,76].

Until 2021, little was known about the genetic landscape of primary cutaneous CD8-positive aggressive epidermotropic cytotoxic T-cell lymphoma. Then a research discovered genetic alterations that appeared specific to this disease subtype [76]. Compared with cases primary cutaneous gamma delta T-cell lymphoma and other presentations of CTCL, NGS revealed fusions of *JAK2* and *ABL1* with several gene partners that were only observed in samples best diagnosed as primary cutaneous aggressive epidermotropic cytotoxic T-cell lymphoma (Fig. 4). The authors surmised that the

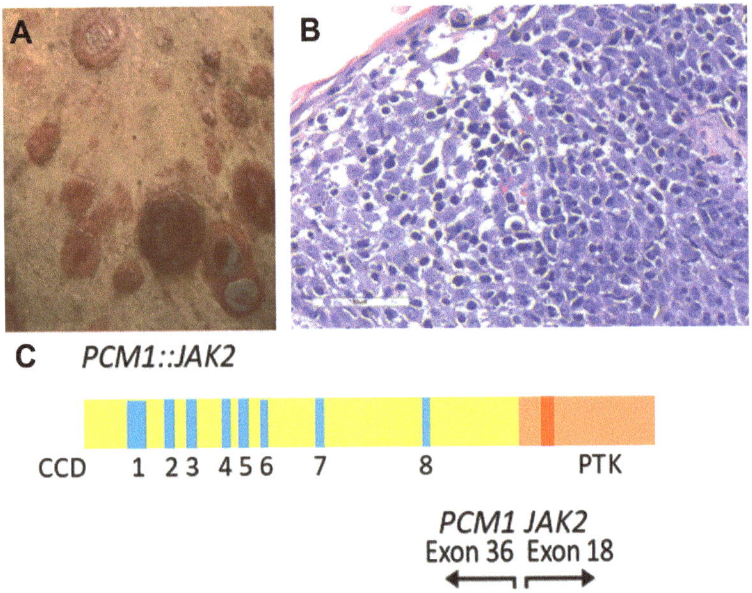

FIG. 4 Important genetic findings in primary cutaneous CD8-positive aggressive epidermotropic cytotoxic T-cell lymphoma. The patient cohort presented by Lee and colleagues [76] included one 72-year-old man with rapidly evolving, ulcerated tumors over his torso and extremities (**A**). Histologically, full-thickness epidermotropism by medium-sized atypical lymphocytes was appreciated, with focal epidermal breakdown (**B**). By immunohistochemistry, the cells were strongly positive for CD2, CD3, CD8, and the cytotoxic markers granzyme B, TIA1, and perforin (not pictured), consistent with the diagnosis of primary cutaneous CD8-positive aggressive epidermotropic cytotoxic T-cell lymphoma. RNA-sequencing detected the *PCM1::JAK2* intergenic fusion, involving exon 36 of *PCM1* and exon 18 of *JAK2*. CCD, coiled coil domain; PTK, protein tyrosine kinase; 1 to 8, eight numerical subdomains of PCM1 (**C**).

fusions, as well the other detected single nucleotide and copy number alterations, would serve as important therapeutic targets for JAK/STAT inhibitors or tyrosine kinase inhibitors. Subsequent in-vitro studies confirmed this hypothesis, as Ba/F3 cells transduced with the gene fusions experienced downregulation of kinase signaling when exposed to varying concentrations of ruxolitinib or imatinib. This discovery of specific, targetable fusion proteins provides new hope for patients diagnosed with primary cutaneous aggressive epidermotropic cytotoxic T-cell lymphoma. Compassionate use of ruxolitinib is currently being investigated in a limited number of patients, and the clinical outcomes are anxiously awaited.

DISCUSSION

Recent molecular and cytogenetic studies have clearly demonstrated a wide variety of genomic alterations contributing to the development of CTCL. Moreover, the molecular signature of certain tumors within the same subtype can even differ between individual patients. As a result, emphasis must be placed on the appropriate selection of personalized therapies, particularly in late-stage, aggressive disease.

Abnormal expression of CCR4 in CTCL directly contributed to the discovery of the anti-CCR4 monoclonal antibody mogamulizumab. A multi-institution clinical trial, mogamulizumab versus vorinostat in previously treated cutaneous T-cell lymphoma showed improved progression free survival for this drug as compared with conventional treatment by an acetone deacetylase inhibitor [77]. As a result, mogamulizumab was approved by the United Stated Food and Drug Administration for the treatment of relapsed/refractory MF and SS.

Primary cutaneous CD30-positive lymphoproliferative disorders, such as LyP and C-ALCL, have benefited from the use of the anti-CD30 brentuximab vedotin [78]. Also, tumors with recurrent JAK/STAT pathway alterations may benefit from the anti-tumor properties of ruxolitinib, or the JAK 1/3 inhibitor tofacitinib that has demonstrated efficacy in CTCL cell lines [20,30,31,43]. Active research continues to explore downregulation of

JAK/STAT signaling, such as targeting two important tumor suppressor genes, *HNRNPK* and *SOCS1*, which are frequently altered in MF [79].

Upregulation of the PI3K/AKT/mTOR signaling pathway has also been implicated in cases of CTCL. Duvelisib has been marketed as a prospective oral inhibitor of phosphatidylinositol 3-kinase (PI3K)-δ/γ isoforms. Inhibition of this protein is thought to interfere with T-cell development, and early clinical trial data seem to advocate for its use in CTCL. A recent phase I open label study of duvelisib for the treatment of T-cell lymphomas, including 19 cases of CTCL, demonstrated a 31.6% response rate [80].

Finally, alterations of the PD1/PD-L1 pathway, which have become important in the pathogenesis of many neoplasms, have also been identified in CTCL. Structural variants involving *CD274*, the gene encoding PD-L1, have been observed as along with recurrent disruption of the 3′ untranslated region of PD ligands. A phase II trial of the PD1 inhibitor pembrolizumab has produced a response rate of 38% in the treatment of MF and SS [81]. We hope that ongoing clinical research will provide additional insight as to whether patients with CTCL will benefit as significantly from PD1 blockade compared with the individuals with different tumor types.

SUMMARY

The broad molecular landscape of CTCL subtypes that has been uncovered in recent years provides strong motivation for new research, which will continue to use state-of-the-art technologies. Recent studies have particularly emphasized important oncogenic changes in chromatin modification, DNA repair, cell cycle control, JAK/STAT pathway activation, TCR/NFκB signaling, and MAPK pathway regulation, many of which serve or could serve as promising targets for new therapies. Upcoming NGS methodologies, including whole-exome/genome and RNA-sequencing, will inevitably lead to the discovery of additional recurrent genetic alterations in CTCL, providing avenues for exploring novel medications. New hope exists in the future, as molecular and cytogenetic testing will ultimately promote the development of unique personalized therapies.

CLINICS CARE POINTS

- Novel therapies should be considered when treating patients diagnosed with late-stage cutaneous T-cell lymphoma (CTCL) with aggressive or recurrent disease.
- State-of-the art molecular and cytogenetic testing should be used in this clinical context as such analyses could demonstrate targetable genetic alterations.
- Targeted systemic therapies that have been proven efficacious in the treatment of CTCL include, but are not limited to, mogamulizumab, brentuximab vedotin, duvelisib, and pembrolizumab.

ACKNOWLEDGMENTS

The authors acknowledge and are grateful for Dr Auri Huen and Kim-Anh Vu, who provided the clinical photographs for this article.

DISCLOSURE

The authors have nothing to disclose.

REFERENCES

[1] Willemze R, Cerroni L, Kempf W, et al. The 2018 update of the WHO-EORTC classification for primary cutaneous lymphomas. Blood 2019;133(16):1703–14 [published correction appears in Blood. 2019 Sep 26;134(13):1112].

[2] Torres-Cabala CA. Diagnosis of T-cell lymphoid proliferations of the skin: putting all the pieces together. Mod Pathol 2020;33(Suppl 1):83–95.

[3] Willemze R, Jaffe ES, Burg G, et al. WHO-EORTC classification for cutaneous lymphomas. Blood 2005;105(10):3768–85.

[4] Agar NS, Wedgeworth E, Crichton S, et al. Survival outcomes and prognostic factors in mycosis fungoides/Sézary syndrome: validation of the revised International Society for Cutaneous Lymphomas/European Organisation for Research and Treatment of Cancer staging proposal. J Clin Oncol 2010;28(31):4730–9.

[5] Whittaker SJ, Cerroni L, Willemze R, et al. Sézary syndrome. In: Swerdlow SH, Campo E, Harris NL, et al, editors. Classification of tumours of haematopoietic and lymphoid tissues, revised. 4th edition. Lyon (France): IARC Press; 2017. p. 90.

[6] Ponti R, Quaglino P, Novelli M, et al. T-cell receptor gamma gene rearrangement by multiplex polymerase chain reaction/heteroduplex analysis in patients with cutaneous T-cell lymphoma (mycosis fungoides/Sézary syndrome) and benign inflammatory disease: correlation with clinical, histological and immunophenotypical findings. Br J Dermatol 2005;153(3):565–73.

[7] Comfere N, Sundram U, Hurley MY, et al. Views of dermatopathologists about clonality assays in the diagnosis

of cutaneous T-cell and B-cell lymphoproliferative disorders. J Cutan Pathol 2018;45:39–47.
[8] Jawed SI, Myskowski PL, Horwitz S, et al. Primary cutaneous T-cell lymphoma (mycosis fungoides and Sézary syndrome): Part I. Diagnosis: clinical and histopathologic features and new molecular and biologic markers. J Am Acad Dermatol 2014;70(205):e201–16.
[9] Xu C, Wan C, Wang L, et al. Diagnostic significance of TCR gene clonal rearrangement analysis in early mycosis fungoides. Chin J Cancer 2011;30:264–72.
[10] Hodges E, Krishna MT, Pickard C, et al. Diagnostic role of tests for T cell receptor (TCR) genes. J Clin Pathol 2003; 56:1–11.
[11] Hsiao PF, Hsiao CH, Lin YC, et al. Histopathologic-molecular correlation in early mycosis fungoides using T-cell receptor gamma gene rearrangement by polymerase chain reaction with laser capture microdissection. J Formos Med Assoc 2007;106:265–72.
[12] Ponti R, Fierro MT, Quaglino P, et al. TCRgamma-chain gene rearrangement by PCR-based GeneScan: diagnostic accuracy improvement and clonal heterogeneity analysis in multiple cutaneous T-cell lymphoma samples. J Invest Dermatol 2008;128:1030–8.
[13] Walia R, Yeung CCS. An update on molecular biology of cutaneous T cell lymphoma. Front Oncol 2020;9:1558.
[14] Sufficool KE, Lockwood CM, Abel HJ, et al. T-cell clonality assessment by next-generation sequencing improves detection sensitivity in mycosis fungoides. J Am Acad Dermatol 2015;73(2):228–36.e2.
[15] Olsen E, Vonderheid E, Pimpinelli N, et al. Revisions to the staging and classification of mycosis fungoides and Sézary syndrome: a proposal of the International Society for Cutaneous Lymphomas (ISCL) and the cutaneous lymphoma task force of the European Organization of Research and Treatment of Cancer (EORTC). Blood 2007;110(6):1713–22.
[16] Weng WK, Armstrong R, Arai S, et al. Minimal residual disease monitoring with high-throughput sequencing of T cell receptors in cutaneous T cell lymphoma. Sci Transl Med 2013;5(214):214ra171.
[17] Hurabielle C, Ingen-Housz-Oro S, Ortonne N, et al. Frequency and prognostic value of cutaneous molecular residual disease in mycosis fungoides: a prospective multicentre trial of the Cutaneous Lymphoma French Study Group. Br J Dermatol 2015;173(4):1015–23.
[18] Massone C, Crisman G, Kerl H, et al. The prognosis of early mycosis fungoides is not influenced by phenotype and T-cell clonality. Br J Dermatol 2008;159(4):881–6.
[19] de Masson A, O'Malley JT, Elco CP, et al. High-throughput sequencing of the T cell receptor β gene identifies aggressive early-stage mycosis fungoides. Sci Transl Med 2018;10(440):eaar5894.
[20] Choi J, Goh G, Walradt T, et al. Genomic landscape of cutaneous T cell lymphoma. Nat Genet 2015;47(9): 1011–9.
[21] Vermeer MH, van Doorn R, Dijkman R, et al. Novel and highly recurrent chromosomal alterations in Sézary syndrome. Cancer Res 2008;68(8):2689–98.
[22] Mao X, Lillington D, Scarisbrick JJ, et al. Molecular cytogenetic analysis of cutaneous T-cell lymphomas: identification of common genetic alterations in Sézary syndrome and mycosis fungoides. Br J Dermatol 2002; 147(3):464–75.
[23] Woollard WJ, Pullabhatla V, Lorenc A, et al. Candidate driver genes involved in genome maintenance and DNA repair in Sézary syndrome. Blood 2016;127(26): 3387–97.
[24] Wang L, Ni X, Covington KR, et al. Genomic profiling of Sézary syndrome identifies alterations of key T cell signaling and differentiation genes. Nat Genet 2015; 47(12):1426–34.
[25] Sekulic A, Liang WS, Tembe W, et al. Personalized treatment of Sézary syndrome by targeting a novel CTLA4: CD28 fusion. Mol Genet Genomic Med 2015;3(2): 130–6.
[26] Prasad A, Rabionet R, Espinet B, et al. Identification of gene mutations and fusion genes in patients with Sézary syndrome. J Invest Dermatol 2016;136(7):1490–9.
[27] Vaqué JP, Gómez-López G, Monsálvez V, et al. PLCG1 mutations in cutaneous T-cell lymphomas. Blood 2014; 123(13):2034–43.
[28] Ungewickell A, Bhaduri A, Rios E, et al. Genomic analysis of mycosis fungoides and Sézary syndrome identifies recurrent alterations in TNFR2. Nat Genet 2015;47(9): 1056–60.
[29] Lee CS, Ungewickell A, Bhaduri A, et al. Transcriptome sequencing in Sézary syndrome identifies Sézary cell and mycosis fungoides-associated lncRNAs and novel transcripts. Blood 2012;120(16):3288–97.
[30] da Silva Almeida AC, Abate F, Khiabanian H, et al. The mutational landscape of cutaneous T cell lymphoma and Sézary syndrome. Nat Genet 2015;47(12):1465–70.
[31] McGirt LY, Jia P, Baerenwald DA, et al. Whole-genome sequencing reveals oncogenic mutations in mycosis fungoides. Blood 2015;126(4):508–19.
[32] Kiel MJ, Sahasrabuddhe AA, Rolland DC, et al. Genomic analyses reveal recurrent mutations in epigenetic modifiers and the JAK-STAT pathway in Sézary syndrome. Nat Commun 2015;6:8470.
[33] Izykowska K, Przybylski GK, Gand C, et al. Genetic rearrangements result in altered gene expression and novel fusion transcripts in Sézary syndrome. Oncotarget 2017;8(24):39627–39.
[34] Damsky WE, Choi J. Genetics of cutaneous T cell lymphoma: from bench to bedside. Curr Treat Options Oncol 2016;17(7):33.
[35] Larocca C, Kupper T. Mycosis fungoides and Sézary syndrome: an update. In: LeBoeuf NR, Larocca C, editors. Cutaneous malignancy. Philadelphia: Elsevier; 2019. p. p113.

[36] Wooler G, Melchior L, Ralfkiaer E, et al. TP53 Gene Status Affects Survival in Advanced Mycosis Fungoides. Front Med (Lausanne) 2016;3:51.

[37] Stolearenco V, Namini MRJ, Hasselager SS, et al. Cellular interactions and inflammation in the pathogenesis of cutaneous T-cell lymphoma. Front Cell Dev Biol 2020; 8:851.

[38] Zhang Y, Wang Y, Yu R, et al. Molecular markers of early-stage mycosis fungoides. J Invest Dermatol 2012;132: 1698–706.

[39] Huang Y, Litvinov IV, Wang Y, et al. Thymocyte selection-associated high mobility group box gene (TOX) is aberrantly over-expressed in mycosis fungoides and correlates with poor prognosis. Oncotarget 2014;5:4418–25.

[40] Yu X, Li Z. TOX gene: a novel target for human cancer gene therapy. Am J Cancer Res 2015;5:3516–24.

[41] Bagot M. New targeted treatments for cutaneous T-cell lymphomas. Indian J Dermatol 2017;62:142–5.

[42] Izban KF, Ergin M, Qin JZ, et al. Constitutive expression of NF-kappa B is a characteristic feature of mycosis fungoides: implications for apoptosis resistance and pathogenesis. Hum Pathol 2000;31(12):1482–90.

[43] Pérez C, González-Rincón J, Onaindia A, et al. Mutated JAK kinases and deregulated STAT activity are potential therapeutic targets in cutaneous T-cell lymphoma. Haematologica 2015;100(11):e450–3.

[44] Pérez C, Mondéjar R, García-Díaz N, et al. Advanced-stage mycosis fungoides: role of the signal transducer and activator of transcription 3, nuclear factor-κB and nuclear factor of activated T cells pathways. Br J Dermatol 2020;182(1):147–55.

[45] Litvinov IV, Netchiporouk E, Cordeiro B, et al. The use of transcriptional profiling to improve personalized diagnosis and management of cutaneous T-cell lymphoma (CTCL). Clin Cancer Res 2015;21:2820–9.

[46] Nebozhyn M, Loboda A, Kari L, et al. Quantitative PCR on 5 genes reliably identifies CTCL patients with 5% to 99% circulating tumor cells with 90% accuracy. Blood 2006;107:3189–96.

[47] Michel L, Jean-Louis F, Begue E, et al. Use of PLS3, Twist, CD158k/KIR3DL2, and NKp46 gene expression combination for reliable Sézary syndrome diagnosis. Blood 2013;121:1477–8.

[48] Ralfkiaer U, Hagedorn PH, Bangsgaard N, et al. Diagnostic microRNA profiling in cutaneous T-cell lymphoma (CTCL). Blood 2011;118:5891–900.

[49] Lindahl LM, Besenbacher S, Rittig AH, et al. Prognostic miRNA classifier in early-stage mycosis fungoides: development and validation in a Danish nationwide study. Blood 2018;131:759–70.

[50] Bekkenk MW, Geelen FA, van Voorst Vader PC, et al. Primary and secondary cutaneous CD30(+) lymphoproliferative disorders: a report from the Dutch Cutaneous Lymphoma Group on the long-term follow-up data of 219 patients and guidelines for diagnosis and treatment. Blood 2000;95(12):3653–61.

[51] Willemze R, Paulli M, Kadin ME. Primary cutaneous CD30-positive lymphoproliferative disorders. In: Swerdlow SH, Campo E, Harris NL, et al, editors. Classification of tumours of haematopoietic and lymphoid tissues. Revised 4th edition. Lyon (France): IARC Press; 2017. p. p395.

[52] Sun J, Yi S, Qiu L, et al. SATB1 defines a subtype of cutaneous CD30+ lymphoproliferative disorders associated with a T-helper 17 cytokine profile. J Invest Dermatol 2018;138(8):1795–804.

[53] Karai LJ, Kadin ME, Hsi ED, et al. Chromosomal rearrangements of 6p25.3 define a new subtype of lymphomatoid papulosis. Am J Surg Pathol 2013;37(1):173–81.

[54] Wada DA, Law ME, Hsi ED, et al. Specificity of IRF4 translocations for primary cutaneous anaplastic large cell lymphoma: a multicenter study of 204 skin biopsies. Mod Pathol 2011;24:596–605.

[55] Laharanne E, Oumouhou N, Bonnet F, et al. Genome-wide analysis of cutaneous T-cell lymphomas identifies three clinically relevant classes. J Invest Dermatol 2010; 130:1707–18.

[56] van Kester MS, Tensen CP, Vermeer MH, et al. Cutaneous anaplastic large cell lymphoma and peripheral T-cell lymphoma NOS show distinct chromosomal alterations and differential expression of chemokine receptors and apoptosis regulators. J Invest Dermatol 2010;130(2): 563–75.

[57] Velusamy T, Kiel MJ, Sahasrabuddhe AA, et al. A novel recurrent NPM1-TYK2 gene fusion in cutaneous CD30-positive lymphoproliferative disorders. Blood 2014; 124:3768–71.

[58] Oschlies I, Lisfeld J, Lamant L, et al. ALK-positive anaplastic large cell lymphoma limited to the skin: clinical, histopathological and molecular analysis of 6 pediatric cases. A report from the ALCL99 study. Haematologica 2013;98(1):50–6.

[59] Wehkamp U, Oschlies I, Nagel I, et al. ALK-positive primary cutaneous T-cell-lymphoma (CTCL) with unusual clinical presentation and aggressive course. J Cutan Pathol 2015;42(11):870–7.

[60] Vasmatzis G, Johnson SH, Knudson RA, et al. Genome-wide analysis reveals recurrent structural abnormalities of TP63 and other p53-related genes in peripheral T-cell lymphomas. Blood 2012;120:2280–9.

[61] Chavan RN, Bridges AG, Knudson RA, et al. Somatic rearrangement of the TP63 gene preceding development of mycosis fungoides with aggressive clinical course. Blood Cancer J 2014;4(10):e253.

[62] Bekkenk MW, Vermeer MH, Jansen PM, et al. Peripheral T-cell lymphomas unspecified presenting in the skin: analysis of prognostic factors in a group of 82 patients. Blood 2009;102:2213–9.

[63] Gaulard P, Berti E, Willemze R, et al. Primary cutaneous peripheral T-cell lymphoma, rare subtypes. In: Swerdlow SH, Campo E, Harris NL, et al, editors. Classification of tumours of haematopoietic and lymphoid

tissues. Revised 4th edition. Lyon (France): IARC Press; 2017. p. p397–402.

[64] Rodríguez Pinilla SM, Roncador G, Rodríguez-Peralto JL, et al. Primary cutaneous CD4+ small/medium-sized pleomorphic T-cell lymphoma expresses follicular T-cell markers. Am J Surg Pathol 2009;33(1):81–90.

[65] Alberti-Violetti S, Torres-Cabala CA, Talpur R, et al. Clinicopathological and molecular study of primary cutaneous CD4+ small/medium-sized pleomorphic T-cell lymphoma. J Cutan Pathol 2016;43(12):1121–30.

[66] Kumar S, Krenacs L, Medeiros J, et al. Subcutaneous panniculitic T-cell lymphoma is a tumor of cytotoxic T lymphocytes. Hum Pathol 1998;29:397–403.

[67] Gonzalez CL, Medeiros LJ, Braziel RM, et al. T-cell lymphoma involving subcutaneous tissue. A clinicopathologic entity commonly associated with hemophagocytic syndrome. Am J Surg Pathol 1991;15:17–27.

[68] Oschlies I, Simonitsch-Klupp I, Maldyk J, et al. Subcutaneous panniculitis-like T-cell lymphoma in children: a detailed clinicopathological description of 11 multifocal cases with a high frequency of haemophagocytic syndrome. Br J Dermatol 2015;172:793–7.

[69] Guitart J. Subcutaneous lymphoma and related conditions. Dermatol Ther 2010;23(4):350–5.

[70] Gayden T, Sepulveda FE, Khuong-Quang DA, et al. Germline HAVCR2 mutations altering TIM-3 characterize subcutaneous panniculitis-like T cell lymphomas with hemophagocytic lymphohistiocytic syndrome. Nat Genet 2018;50(12):1650–7.

[71] Willemze R, Jansen PM, Cerroni L, et al. Subcutaneous panniculitis-like T-cell lymphoma: definition, classification, and prognostic factors: an EORTC Cutaneous Lymphoma Group Study of 83 cases. Blood 2008;111:838–45.

[72] Guitart J, Weisenburger DD, Subtil A, et al. Cutaneous γδ T-cell lymphomas: a spectrum of presentations with overlap with other cytotoxic lymphomas. Am J Surg Pathol 2012;36:1656–65.

[73] Daniels J, Doukas PG, Escala MEM, et al. Cellular origins and genetic landscape of cutaneous gamma delta T cell lymphomas. Nat Commun 2020;11(1):1806.

[74] Merrill ED, Agbay R, Miranda RN, et al. Primary cutaneous T-cell lymphomas showing gamma-delta (γδ) phenotype and predominantly epidermotropic pattern are clinicopathologically distinct from classic primary cutaneous γδ T-cell lymphomas. Am J Surg Pathol 2017;41(2):204–15.

[75] Robson A, Assaf C, Bagot M, et al. Aggressive epidermotropic cutaneous CD30(+) lymphoma: a cutaneous lymphoma with distinct clinical and pathological features. Report of an EORTC Cutaneous Lymphoma Task Force Workshop. Histopathology 2015;67:425–41.

[76] Lee K, Evans MG, Yang L, et al. Primary cutaneous cytotoxic T-cell lymphomas harbor recurrent targetable alterations in the JAK-STAT pathway. Blood 2021;138(23):2435–40.

[77] Kim YH, Bagot M, Pinter-Brown L, et al. Mogamulizumab versus vorinostat in previously treated cutaneous T-cell lymphoma (MAVORIC): an international, open-label, randomised, controlled phase 3 trial. Lancet Oncol 2018;19:1192–204.

[78] Prince HM, Kim YH, Horwitz SM, et al. Brentuximab vedotin or physician's choice in CD30-positive cutaneous T-cell lymphoma (ALCANZA): an international, open-label, randomised, phase 3, multicentre trial. Lancet 2017;390(10094):555–66.

[79] Bastidas Torres AN, Cats D, Mei H, et al. Genomic analysis reveals recurrent deletion of JAK-STAT signaling inhibitors HNRNPK and SOCS1 in mycosis fungoides. Genes Chromosomes Cancer 2018;57:653–64.

[80] Horwitz SM, Koch R, Porcu P, et al. Activity of the PI3K-δ,γ inhibitor duvelisib in a phase 1 trial and preclinical models of T-cell lymphoma. Blood 2018;131(8):888–98.

[81] Khodadoust MS, Rook AH, Porcu P, et al. Pembrolizumab in relapsed and refractory mycosis fungoides and Sézary syndrome: a multicenter phase II study. J Clin Oncol 2020;38(1):20–8.

Advances in Molecular Pathology 5 (2022) 41–50
ADVANCES IN MOLECULAR PATHOLOGY

High-Grade B-cell Lymphomas

Anna Shestakova, MD, PhD[a,*], Kristin H. Karner, MD[b]
[a]ARUP Laboratories/University of Utah, 500 Chipeta Way, Mail Code 115-J13, Salt Lake City, UT 84108-1221, USA; [b]Department of Pathology, University of Utah/ARUP Laboratories, 500 Chipeta Way, Mail Code 115-J13, Salt Lake City, UT 84108-1221, USA

KEYWORDS
• HGBL • High-grade B-cell lymphoma • Double-hit lymphoma • Triple-hit lymphoma • MYC • BCL2 • 11q aberration • Burkitt-like lymphoma

KEY POINTS

- The 5th edition of the World Health Organization classification recognizes 3 major groups of high grade B-cell lymphomas: 1. High grade B-cell lymphoma with MYC and BCL2 rearrangements; HGBL with rearrangements of MYC, BCL2 and BCL6 (known as triple-hit (TH) lymphoma); and HGBL with rearrangements of MYC and BCL2 (with/without BCL6 rearrangement) and TdT expression); 2. High grade B-cell lymphoma, not otherwise specified (NOS) - a diagnosis of exclusion; 3. High grade B-cell lymphoma with 11q aberration.
- The International consensus classification (ICC 2022) recognizes four distinct entities: 1. Large B-cell lymphoma with 11q aberration 2. High-grade B-cell lymphoma, with MYC and BCL2 rearrangements 3. High-grade B-cell lymphoma with MYC and BCL6 rearrangements 4. High-grade B-cell lymphoma, NOS.
- Double-hit molecular signature portends a poor prognosis.

INTRODUCTION

Accurate classification of mature B-cell lymphomas is clinically relevant in order to determine the most appropriate treatment and long-term prognosis. Historically, the third edition of the World Health Organization (WHO) classification had a category of B-cell lymphoma, unclassifiable [BCL-U], with features intermediate between Burkitt lymphoma (BL) and diffuse large B-cell lymphoma (DLBCL), that were reclassified as high-grade B-cell lymphoma (HGBL) under the current fourth edition of the WHO. There are 2 groups in HGBL: HGBL with *MYC* and *BCL2* and/or *BCL6* rearrangements (double-hit or triple-hit) and HGBL, not otherwise specified (NOS) [1]. Recently two classifications have been released – The 5th edition of the WHO [2] and The International Consensus Classification (ICC) 2022 [3]. Both classifications recognize HGBL with MYC and BCL2 rearrangements (with or without BCL6 rearrangement). ICC 2022 recognizes the distinct entity HGBL with MYC and BCL6 rearrangements. This distinction is made based on the poor outcomes in patients with HGBL with MYC and BCL6 rearrangements [4][5–8]. Both classifications recognize HGBL, NOS, which is a diagnosis of exclusion. These categories represent 1% to 2% of patients with non-Hodgkin lymphomas and are usually refractory to R-CHOP therapy with a more aggressive clinical course [9]. Due to the distinct mutational landscape and clinical management, they should not be diagnosed as DLBCL, NOS, or BL [10,11]. The same holds true for High grade B-cell lymphoma with 11q aberration, which also has a distinct mutational landscape and should not be diagnosed as BL.

HGBL with *MYC* and *BCL2* encompasses a group of B-cell lymphomas that have a *MYC* (8q24.2) rearrangement in combination with a *BCL2* (18q21.3). In addition to MYC and BCL2 gene rearrangements, these lymphomas can also present with *BCL6* (3q27.3). rearrangement, resulting in a triple hit rearrangement in *MYC, BCL2*

*Corresponding author, *E-mail address:* ania.shestakova@hsc.utah.edu

https://doi.org/10.1016/j.yamp.2022.06.001
2589-4080/22/

and *BCL6* genes. Notably, in comparison to HGBL with *MYC* and *BCL2* rearrangements, HGBL with *MYC* and *BCL6* rearrangements have an adverse outcome, therefore ICC 2022 recognizes the distinct entity of HGBL with *MYC* and *BCL6* rearrangements. Common morphologies resemble either DLBCL or have features intermediate between BL and DLBCL. Sometimes, a blastoid appearance is seen that resembles lymphoblastic lymphoma or the blastoid variant of mantle cell lymphoma.

HGBL, NOS is morphologically indistinguishable from cases that are either blastoid or have features intermediate between DLBCL and BL but do not have a DH or TH genetic signature. Morphology that is typical of DLBCL in this context excludes the diagnosis of HGBL, NOS.

High grade B-cell lymphoma with 11q aberration can be morphologically and immunophenotypically indistinguishable from BL but it does not have *MYC* gene rearrangement and harbors a distinct chromosome 11q aberration characterized by proximal gain and terminal loss.

High-Grade B-Cell Lymphoma with *MYC* and *BCL2* with/without *BCL6* Rearrangements

WHO 5th edition recognizes a group of High grade B-cell lymphomas with MYC and BCL2 rearrangements. This group is subdivided into three subgroups: 1. HGBL with rearrangements of MYC and BCL2 without BCL6 rearrangement; 2. HGBL with rearrangements of MYC and BCL2 with BCL6 rearrangement, and 3. HGBL with rearrangements of MYC and BCL2 (with/without BCL6 rearrangement) and TdT expression. ICC 2022 recognizes a distinct entity of HGBL with MYC and BCL6 rearrangements. ICC 2022 acknowledges TdT expression in HGBL, but does not recognize it as a distinct entity. Both classifications recognize HGBL, NOS, as a diagnosis of exclusion. Structural chromosomal aberrations with breakpoints in both MYC and BCL2 genes define HGBL with *MYC* and *BCL2* and/or *BCL6* rearrangements. In addition to MYC and BCL2 gene rearrangements these lymphomas may harbor BCL6 rearrangements (also known as DH or TH lymphoma). These lymphomas are commonly seen in elderly patients, with male predominance. The frequency may vary in populations depending on ethnicity [12], and is reported to comprise 4-9% of patients initially diagnosed with DLBCL [7,13]. It is an aggressive mature B-cell lymphoma that has a *MYC* gene rearrangement at chromosome 8q24 and a rearrangement in *BCL2* (at chromosome 18q21.3) with/without in *BCL6* (at chromosome 3q27.3). DH refers to the rearrangement of 2 genes, including *MYC* accompanied by *BCL2* and/or *BCL6*. TH lymphomas harbor rearrangements of *MYC*, *BCL2*, and *BCL6* genes. Although overexpression of MYC and BCL2 proteins also correlates with an adverse clinical outcome and is known as a "double expressor" phenotype, overexpression cannot be used as a surrogate for the rearrangement of corresponding genes [14]. Notably, lymphomas with rearrangements of the *MYC* gene in addition to other genes (for instance, *CCND1* seen in mantle cell lymphoma) are excluded from the category of HGBL with *MYC* and *BCL2* and/or *BCL6* rearrangements. Grade 3 B follicular lymphomas that have a completely follicular architectural pattern without significant diffuse areas, harboring *IGH-BCL2* and *MYC* rearrangements, should be diagnosed as follicular lymphoma. Rare cases of B-lymphoblastic leukemia/lymphoma harboring *IGH-BCL2* and *MYC* rearrangements are also excluded from this category.

Clinical features. According to one of the large studies of patients with DH lymphomas, the median age was 67 years (range 17–89 years) with a slight male predominance [15,16]. In one study of TH lymphomas, all patients were men [17]. Patients with HGBL with *MYC* and *BCL2* and/or *BCL6* rearrangements benefit from high-intensity therapies such as R-EPOCH (rituximab, etoposide, prednisone, vincristine, cyclophosphamide, doxorubicin) rather than R-CHOP therapy (rituximab, cyclophosphamide, doxorubicin, vincristine, prednisone) with 2-year event-free survival of 67% compared with 33% with R-CHOP. A subset of patients may completely respond to the treatment followed by stem cell transplant [17,18]. Interestingly, patients with DH/TH have a similar prognosis to all patients affected by DLBCL when given CAR-T therapy in the JULIET trial (Schuster and colleagues 2019).

Morphology and immunophenotype. Morphology ranges from DLBCL to a more blastoid appearance that resembles BL. Immunophenotype is often of germinal center B-cell type (GCB) [15,19,20]. Expression of MYC, BCL2, and BCL6 proteins can be assessed by immunohistochemical analysis but expression cannot be used as a surrogate for the gene rearrangement. Cases that are "double-expressor" lymphomas are characterized by the increased expression of MYC (>40%) and BCL2 (>50%) proteins that are not related to the underlying chromosomal rearrangement. Double-expressor lymphomas serve as markers of inferior clinical outcome in patients with DLBCL. Patients with double-expressor lymphoma seem to have a favorable clinical course in comparison to patients with DH lymphoma. There is an evidence to suggest that patients with double-expressor lymphoma might benefit from intensive induction therapy [21,22]. Approximately 2% of HGBL with MYC and BCL2 rearrangements express terminal deoxynucleotide transferase

(TdT). TdT can be variable intensity and correlates with immature immunophenotype. Although TdT expression is documented in mature B-cell lymphomas, these cases need to be differentiated from B-lymphoblastic leukemia/lymphoma (B-ALL) with MYC and BCL2 double rearrangements, especially in young patients [22,23].

Karyotype. DH HGBLs often have complex karyotypes, defined by 3 or greater numerical or structural aberrations. Frequently, aberrations involve *MYC* (8q24), and *BCL2* (18q21) and *BCL6* (3q27) genes [24]. Some of the other observed abnormalities include t(14;18) (q32;q21.3) and abnormalities of chromosomal region 1p36 [25].

Cytogenetics. Fluorescence in situ hybridization (FISH), conventional karyotyping or other molecular genetic methods are required to demonstrate rearrangement in *MYC*, *BCL2*, and *BCL6* genes. *MYC* and *BCL2* rearrangements dominate DH lymphomas (ranging from 45% to 72%) *MYC* and *BCL6* constitute from 9% to 36% of double-hit cases, and TH cases account for approximately 19% [16,19]. There is a concordance between conventional karyotype and FISH involving 8q24 (*MYC* gene), 3q27 (*BCL6*), and *BCL2* (18q21). Interestingly, approximately 10% of cases show aberrations of the 18q21 region but test negative for *BCL2* rearrangement by FISH [24]. Most follicular lymphomas have *IGH-BCL2* translocation, t(14;18), therefore it is feasible to suggest that HGBL with *MYC* and *BCL2* rearrangement might represent transformed follicular lymphomas. Although earlier studies identified only 11% of cases with an underlying follicular lymphoma, more recent studies argue that most lymphomas with both *MYC* and *BCL2* rearrangements are the result of transformation from an underlying follicular lymphoma [15,16].

MYC translocation partners. The *MYC* gene can be juxtaposed to one of the immunoglobulin (IG) genes or a non-IG gene. It is usually *IGH* (heavy chain on chromosome 14q32), less frequently *IGK* (kappa light chain on chromosome 2p11), or *IGL* (lambda light chain on chromosome 22q11). HGBL DH/TH is reported to have somewhat conflicting data on the relative distribution of *MYC* gene translocation partners. Kim and colleagues report more than 80% of HGBL DH/TH harbor juxtaposition of the *MYC* gene to IG loci. The majority (80%) of the MYC-IG translocations juxtapose *MYC* to *IGH* (14q32), 15%—*MYC* to *IGK* (2p12), and 5%—*MYC* to *IGL* (22q11.2). Chong and colleagues reports that 65% of HGBL DH/TH harbor a *MYC* translocation with a non-IG partner, followed by 28% of *MYC-IGH* translocation, and 7% *MYC-IGK/IGL* translocation. A similar trend is observed in patients with GCB-DLBCL [26]. In contrast, approximately 50% of patients with DLBCL harbor a *MYC-IG* translocation, and the remaining cases have *MYC* translocated to a non-IG partner, such as at 9p13 (gene unknown), 3q27 (*BCL6*), or other loci [27]. False-negative results from FISH *MYC* break-apart probes might result from a cryptic insertion of the *IGH* promoter into the *MYC* gene. Therefore, it might be useful to follow up with MYC/IGH fusion probes to help identify a wider range of rearrangements. Similar to patients with DLBCL, *MYC-IG* translocation is reported to confer an inferior outcome in patients with HGBL DH when compared with cases in which *MYC* has a non-IG translocation partner [27]. The clinical significance of the MYC partner gene, including non-IG *MYC*-translocation partners needs to be further elucidated [7,28].

Copy number alterations. Whole exome sequencing identified recurrent copy number gains in protooncogenes *MEF2B* and *CSFR1* and copy number losses in tumor suppressors including *NPM1* [16]. There was no difference in copy number variations between HGBL DH *BCL2*-rearranged, HGBL-DH *BCL6*-rearranged, and HGBL-THL [16].

Sequencing studies. Morphology, to some extent, is defined by the mutational landscape. For instance, it is interesting to note that HGBL DH/TH with Burkitt-like morphology is enriched with *TP53* and *CCND3* mutations, a known driver in BL [16].

In comparison to germinal center-type DLBCL, DH and TH HGBL are enriched in mutations affecting apoptosis and cell cycle genes (*BCL2*, *KMT2D*, *MYC*, *NOTCH1*, *EZH2*, and *FOXO1*) and epigenetic regulation genes (*CREBBP1*), and are known to carry an adverse prognosis (Table 1) [20]. In contrast, mutations in EZH2 and IRF8 were found in HGBL DT/TH and GCB-type DLBCL, suggesting their common origin [16]. Whole exome sequencing and targeted amplicon sequencing of 47 cases of HGBL-DH/TH demonstrated an accumulation of oncogenic mutations in NOTCH, IL6/JAK/STAT, and NFκB signaling pathways [16]. The heterogenous mutational landscape results in presumably constitutively active NOTCH signaling in 74% of HGBL DH/TH, including variants in *NCOR1* and *DTX1*. Interestingly, previous studies conducted by Karube and colleagues did not identify mutations in exon 34 of *NOTCH1 and NOTCH2* genes in HGBL DH/TH. This negative finding might be due to the targeted region of the study [29]. *MYD88* mutations are rare in HGBL DH, as compared with DLBCL where they are quite common [16,30].

There are striking differences in mutational signatures in *BCL2*-rearranged and *BCL6*-rearranged HGBL that highlight their divergent pathogenesis. For instance, *TP53* mutations are frequent in HGBL DH with *MYC* and *BCL2* but not *MYC* and *BCL6*

TABLE 1
Signaling Pathways and Gene Mutations Found in High-Grade B-Cell Lymphoma Double-Hit and Triple-Hit (HGBL DH/TH)

Pathways								
	NOTCH1	**IL6/JAK/STAT**	**NF-kB**	**Apoptosis/Cell Cycle**	**Epigenetics**	**Immunity**	**AID and SHM Targets**	**MAPK**
HGBL DH/TH	74%—*28* genes, most are gain of function [16]	74%—*PIM1* and *SOCS1*—most frequent [16]	62% [16] 7%—*PIM1*, *PRDM1*, *TNFAIP3*, *BTK*, *CARD11*, *MYD88* [20]	35%—*BCL2*, *MYC*, *TP53*, *FOXO1*, *GNA13*, *MFHAS1*, *BIRC3* [20]	32%—*KMT2D*, *EZH2*, *MEF2B*, *HIST1H1C*, *EP300*, *KMT2A*	15%—*CIITA*, *IGLL5*, *B2M*, *BCL6*, *TNFRSF14* [20]	*PIM1*, *SOCS1* [16,20] *IGL5* [20]	3%—*DUSP2*, *BRAF* [16]

	Genes, Mutations										Molecular Signatures		Molecular Cluster
	CREBBP[a]	**BCL2**	**KMT2D**	**TP53**	**MYC**	**EZH2**	**FOXO1**	**SOCS1**	**IGL5**	**ARID1A**	**CCND3**	**SBS5**	**SBS6**	
HGBL DH/TH	[a,c] [16,20]	[b] [9]	[b] [16,20]	[b] [20]	[b] [20]	- [20]	[b] [20]	[b] [20]	[b] [20]	[b] [20]	[b] [20]	[b] [16]		
BCL2-rearranged	[c] [16,20]	[c] [20]	[c] [16,20]	[c] [16]	[c] [16]	[c] Y646 [20] [d]	[c] Hot spot R19, R21, T24 [20] [d]	[c] [20]	[c] [20]	[b] [16]	[b] [16]	[c] [16]		C3/EZB [16]
BCL6-rearranged	- [20]	- [20]	[b] [16,20]	[b] [20]	[b] [20]	- [20]	- [20]	- [20]	[b] [20]	[c] [16]	[b] [16]		c [16]	Decrease C3 genes, increase BN2 cluster [16]
Triple-hit	100% [20]	[b] [16]	[b] [16]	[b] [16]	[b] [16]	[b] [16]	[b] [16]	[b] [16]	[b] [16]	[b] [16]	[b] [16]	SBS5 and SBS6 [16]		EZB [16]

Burkitt-like morphology–enriched with mutations in *TP53*, *CCND3*, and *CDKN2A* genes [16,20].

High-grade transformation–enriched with mutations in *TP53* gene [16,20].

Hans algorithm—germinal center B-cell type vast majority of HGBL with *MYC* and *BCL2*-rearranged; nongerminal center B-cell in ~50% HGBL with *MYC* and *BCL6*-rearranged [20]; Karyotype is complex in vast majority of cases.

Abbreviation: HGBL DH/TH, high-grade B-cell lymphoma, double-hit/triple-hit.

[a] Most frequently mutated gene.
[b] Present.
[c] Enriched.
[d] Exclusive.

rearrangements [31]. In addition to the gene rearrangements, gene sequence mutations are frequently identified in *MYC* (45% cases) and *BCL2* (60% cases) in *BCL2*-rearranged HGBL DH cases [20]. *BCL2*-rearranged HGBL DH cases are enriched for mutations in *CREBBP, KMT2A, EZH2, FOXO1*, and *SOCS1* genes [16]. *CREBBP* is the most frequently mutated gene in *BCL2*-rearranged cases. Predominantly missense mutations are described; resulting in the loss of *CREBBP* acetyltransferase activity, activation of *BCL6*, and reduction in *TP53* activity [16,20]. Notably, *EZH2* and *FOXO1* mutations seem exclusive to *MYC/BCL2* HGBL DH. Codon Y646 seems to be an *EZH2* mutational hotspot. *FOXO1* mutations (30% of cases), exclusive to *BCL2*-rearranged cases, also had mutational hotspots (codons R19, R21, and T24), and these clustered in the N-terminal domain.

Cases with *BCL6* rearrangement showed enrichment for *ARID1A* gene variants, and alterations of E2F targets. There is an enrichment in SBS6 molecular signature (implicated in defective DNA mismatch repair) in *BCL6*-rearranged cases (see Table 1).

The most frequently mutated gene in DH and TH HGBL is *CREBBP1* [16]. In addition, TH HGBL cases are enriched in E2F targets and mutations in *CDKN2A, LNP1*, and *CCND3* genes [16]. KMT2D mutations are detected in both DH and TH HGBL and are mostly frameshift deletions or stop gains that result in a loss of protein function [20].

Mutations in *CREBBP, FOXO1*, and *ARID1A* are associated with a worse prognosis and might be used for clinical management [16,20].

DH molecular signature. Recently, an RNA-based 104 gene DH molecular signature (DHITsig) was developed based on the gene expression profile of HGBL DH, TH, and GCB DLBCL [32]. Patients with the DH molecular signature had inferior outcomes after chemoimmunotherapy in comparison to the patients negative for the DH molecular signature (5-year time to progression rate 57% and 81%, respectively). Almost one-third of germinal center type DLBCL were classified as positive for DH molecular signature. Strikingly, only 50% of those had *MYC* and *BCL2* rearrangements identifiable by conventional interphase FISH. Subsequent whole genome sequencing studies identified that more than 25% of these cases indeed had a *MYC* and *BCL2* rearrangement that were cryptic to FISH [32]. Although FISH is currently the gold standard test for *MYC, BCL2*, and *BCL6* rearrangements, it is feasible to suggest that the whole genome or focused gene expression studies might be a preferred testing modality in the future.

The molecular high-grade (MHG) gene expression (70 genes) signature is enriched in cases of *BCL2*-rearranged HGBL-DH. Notably, a proportion of cases that are *MYC*-rearranged and *BCL2*-rearranged by FISH do not show MHG, and these cases have comparable survival to conventional GCB DLBCL [33]. An MYC sequence variant hot spot (at phosphorylation site T58) has been described in the high-risk molecular group, associated with DH with IG as the MYC partner, and portends poor survival [33].

High-Grade B-Cell Lymphoma, Not Otherwise Specified

HGBL, NOS is an aggressive B-cell lymphoma that can seem blastoid or with features intermediate between DLBCL and BL. Cases that have a DLBCL morphology and harbor *MYC* rearrangement are excluded from this category. Genetically, it lacks *MYC, BCL2*, and/or *BCL6* gene rearrangements and therefore cannot be classified as DH or TH lymphoma. BL-like cases with 11q aberrations are also excluded.

Clinical features. HGBL, NOS are rare and comprise less than 1% to 2% of all non-Hodgkin mature B-cell lymphomas [9]. A recent study of 41 cases showed male predominance with median age 41 years (ranging from 12 to 79 years). Patients with HGBL, NOS benefit from an intensive chemotherapy regimen (for instance DA-EPOCH-R) in comparison to R-CHOP. Median overall survival is short, at 18 months [34]. There seems to be a better prognosis of HGBL, NOS in comparison to DH/TH (75% vs 43% 3-year overall survival) [35].

Morphology and immunophenotype. Morphology is dominated by medium-sized more uniform lymphoma cells, some with BL-like morphology, and numerous tingible body macrophages imparting a "starry sky" appearance.[24] Most cases (approximately 80%) have a GCB immunophenotype, based on the Hans algorithm, and a high proliferative rate [36]. Shamana and colleagues reported that a GCB cell immunophenotype was as high as 89% in one study. Another study showed that 65% of HGL, NOS were CD10+, 91% were BCL6+, and 65% expressed the BCL2 protein [37]. Recent work on mutational landscape of TdT-positive HGBL suggests that TdT expression can be seen in mature B-cell lymphomas, and therefore does not exclude the diagnosis of HGBL, NOS [38,39].

Karyotype. The karyotype is often complex ($\geq$3 abnormalities) and has no evidence of double or triple rearrangement involving *MYC, BCL2*, and/or *BCL6* genes [34]. The following is an example complex karyotype found in HGBL, NOS that includes rearrangement of the *MYC* gene: 51,XX,+1,i(1) (q10),+7,add(8) (q24.1),t(8;14) (q24.1;q32),del(9) (p21p24),del(13) (q12q22),+19,+21,+21[19] [25]. Rearrangements of the *MYC* gene are reported in 17% (Perry and colleagues), and up to 35% of cases.[27 28]

Cytogenetics and molecular landscape. Interphase FISH is used routinely to detect rearrangements in *MYC*, *BCL2*, and *BCL6* genes. Usually, break-apart FISH probes to target *MYC, BCL2, and BCL6* are used. Up to approximately one-third of HGBL, NOS cases harbor only a *MYC* gene rearrangement, 5% to 14% show *BCL2*, and 3% to 7% had *BCL6* gene rearrangements.[28 24] A recent study showed that 13% (4/32 cases) had a single *MYC* gene rearrangement [37]. None of the patients with HGBL, NOS had both *BCL2* and *BCL6* rearrangements. Cases with blastoid morphology reportedly have fewer *MYC* or *BCL2* translocations.[28 27] *BCL2* and *BCL6* rearrangements are reported in 14% and 3% of HGBL, NOS, respectively [40]. Interestingly, approximately 20% to 25% of cases do not have notable cytogenetic abnormalities.[28, 24] Less than 10% of patients have numerical or copy number variations in addition to the rearrangements [34]. About 14% of patients reportedly had copy number changes without rearrangements [40]. HGBL, NOS has been reported to have a high genetic complexity with 8 copy number variations in an OncoScan (chromosomal microarray) assay [37]. Copy number variations cannot be used as an evidence of gene rearrangement and therefore cannot be used to diagnose DH or TH lymphomas. Recently, a few cases of HGBL, NOS with *MYC* rearrangement and 11q aberration were discovered [41]. These cases cannot be classified as BLL-11q because they carry a *MYC* rearrangement. One hypothesis is that an 11q aberration may enhance the effect of the *MYC* rearrangement and contribute to *MYC*-positive lymphoma pathogenesis. Although a recent study reported mutations in *TP53* and *PRDM1* genes, there is very little literature available to characterize the genetic mutational landscape of HGBL, NOS, perhaps, because it is such a rare, and somewhat ambiguous category [37].

High grade B-cell Lymphoma with 11q Aberrations

It is seen in younger patients, resembles Burkitt lymphoma by morphology and immunophenotype, but instead of a MYC gene rearrangement, it harbors aberrations of chromosome 11. It was initially recognized as a provisional Burkitt-like lymphoma with 11q aberration (BLL-11q) the fourth edition of the WHO. Current knowledge on mutational landscape shows that it is different from Burkitt lymphoma and is more related to germinal B-cell origin DLBCL. In addition, subsequent studies identified variable morphology with frequent large cells. As a consequence, this provisional entity was renamed as High grade B-cell lymphoma with 11q aberration (WHO 5th edition [2] and Large B-cell lymphoma with 11q aberration (International Consensus Classification 2022) [3].

Clinical features. Patients with a diagnosis of High grade B-cell lymphoma with 11q aberrations tend to be younger, with a mean age of 15 years (range 8–37 years), and with male predominance [52]. This disease most commonly presents in lymph nodes, commonly in a head and neck distribution. Extranodal sites are rare [52]. Based on the limited number of cases, the clinical course seems to be similar to BL [42]. The prognosis is generally favorable with 5-year overall survival of 80% [51]. Treatment consists of aggressive chemoimmunotherapy with central nervous system prophylaxis [52]. High grade B-cell lymphoma with 11q aberrations has been reported in both immunocompetent [51] and immunocompromised patients [44].

Morphology and immunophenotype. The morphology resembles BL Burkitt lymphoma with a more nodular/follicular growth pattern [42]. In addition, it can present with large centroblastic cells [45–47].

Karyotype. Cases of High grade B-cell lymphoma with 11q aberrations have more complex karyotypes and more frequent nodal presentation than BL but the clinical course and prognosis seem to be similar. Although the 11q aberration can be identified by conventional karyotype or FISH, the preferred method to identify 11q aberration is by chromosomal microarray.

Cytogenetics. For diagnostic purposes, chromosome 11q gains and losses can be identified using FISH strategies or, if FISH is equivocal, chromosomal microarray [46]. These abnormalities include 11q proximal gains and telomeric losses; specifically, interstitial gains including a minimal region of gain in 11q23.2-23.3 and telomeric losses of 11q24.1-qter [48,49,50] (Figure 1A). This peculiar aberration is presumed to originate from the duplication and inversion of the q (long) arm of the chromosome 11 (Fig. 1B). The 11q aberration can be identified by conventional karyotype or FISH. FISH probes that might be useful to identify 11q aberration are designed to target CEN 11 (11p11.1-q11), KMT2A (11q23), 11qTel (11q25). SNP array is a widely available methodology in the clinical laboratory, where formalin-fixed paraffin-embedded tissue can be used. There is a reported spectrum of the breakpoints spanning the q arm of chromosome 11 that results in the pattern of proximal gain and terminal loss [51,51]. Massively parallel sequencing techniques, such as whole genome or transcriptome sequencing, can be instrumental in detecting copy number variations but are usually used in the research setting.

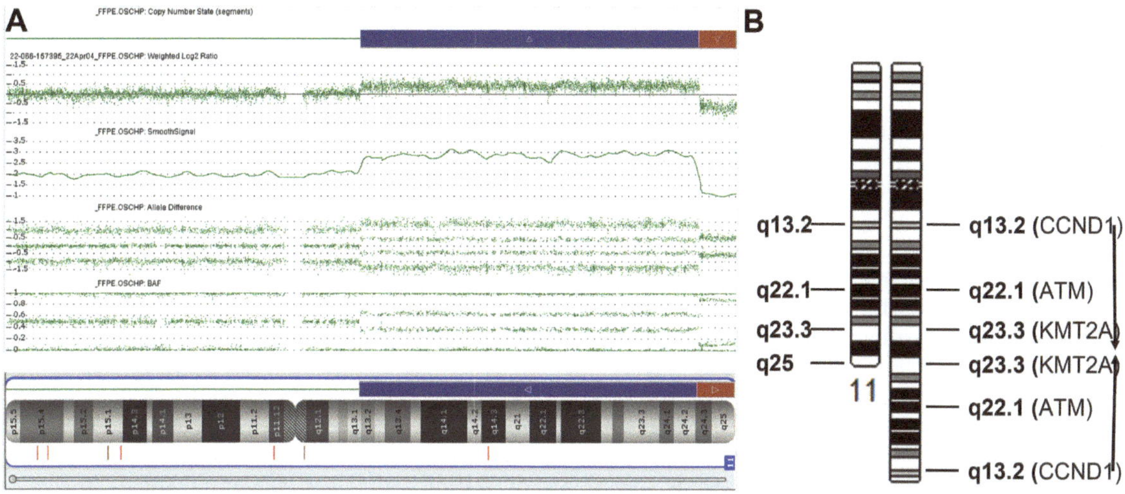

FIG. 1 11q aberration with proximal gain and terminal loss. (**A**) Cytogenomic molecular inversion probe array shows duplication (gain) within 11q13.1q24.3 (11q13.1q24.3, 685 genes) and deletion (loss) within 11q24.3q25 (6.8 Mb, 51 genes). (**B**) Graphic depiction of the possible mechanism of duplication and inversion of 11q.

It is important to note that an isolated 11q proximal gain or terminal loss is not diagnostic of 11q aberration.

High grade B-cell lymphoma with 11q aberration cases are negative for *MYC* rearrangement. High grade B-cell lymphoma with 11q aberration is negative for 1q gains (seen in *MYC*-positive BL), 2p16.1 and 7p and losses of 1p36.32 (seen in DLBCL, germinal center type). High grade B-cell lymphoma with 11q aberration is positive for aberration of chromosome 11q characterized by proximal gain and distal loss, which is mainly absent in other lymphomas, including transformed follicular lymphoma, a few cases of *MYC*-rearranged BL, and *MYC*-rearranged HGBL, NOS [48,52]. In contrast to BL, High grade B-cell lymphoma with 11q aberration lacks 1q gain, has a more complex karyotype, and frequently presents with a follicular pattern with nodal involvement [53].

Molecular profile. High grade B-cell lymphoma with 11q aberration has a unique microRNA and gene expression profile that suggests synchronous upregulation of oncogenes (PAFAH1B2/*11q23.3*) and downregulation of tumor suppressor genes (FLI1 and ETS1/11q24 microdeletion) [43]. Although BL and High grade B-cell lymphoma with 11q aberration share morphologic, immunophenotypic, and certain gene expression profile features, their mutational landscape differs [54]. High grade B-cell lymphoma with 11q aberration has higher chromosomal complexity and an absence of the ID3, TCF3, or CCND3 mutations that are typical for BL. The 11q-gain/loss aberration has been found not only in *MYC*-negative Burkitt-like lymphoma but also in some cases of *MYC*-positive BL. Three cases of *MYC*-rearranged BL were reported to harbor the 11q aberration [48]. In addition, *MYC*-rearranged aggressive B-cell lymphomas including HGBL, NOS, and Burkitt-lymphoma were demonstrated to harbor the 11q aberration in some cases [48,50]. Attempts have been made to identify the genes that are dysregulated in the 11q aberrations. The region that involves 11q proximal gain and telomeric loss was implicated in coordinated upregulation of oncogenes (*PAFAH1B2*) and deletion of tumor suppressor genes (*FLI1, ETS1*) [51]. All cases of High grade B-cell lymphoma with 11q aberration aberration lacked mutations in both *TCF3* and its negative regulator *ID3*. Mutations in *TCF3* and/or *ID3* are identified in 70%, 67%, and 40% of sporadic BL, HIV-associated BL, and endemic BL, respectively. Oncogenic mutations in *CCND3* are identified in 38% of sporadic BL cases, producing highly stable cyclin D3 isoforms that drive cell cycle progression. Interestingly, one case of High grade B-cell lymphoma with 11q aberration had a mutational profile characteristic of BL including *MYC, DDX3X, SMARC4, CCND3,* and *TP53* mutations [52].

DISCUSSION AND FUTURE DIRECTIONS

Recently, gene expression profiling of 104 genes identified a molecular DH signature that correlated with clinical outcomes similar to HGBL DH/TH. Half of the cases that were positive for the DH signature were negative for *MYC* and *BCL2* genes rearrangement by FISH [32] but 30% of these cases were later found to carry FISH-cryptic rearrangements by whole-genome sequencing [32]. Although a break-apart FISH probe detection scheme fails to detect up to 4% of *MYC* rearrangements,

FISH break-apart probes for *MYC* gene rearrangement is still standardly used to diagnose HGBL DH/TH [55]. Massively parallel DNA and RNA sequencing provides additional insights into the understanding of genomes and transcriptomes of HGBL and may be a valuable addition in the diagnosis of HGBL DH/T.

Although mutational landscapes vary in HGBL DH/TH, depending on the *BCL2* or *BCL6* rearrangements, common alterations are present in HGBL DH/TH. Commonly described gene sequence alterations include single nucleotide variants and insertion/deletions, with the most frequent type of alteration being a missense mutation. For instance, aberrant NOTCH signaling seems to be a frequently shared pathway in HGBL DH/TH. Most of the NOTCH pathway mutations are activating, with mutations in *NCOR1* and *DTX1* portending a worse clinical outcome [16]. HGBL DH/TH is enriched in alterations that are hypothesized to result in the activation of IL6/JAK/STAT pathway (74% of cases) [16]. Cases that have Burkitt-like morphology seem to be enriched with *CCND3* and *TP53* mutations [16].

TP53 and *MYC* mutations are more frequent in *BCL2*-rearranged cases of HGBL DH but not in *BCL6*-rearranged HGBL DH cases. *BCL2*-rearranged cases more commonly carried mutations in CREBBP and KMT2D, whereas BCL6-rearranged cases were enriched for mutations in ARID1A and E2F targets [16]. Mutations in *ARID1A* have been associated with the worst clinical outcomes, suggesting that HGBL with *MYC* and *BCL6* rearrangements may have a worse prognosis than HGBL with *MYC* and *BCL2* rearrangements [16]. HGBL TH displays intermediate mutational features, including mutations in *CREBBP, CDKN2A, LNP1*, and *CCND3* genes [16,20].

Genomic studies have identified mutations in numerous key molecular drivers in HGBL DH/TH, such as *TP53, CREBBP, CCND3, BCL2, KMT2D, NOTCH1/2MYC, EZH2*, and *FOXO1*. Mutations in *CREBBP, FOXO1*, and *ARID1A* are associated with a worse prognosis [16,20]. *BCL2*-rearranged cases showed alterations in p53 and MYC pathways, whereas *BCL6*-rearranged cases showed alterations of E2F targets. There are some discrepancies in the mutational landscape of HGBL DH/TH, for instance NOTCH pathway, that were reported recently. One group that used a more targeted analytical approach failed to identify mutations in the *NOTCH1* gene, whereas study that used whole exome sequencing identified numerous mutations in genes associated with NOTCH pathway signaling [16,20]. HGBL, NOS is a rare entity and more studies on its mutational landscape are warranted in the future.

Minimal or measurable residual disease testing (MRD) has recently emerged as an indicator of a disease progression in patients with CLL/SLL [56]. MRD use is not yet established for HGBL. However, there is evidence to suggest that circulating cell-free tumor DNA might be a prognostic tool in patients with DLBCL who underwent treatment with anti-CD19 chimeric antigen receptor (CAR) T cell therapy (CAR-T) [57].

Massively parallel sequencing methods will soon be incorporated into routine daily clinical practice, enabling more accurate classification of HGBL, and allowing patients to receive optimal treatment [58]. Patients with HGBL DH/TH are treated with intensive chemotherapy regimens (eg, DA-EPOCH-R) as outcomes with R-CHOP are suboptimal. There is currently no molecularly targeted therapy available for patients with HGBL DH/TH. Considering the aggressive clinical course in patients with HGBL DH/TH, it will be important to discover novel drivers of disease that can be efficiently molecularly targeted as part of the treatment regimen.

CLINICS CARE POINTS

- Choice of treatment regimen depends on the World Health Organization- and/or International Consensus Classification-defined diagnostic entity
- Testing for 11q aberration by Fluorescence in situ hybridization, chromosomal microarray, or massively parallel sequencing is required to diagnose High grade B-cell lymphoma with 11q aberration
- High grade B-cell lymphoma with 11q aberration has a good prognosis when treated with intense chemo-immunotherapy with central nervous system prophylaxis
- High-grade B-cell lymphoma with *MYC* and *BCL2* with/without *BCL6* rearrangements is treated with more intense chemoimmunotherapy than diffuse large B-cell lymphoma

ACKNOWLEDGMENTS

Authors are grateful to Dr Erica Anderson (University of Utah) and Dr Makenzie Fulmer (University of Utah) for the help with obtaining and interpreting microarray data.

DISCLOSURE

The authors have nothing to disclose.

REFERENCES

[1] Swerdlow S, Campo E, Harris N, et al. WHO classification of tumours of haematopoietic and lymphoid tissues. Lyon, France: IARC Press; 2017.

[2] Alaggio R, Amador C, Anagnostopoulos I, et al. The 5th edition of the World Health Organization Classification of Haematolymphoid Tumours: Lymphoid Neoplasms. Leukemia 2022;36(7):1720–48.

[3] Campo E, Jaffe ES, Cook JR, et al. The International Consensus Classification of Mature Lymphoid Neoplasms: a report from the Clinical Advisory Committee. Blood 2022;140(11):1229–53.

[4] Ennishi D, Jiang A, Boyle M, et al. Double-Hit Gene Expression Signature Defines a Distinct Subgroup of Germinal Center B-Cell-Like Diffuse Large B-Cell Lymphoma. J Clin Oncol Off J Am Soc Clin Oncol 2019;37(3):190–201.

[5] Li S, Desai P, Lin P, et al. MYC/BCL6 double-hit lymphoma (DHL): a tumour associated with an aggressive clinical course and poor prognosis. Histopathology 2016;68(7):1090–8.

[6] Pillai RK, Sathanoori M, Van Oss SB, Swerdlow SH. Double-hit B-cell lymphomas with BCL6 and MYC translocations are aggressive, frequently extranodal lymphomas distinct from BCL2 double-hit B-cell lymphomas. Am. J. Surg. Pathol. 2013;37(3):323–32.

[7] Rosenwald A, et al. Prognostic Significance of MYC Rearrangement and Translocation Partner in Diffuse Large B-Cell Lymphoma: A Study by the Lunenburg Lymphoma Biomarker Consortium. J. Clin. Oncol. Off. J. Am. Soc. Clin. Oncol. 2019;37(35):3359–68.

[8] Ye Q, et al. Prognostic impact of concurrent MYC and BCL6 rearrangements and expression in de novo diffuse large B-cell lymphoma. Oncotarget 2016;7(3):2401–16.

[9] Li S, Lin P, Medeiros LJ. Advances in pathological understanding of high-grade B cell lymphomas. Expert Rev Hematol 2018;11(8):637–48.

[10] Haralambieva E, Boerma EJ, van Imhoff GW, et al. Clinical, immunophenotypic, and genetic analysis of adult lymphomas with morphologic features of Burkitt lymphoma. Am J Surg Pathol 2005;29(8):1086–94.

[11] Swerdlow SH. Diagnosis of "double hit" diffuse large B-cell lymphoma and B-cell lymphoma, unclassifiable, with features intermediate between DLBCL and Burkitt lymphoma: when and how, FISH versus IHC. Hematol Am Soc Hematol Educ Program 2014;2014(1):90–9.

[12] Zhang J, et al. High-grade B-Cell Lymphoma With MYC, BCL2, and/or BCL6 Translocations/Rearrangements: Clinicopathologic Features of 51 Cases in a Single Institution of South China. Am. J. Surg. Pathol. 2020;44(12):1602–11.

[13] Scott DW, et al. High-grade B-cell lymphoma with MYC and BCL2 and/or BCL6 rearrangements with diffuse large B-cell lymphoma morphology. Blood 2018;131(18):2060–4.

[14] Johnson NA, Slack GW, Savage KJ, et al. Concurrent Expression of MYC and BCL2 in Diffuse Large B-Cell Lymphoma Treated With Rituximab Plus Cyclophosphamide, Doxorubicin, Vincristine, and Prednisone. J Clin Oncol 2012; 30(28):3452–9.

[15] Oki Y, Noorani M, Lin P, et al. Double hit lymphoma: the MD Anderson Cancer Center clinical experience. Br J Haematol 2014;166(6):891–901.

[16] Künstner A, Witte HM, Riedl J, et al. Mutational landscape of high-grade B-cell lymphoma with MYC-, BCL2 and/or BCL6 rearrangements characterized by whole-exome sequencing. Haematologica 2021;18. https://doi.org/10.3324/haematol.2021.279631.

[17] Wang W, Hu S, Lu X, et al. Triple-hit B-cell Lymphoma With MYC, BCL2, and BCL6 Translocations/Rearrangements: Clinicopathologic Features of 11 Cases. Am J Surg Pathol 2015;39(8):1132–9.

[18] Landsburg DJ, Falkiewicz MK, Maly J, et al. Outcomes of patients with double-hit lymphoma who achieve first complete remission. J Clin Oncol Off J Am Soc Clin Oncol 2017;35(20):2260–7.

[19] Aukema SM, Siebert R, Schuuring E, et al. Double-hit B-cell lymphomas. Blood 2011;117(8):2319–31.

[20] Evrard SM, Péricart S, Grand D, et al. Targeted next generation sequencing reveals high mutation frequency of CREBBP, BCL2 and KMT2D in high-grade B-cell lymphoma with MYC and BCL2 and/or BCL6 rearrangements. Haematologica 2019;104(4):e154–7.

[21] Riedell PA, Smith SM. Double hit and double expressors in lymphoma: Definition and treatment. Cancer 2018; 124(24):4622–32.

[22] Reagan PM, Davies A. Current treatment of double hit and double expressor lymphoma. Hematol Am Soc Hematol Educ Program 2017;2017(1):295–7.

[23] Wagener R, et al. IG-MYC + neoplasms with precursor B-cell phenotype are molecularly distinct from Burkitt lymphomas. Blood 2018;132(21):2280–5.

[24] Kim H, Kim HJ, Kim SH. Diagnostic Approach for Double-Hit and Triple-Hit Lymphoma Based on Immunophenotypic and Cytogenetic Characteristics of Bone Marrow Specimens. Ann Lab Med 2020;40(5):361–9.

[25] Kanagal-Shamanna R, Medeiros LJ, Lu G, et al. High-grade B cell lymphoma, unclassifiable, with blastoid features: an unusual morphological subgroup associated frequently with BCL2 and/or MYC gene rearrangements and a poor prognosis. Histopathology 2012;61(5):945–54.

[26] Chong LC, Ben-Neriah S, Slack GW, et al. High-resolution architecture and partner genes of MYC rearrangements in lymphoma with DLBCL morphology. Blood Adv 2018;2(20):2755–65.

[27] Copie-Bergman C, Cuillière-Dartigues P, Baia M, et al. MYC-IG rearrangements are negative predictors of survival in DLBCL patients treated with immunochemotherapy: a GELA/LYSA study. Blood 2015;126(22):2466–74.

[28] McPhail ED, et al. Inferior survival in high-grade B-cell lymphoma with MYC and BCL2 and/or BCL6 rearrangements is not associated with MYC/IG gene rearrangements. Haematologica 2018;103(11):1899–907.

[29] Karube K, Enjuanes A, Dlouhy I, et al. Integrating genomic alterations in diffuse large B-cell lymphoma identifies new relevant pathways and potential therapeutic targets. Leukemia 2018;32(3):675–84.

[30] Gebauer N, Bernard V, Thorns C, et al. Oncogenic MYD88 mutations are rare events in double-hit B-cell lymphomas. Acta Haematol 2015;133(1):113–5.

[31] Gebauer N, Bernard V, Gebauer W, et al. TP53 mutations are frequent events in double-hit B-cell lymphomas with

MYC and BCL2 but not MYC and BCL6 translocations. Leuk Lymphoma 2015;56(1):179–85.

[32] Hilton LK, Tang J, Ben-Neriah S, et al. The double-hit signature identifies double-hit diffuse large B-cell lymphoma with genetic events cryptic to FISH. Blood 2019;134(18):1528–32.

[33] Cucco F, Barrans S, Sha C, et al. Distinct genetic changes reveal evolutionary history and heterogeneous molecular grade of DLBCL with MYC/BCL2 double-hit. Leukemia 2020;34(5):1329–41.

[34] Li J, Liu X, Yao Z, et al. High-Grade B-Cell Lymphomas, Not Otherwise Specified: A Study of 41 Cases. Cancer Manag Res 2020;12:1903–12.

[35] Baryakh EA, Misyurina AE, Kovrigina AM, et al. [Diagnosis and treatment in patients with B-cell lymphoma unclassified that is intermediate between diffuse large B-cell lymphoma and Burkitt's lymphoma]. Ter Arkh 2015;87(8): 77–85.

[36] Hans CP, Weisenburger DD, Greiner TC, et al. Confirmation of the molecular classification of diffuse large B-cell lymphoma by immunohistochemistry using a tissue microarray. Blood 2004;103(1):275–82.

[37] Hüttl KS, Staiger AM, Richter J, et al. The "Burkitt-like" immunophenotype and genotype is rarely encountered in diffuse large B cell lymphoma and high-grade B cell lymphoma, NOS. Virchows Arch Int J Pathol 2021;479(3):575–83.

[38] Bhavsar S, Liu Y-C, Gibson SE, Moore EM, Swerdlow SH. Mutational Landscape of TdT+ Large B-cell Lymphomas Supports Their Distinction From B-lymphoblastic Neoplasms: A Multiparameter Study of a Rare and Aggressive Entity. Am. J. Surg. Pathol. 2022;46(1):71–82.

[39] Khanlari M, et al. Blastoid high-grade B-cell lymphoma initially presenting in bone marrow: a diagnostic challenge. Mod. Pathol. Off. J. U. S. Can. Acad. Pathol. Inc 2022;35(3):419–26.

[40] Perry AM, Crockett D, Dave BJ, et al. B-cell lymphoma, unclassifiable, with features intermediate between diffuse large B-cell lymphoma and burkitt lymphoma: study of 39 cases. Br J Haematol 2013;162(1):40–9.

[41] Grygalewicz B, Woroniecka R, Rymkiewicz G, et al. The 11q-Gain/Loss Aberration Occurs Recurrently in MYC-Negative Burkitt-like Lymphoma With 11q Aberration, as Well as MYC-Positive Burkitt Lymphoma and MYC-Positive High-Grade B-Cell Lymphoma, NOS. Am J Clin Pathol 2018;149(1):17–28.

[42] Gonzalez-Farre B, Ramis-Zaldivar JE, Salmeron-Villalobos J, et al. Burkitt-like lymphoma with 11q aberration: a germinal center-derived lymphoma genetically unrelated to Burkitt lymphoma. Haematologica 2019;104(9):1822–9.

[43] Salaverria I, Martin-Guerrero I, Wagener R, et al. A recurrent 11q aberration pattern characterizes a subset of MYC-negative high-grade B-cell lymphomas resembling Burkitt lymphoma. Blood 2014;123(8):1187–98.

[44] Ferreiro JF, Morscio J, Dierickx D, et al. Post-transplant molecularly defined Burkitt lymphomas are frequently MYC-negative and characterized by the 11q-gain/loss pattern. Haematologica 2015;100(7):e275–9.

[45] Gebauer N, et al. Aggressive B-cell lymphoma cases with 11q aberration patterns indicate a spectrum beyond Burkitt-like lymphoma. Blood Adv 2021;5(23):5220–5.

[46] Horn H, et al. A Diagnostic Approach to the Identification of Burkitt-like Lymphoma With 11q Aberration in Aggressive B-Cell Lymphomas. Am. J. Surg. Pathol. 2021;45(3):356–64.

[47] Au-Yeung RKH, et al. Experience with provisional WHO-entities large B-cell lymphoma with IRF4-rearrangement and Burkitt-like lymphoma with 11q aberration in paediatric patients of the NHL-BFM group. Br. J. Haematol. 2020;190(5):753–63.

[48] Grygalewicz B, Woroniecka R, Rymkiewicz G, et al. The 11q-Gain/Loss Aberration Occurs Recurrently in MYC-Negative Burkitt-like Lymphoma With 11q Aberration, as Well as MYC-Positive Burkitt Lymphoma and MYC-Positive High-Grade B-Cell Lymphoma, NOS. Am J Clin Pathol 2017;149(1):17–28.

[49] Pienkowska-Grela B, Rymkiewicz G, Grygalewicz B, et al. Partial trisomy 11, dup(11)(q23q13), as a defect characterizing lymphomas with Burkitt pathomorphology without MYC gene rearrangement. Med Oncol Northwood Lond Engl 2011;28(4):1589–95.

[50] Havelange V, Ameye G, Théate I, et al. The peculiar 11qgain/loss aberration reported in a subset of MYCnegative high-grade B-cell lymphomas can also occur in a MYC-rearranged lymphoma. Cancer Genet 2016;209(3):117–8.

[51] Rymkiewicz G, Grygalewicz B, Chechlinska M, et al. A comprehensive flow-cytometry-based immunophenotypic characterization of Burkitt-like lymphoma with 11q aberration. Mod Pathol 2018;31(5):732–43.

[52] Bouska A, McKeithan TW, Deffenbacher KE, et al. Genome-wide copy-number analyses reveal genomic abnormalities involved in transformation of follicular lymphoma. Blood 2014;123(11):1681–90.

[53] Zajdel M, Rymkiewicz G, Chechlinska M, et al. miR expression in MYC-negative DLBCL/BL with partial trisomy 11 is similar to classical Burkitt lymphoma and different from diffuse large B-cell lymphoma. Tumour Biol J Int Soc Oncodevelopmental Biol Med 2015;36(7):5377–88.

[54] Wagener R, Seufert J, Raimondi F, et al. The mutational landscape of Burkitt-like lymphoma with 11q aberration is distinct from that of Burkitt lymphoma. Blood 2019; 133(9):962–6.

[55] King RL, McPhail ED, Meyer RG, et al. False-negative rates for MYC fluorescence in situ hybridization probes in B-cell neoplasms. Haematologica 2019;104(6):e248–51.

[56] Wierda WG, Rawstron A, Cymbalista F, et al. Measurable residual disease in chronic lymphocytic leukemia: expert review and consensus recommendations. Leukemia 2021;35(11):3059–72.

[57] Galimberti S, Genuardi E, Mazziotta F, et al. The Minimal Residual Disease in Non-Hodgkin's Lymphomas: From the Laboratory to the Clinical Practice. Front Oncol 2019;9:528.

[58] Chiappella A, Crombie J, Guidetti A, et al. Are We Ready to Treat Diffuse Large B-cell and High-Grade Lymphoma According to Major Genetic Subtypes? HemaSphere 2019;3(5):e284.

Advances in Molecular Pathology 5 (2022) 51–58
ADVANCES IN MOLECULAR PATHOLOGY

Molecular Advances in Nodal Peripheral T-Cell Lymphoma

Safina Hafeez, MD*, Allison M. Cushman-Vokoun, MD, PhD
University of Nebraska Medical Center, 985454 Nebraska Medical Center, Omaha, NE 68105-5454, USA

KEYWORDS

• Gene • Mutation • PTCL • PTCL-GATA3 • PTCL-TBX21 • *RHOA* • *TP63* • *DUSP22*

KEY POINTS

- Peripheral T-cell lymphoma (PTCL)-GATA binding protein-3 (GATA3) subtype is associated with unfavorable prognosis.
- PTCL-T-box transcription factor 21 (TBX21) subtype carries favorable prognosis.
- *Ras Homology Family Member A (RHOA)*^{G17V} is commonly mutated in angioimmunoblastic T-cell lymphoma.
- The 5-year overall survival of *Dual specificity phosphatase 22 (DUSP22)* rearranged Anaplastic lymphoma kinase (ALK)-anaplastic large cell lymphoma (ALCL) is comparable with Anaplastic lymphoma kinase (ALK) + ALCL.
- Mutations in genes associated with epigenetic regulation are commonly identified in PTCL.

INTRODUCTION

Peripheral T-cell lymphoma (PTCL) is a rare and heterogeneous group of mature T-cell malignancies, comprising 10% to 15% of all cases of non-Hodgkin lymphoma in the western countries, with a higher incidence in parts of Asia (20%–30%) [1,2]. PTCL is derived from post-thymic T-cells. These are an aggressive set of diseases, which are frequently associated with poor prognosis. The revised 2016 World Health Organization (WHO) classification recognizes at least 29 subtypes of PTCL, subdivided into four major categories based on the clinical presentation and location of the disease: nodal, extranodal, cutaneous, and leukemic [3] and the entities described here are based on this classification. The diagnostic approach in PTCL is based mostly on a combination of multiple features such as clinical presentation, morphology, immunophenotype, cytogenetics, and molecular genetic findings. An alternative paradigm is to view PTCL in the context of the two main components of the normal immune system: the innate immune system, which is the first line of defense, and the adaptive immune system [4]. The adaptive system is a more complex process, mediated by antigen receptor and antigen-presenting cells characterized by both memory and specialized cells [5]. Nodal PTCLs account for over half of all mature T cell neoplasms and include PTCL-not otherwise specified (PTCL-NOS), angioimmunoblastic T-cell lymphoma (AITL), nodal PTCL with a T follicular helper (TFH) phenotype, follicular T-cell lymphoma (FTCL), anaplastic large cell lymphoma (ALCL)-ALK positive (ALK+), and ALCL-ALK negative (ALK−).

Among all nodal PTCL, PTCL-NOS is the most common subtype followed by angioimmunoblastic T-cell lymphoma. The 5-year overall survival (OS) of T-cell lymphoma, in general, is less than 30% [6]. Diagnosing PTCL-NOS is challenging due to its infrequent occurrence and some discomfort on the pathologists' part in interpreting ancillary studies in the context of morphology. For instance, molecular analysis may reveal a clonal T-cell gene rearrangement in a benign/reactive condition, although T-cell lymphomas may lack a demonstrable clonal rearrangement [7,8]. Moreover, PTCLs have a wide morphologic spectrum within

*Corresponding author, *E-mail address:* Shafeez@unmc.edu

https://doi.org/10.1016/j.yamp.2022.05.002
2589-4080/22/ Published by Elsevier Inc.

a single diagnostic entity, and the microscopic appearance can overlap with what may be seen in reactive proliferations. However, recent advances in gene expression profiling (GEP) and next-generation sequencing (NGS) technologies have provided new insight into the different subtypes of PTCL. In this review article, we focus on nodal PTCL.

PERIPHERAL T-CELL LYMPHOMA—NOT OTHERWISE SPECIFIED

PTCL-NOS is one of the most common types of PTCL, accounting for about 25% to 30% of all cases [9]. It is a heterogeneous category that does not correspond to any specifically defined entity and is typically a diagnosis of exclusion. Lymphomas with TFH phenotype are excluded from this category. GEP studies have been used to refine the subclassification of PTCL-NOS, leading to the identification of two major subgroups [10,11]. One subgroup is characterized by the expression of *TBX21* and its target genes such as *CXCR3, IL2RB, CCL3,* and *IFNG,* designated as PTCL-TBX21. The other subgroup is characterized by the expression of *GATA3* and its target genes such as *CCR4, IL18RA, CXCR7* and *IK,* designated as PTCL-GATA3. *TBX21* and *GATA3* are the master regulators of Th1 and Th2 differentiation [12]. Amador and colleagues applied this principle to immunohistochemistry (IHC) using a commercially available four-antibody panel specific for GATA3, CCR4, TBX21, and CXCR3, as a more practical approach for subclassification [12]. This study also demonstrated a worse prognosis in the PTCL-GATA3 subgroup, confirming the GEP findings. Of note, although the PTCL-TBX21 subgroup is generally described to have better outcomes, a subset of cases within this group was identified as having high cytotoxic T-cell signatures and worse outcomes [10,11].

NGS has further unraveled the mutational landscape in PTCL-NOS, leading to progress in the understanding of its biology (Fig. 1). PTCL-GATA3 shows high genomic complexity characterized by frequent loss-of-function alterations (eg, biallelic deletions/mutations) of tumor suppressor genes such as *TP53, PTEN,* and *CDKN2A* [13]. These aberrations are associated with a poorer prognosis. Deletion of *PTEN* and *CDKN2A* are frequently identified in PTCL-NOS in both sequencing and FISH analysis, and co-deletion of *PTEN* and *CDKN2A* has been reported to be highly specific for PTCL-NOS [14]. The PTCL-GATA3 subgroup expression signature has previously been associated with *MYC* overexpression, and a more recent study has reported frequent co-occurrence of gains and amplification of *MYC* and *STAT3* [13]. This study also provided further evidence that these two subgroups are dependent on distinct signaling pathways; the PTCL-GATA3 subtype is associated with altered PI3K-mTOR signaling, and the PTCL-TBX21 subtype is associated with dysregulated Nuclear factor-kappa B (NF-kB) pathway signaling. Watatani and colleagues studied the molecular heterogeneity in PTCL-NOS, identifying a distinct subgroup with mutations and deletions in *TP53* and *CDKN2A* showing marked chromosomal instability, mutations in *IKZF2,* and frequent genetic alteration involving immune surveillance pathways (eg, *HLA-A, HLA-B, CIITA, CD274, CD58,* and *FAS*). This study reported that these aberrations correlated with a poor prognosis [15].

Additional molecular variants have been identified in both epigenetic and T-cell signaling pathways. Although less frequent than in PTCL with a TFH phenotype, mutation of epigenetic regulator genes such as *DNMT3A* and *TET2* do occur in PTCL-NOS [13,15,16]. *TET2* mutations occur more frequently (38%–49%) than *DNMT3A* (5%–36%) in PTCL-NOS [6,15–17]. Mutations in epigenetic regulator/chromatin remodeling genes such as *KMT2C, KMT2D, KMT2A, SETD2,* and *CHD1* showed no prognostic effect in one study, although another study indicated a possible association with inferior progression-free survival and increased responsiveness to histone deacetylase inhibitors [18,19].

Mutations in T-cell receptor (TCR) signaling/NF-KB pathway genes have been reported in *VAV1, RHOA, CARD11, FYN, PLCG1, CD28,* and *PTPRC* in comprehensive genetic profiling of PTCL-NOS [15]. New in-frame fusion transcripts involving TCR signaling genes have been identified in PTCL-NOS, including *FYN::TRAF3IP2, KHDRBS1::LCK,* and *SIN3A::OXO1,* with *FYN::TRAF3IP2* found as a recurrent fusion in a subset of cases [20]. This study also demonstrated that *FYN::TRAF3IP2* and *KHDRBS1::LCK* activate signaling pathways downstream of the TCR complex, suggesting potential for therapy with tyrosine kinase inhibitors. Fusions involving the guanine nucleotide exchange factor, *VAV1,* have been found with a variety of fusion partners including *MYO1F, THAP4,* and S100A7 [21]. These fusions result in the activation of VAV1-dependent signaling pathways. Finally, recurrent mutations in another tumor suppressor, the *FAT1* gene, have been notably found in ~39% of PTCL-NOS cases, leading to an unfavorable outcome [18]. Recurrent structural abnormalities of TP63 and other p53-related genes have also been identified in PTCL, including a *TBL1XR1::TP63* fusion [20–22].

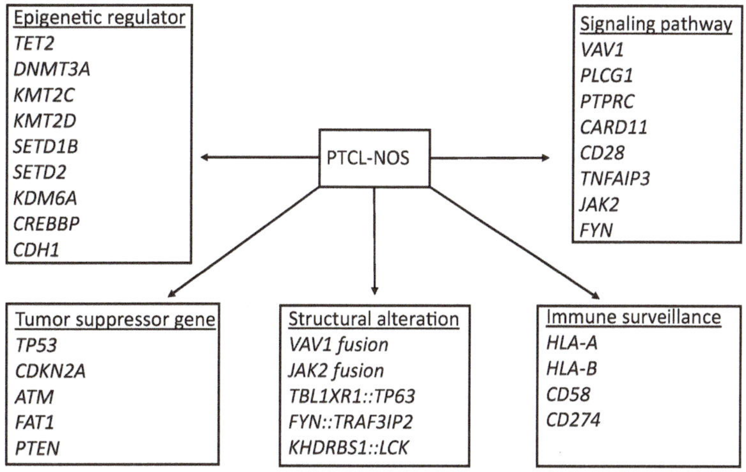

FIG. 1 Genetics pathway components involved in PTCL-NOS.

NODAL LYMPHOMA OF T FOLLICULAR HELPER CELL ORIGIN

There are three nodal lymphomas of TFH cell origin: AITL, FTCL, and nodal PTCL with a TFH phenotype. These lymphomas are the neoplastic counterpart of normal TFH cells, and they share some similar mutational profiles (Fig. 2). Lymphomas with a TFH phenotype should express, at least two, and ideally three TFH-related antigens by IHC (eg,.CD10, BCL6, PD1/CD279, and CXCL13), in addition to CD4. GEP and mutational analysis have helped to clarify the interrelationship among nodal T-cell lymphomas of TFH origin.

ANGIOIMMUNOBLASTIC T-CELL LYMPHOMA

AITL is relatively common among all T-cell neoplasms, being the second most common type of PTCL [23]. As per the WHO 2017, AITL is a "neoplasm of mature TFH cells characterized by systemic disease and a polymorphous infiltrate involving lymph nodes, with a prominent proliferation of high endothelial venules and follicular dendritic cells." Initially, it was thought to be a disorder of immune regulation or a reactive process, but later recognized as a mature T-cell NHL (PTCL). The clinical syndrome is a nearly universal part of the disease. It is commonly seen in older individuals with diverse constitutional signs and symptoms. At an advanced stage, patients commonly present with generalized lymphadenopathy and hepatosplenomegaly. Skin and bone marrow are also commonly involved. Evidence of immune dysfunction such as polyclonal hypergammaglobulinemia, circulating immune complexes, cold agglutinins with hemolytic anemia, positive rheumatoid factor, and anti-smooth muscles antibodies are also present. Epstein-Barr virus (EBV)-positive B-immunoblasts are nearly always present but the neoplastic T-cells are negative for EBV. Both clonal TCR and IGH gene rearrangements may be present (WHO 2017).

AITL has a distinct gene expression profile and the least complex genomic variation profile, when compared with other PTCLs. However, there have been some significant findings with potential therapeutic and diagnostic implications. Epigenetic regulator genes are recurrently affected: *TET2* in 50% to 90% of cases and *DNMT3A* and $IDH2^{R172}$ in ~20% to 50% of cases [24]. The mutation of codon 172 in IDH2 is more specific for AITL [24]. A recurrent inactivating *RHOA* p.G17 V missense has also been found in ~70% of AITL and usually co-occurs with *TET2* mutations [25,26]. $RHOA^{G17V}$-mutated AITLs have the classic clinical and histologic features of AITL compared with *RHOA* wild-type cases, with a higher incidence of splenomegaly and B symptoms, increased microvascular density, and greater expression of TFH markers [27,28]. A variety of other signaling pathway mutations frequently occur in $RHOA^{G17V}$ positive and negative AITLs, including in *CD28, VAV1, PLCG1, STAT3, JAK2,* and *FYN* [29]. In one study, Steinhilber and colleagues suggested that $IDH2^{R172}$ mutation defines a histologically distinct subgroup within AITL, characterized by medium to large clear cells with strong CD10 and CXCL13 expression. They also identified co-mutation of $IDH2^{R172}$, $RHOA^{G17V}$, and *TET2* in 38% of cases, co-mutation of $RHOA^{G17V}$, and *TET2* in *26%* of cases,

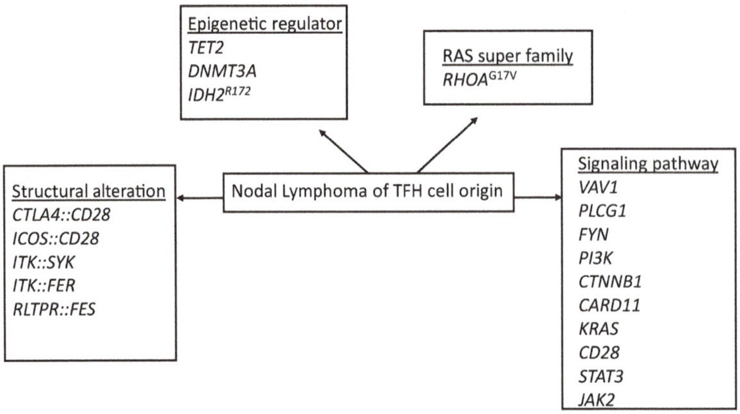

FIG. 2 Genetic pathway components involved in nodal lymphoma of TFH cell origin.

and *DNMT3A* mutation in various cases with and without mutation of these other genes [30]. *TET2* and *DNMT3A* mutations may be found in the neoplastic T-cells, the admixed B-cells, and the hematopoietic stem cells in AITL, whereas *IDH2*^{R172} and *RHOA*^{G17V} are restricted only to the neoplastic T-cells [31–33]. Lastly, *CTLA4::CD28* (58%) and *ICOS::CD28* (rare) fusion genes have also been reported in AITL but also identified in other T-cell lymphomas [34,35]. The *CTLA4::CD28* fusion gene alteration has been shown to activate CD28 downstream intracellular signaling pathways (via Protein kinase B/AKT serine/threonine kinase (AKT) and Extracellular signal-regulated kinases (ERK) phosphorylation), resulting in increased IL-2 production, survival, and proliferation of T-cells, and may represent a potential target for anti-CTLA4 cancer immunotherapy [34]. *CD28* mutations are observed in ~10% of AITL, which is more frequent than in PTCL-NOS, and have been associated with a poor prognosis [35,36].

FOLLICULAR T-CELL LYMPHOMA

FTCL predominantly has a follicular growth pattern and lacks the classical morphologic features of AITL. The neoplastic T-cells that express TFH markers reside within the nodules. FTCL shares similar phenotypic and clinical features, as well as genetic events and mutational profiles with AITL and nodal PTCL with TFH phenotype [16].

A t(5;9) (q33;q22) *ITK::SYK* translocation has been reported in approximately 15% to 20% of FTCL, which preserves the C-terminus (kinase domain) of *SYK* and results in constitutive SYK kinase activation [37–39]. This translocation seems to be more specific for FTCL, though it is also rarely identified in AITL [40]. Additionally, fusions involving the tyrosine kinase-encoding genes *FER* and *FES* have also been identified in FTCL, resulting in abnormally increased STAT3 phosphorylation [37].

Finally, mutations involving epigenetic modifiers (*TET2*, *DNMT3A*, and *IDH2*^{R172}) and *RHOA*^{G17V} have been identified in FTCL [37].

NODAL PERIPHERAL T-CELL LYMPHOMA WITH A T FOLLICULAR HELPER PHENOTYPE

Nodal PTCLs with TFH phenotype frequently show an infiltrative growth pattern and lack classical morphologic features of AITL, such as a vascular proliferation and a prominent polymorphic inflammatory background. These also have a TFH cell phenotype, with the expression of several TFH markers.

The mutational profile of nodal PTCL with TFH phenotype is similar to AITL. Mutations including *TET2*, *DNMT3A*, *IDH2*^{R172}, and *RHOA*^{G17V} are frequently identified [17,41]. Mutations in TCR-signaling-related genes, such as *PLCG1*, *PIK3R1*, *CARD11*, *CTNNB1*, and *KRAS* have also been reported in nodal TFH-like PTCL [41].

ANAPLASTIC LARGE CELL LYMPHOMA

ALK Positive Anaplastic Large Cell Lymphoma

ALK + ALCL is a T-cell lymphoma with characteristic morphologic features including large and pleomorphic

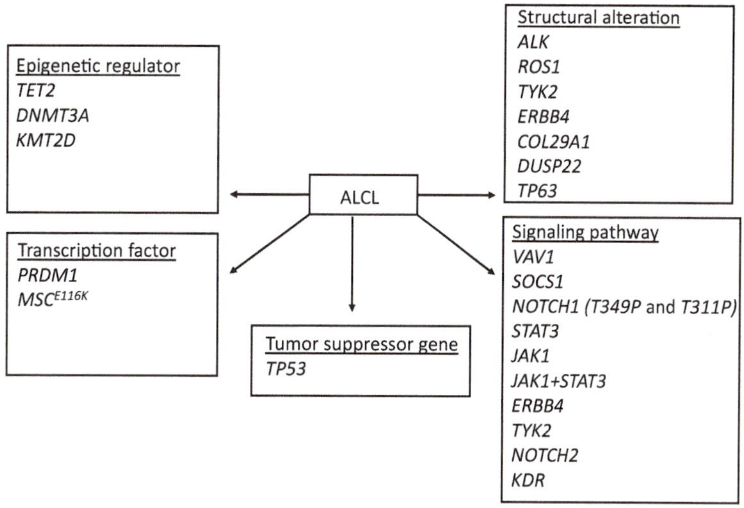

FIG. 3 Genetic pathway components involved in anaplastic large cell lymphoma.

neoplastic cells, often with horseshoe-shaped nuclei (hallmark cells). The neoplastic cells uniformly express CD30 and ALK by IHC [42]. This entity is associated with translocation involving the *ALK* gene on chromosome 2p23.2-p23.1, most commonly t(2;5) (p23;q35) [43]. Frequent loss of one or more T-cell markers is not uncommon. Most cases are associated with favorable outcomes.

ALK is a promiscuous gene with several fusion partners, the most common being *NPM1* located on chromosome 5q35.1. As the NPM1 protein is an important nucleo-cytoplasmic shuttling protein, *NPM1::ALK* fusion-positive cells show nuclear, nucleolar, and cytoplasmic IHC staining with anti-ALK antibodies, whereas non-*NPM1* partners typically lack ALK nuclear staining. *ALK* rearrangements result in gene fusions that lead to constitutive activation of ALK and multiple intracellular signal transduction pathways including the JAK-STAT3 pathway [44]. There are multiple non-*NPM1* partners of *ALK*, including *TPM3, TFG, ATIC, CLTC, TPM4, MSN, ALO17, MYH9,* and *TRAF1*, which are well recognized in ALK + ALCL, and various cell-staining patterns have been described [44–46].

A recent analysis was performed on a cohort of systemic ALK+ and ALK− ALCL cases ($n = 82$ patients, six cell lines) using deep NGS of 275 genes [47]. In this study, *TP53* was shown to be the most frequently mutated gene in ALCL (16%); however, the incidence was lower in ALK + ALCL cases (11%) [47]. Interestingly, *TP53* mutation was more frequently seen in younger patients in ALK + ALCL [47]. The *LRP1B* gene was frequently mutated in ALCL (19% in ALK positive and 9% in ALK negative cases) but did not affect outcomes in ALK + cases [47]. Additionally, in this study, mutations in *EP300* and *KMT2C* have exclusively identified in ALK + ALCL cases. Other recurrently mutated genes belong to epigenetic regulators (*TET2, KMT2D*), DNA damage repair (*ATR* and *MSH6*), chromatin remodeling (*ARID1A*), and signaling pathways (*NOTCH2, KDR, SOCS1*) (Fig. 3) [47,48]. An exome-based study of ALCL ALK + identified *NOTCH1* p.T349P and p.T311P extracellular domain missense mutations in approximately 20% of their cases, which were found to confer a growth advantage to cells [48].

ALK-Negative Anaplastic Large Cell Lymphoma

ALK− ALCL is a CD30+ T-cell neoplasm that is morphologically similar to ALK + ALCL but lacks expression of ALK protein and *ALK* gene rearrangement. ALK− ALCL has a more aggressive clinical course than ALK + disease, and the ultimate prognosis depends on the genetic profile.

Two recurrent and often mutually exclusive rearrangements have been identified. The first group is characterized by rearrangement of *DUSP22*, located on chromosome 6p25.3. This may be found in 30% of cases with a good overall 5-year survival rate that is comparable to ALK + ALCL [49,50]. The second group is characterized by *TP63* rearrangement, located on chromosome 3q28. *TP63* rearrangement occurs in only 8% of cases and is associated with an extremely poor prognosis [49]. In a recent case report of ALK– ALCL, FISH identified the rearrangements of both *DUSP22* and *TP63* genes. The lymphoma was characterized by an immunophenotype of both molecular subtypes and the patient achieved complete remission after chemotherapy [51]. Other genes that have been found to be involved in rearrangements include the kinases *ROS1 and TYK2* [52]. Finally, a new subclass of ALK negative ALCL was identified, in which truncated ERBB4 transcripts with an intronic transcription start were present in 24% of cases [53]. These transcripts demonstrated oncogenicity with potential therapeutic implications.

With regard to mutational signatures in ALK– ALCL: *TP53, STAT3, JAK1, TET2, KMT2D, NOTCH2, SOCS1,* and *PRDM1* are mutated more often in ALK– ALCL than in ALK + ALCL [47]. *TP53* and *STAT3* mutation portend a poor prognosis [47]. *JAK1* mutations often occur in the highly conserved JH1 kinase domain, and *STAT3* mutations occur mainly in the SH2 domain. Both *JAK1* and *STAT3* mutations are reported to cause activation of the STAT pathway, with synergism in double mutants [52]. In systemic ALCL ALK– cases, double mutations can occur in 38% of cases [52]. Other recurrently altered genes include *JAK1, STAT3, NOTCH1, VAV1, KMT2D, TET2,* and *DNMT3A* (see Fig. 3) [6,48,52,54]. A comprehensive NGS assay identified recurrent *JAK2* rearrangement in a spectrum of PTCL-NOS and ALK– ALCL cases showing Hodgkin-like morphology that expressed CD30 by IHC, offering a potential therapeutic target for this aggressive disease. Five different fusion partners, including *TFG, PABPC1, ILF3, MAP7,* and *PCM1* were identified [55]. A recent study identified a highly recurrent missense mutation of MSC^{E116K} in *DUSP22* rearranged ALK– ALCL [56]. *MSC* encodes musculin; a basic helix-loop-helix transcription factor initially demonstrated in skeletal muscle and activated B cells [57]. MSC^{E116K} was found to induce expression of the CD30–IRF4–MYC axis, drive cell cycle progression, and may be targetable with BET inhibitors.

DISCLOSURE

The authors have nothing to disclose.

REFERENCES

[1] Armitage JO. The aggressive peripheral T-cell lymphomas: 2012 update on diagnosis, risk stratification, and management. Am J Hematol 2012;87(5):511–9.

[2] Vega F, Amador C, Chadburn A, et al. Genetic profiling and biomarkers in peripheral T-cell lymphomas: current role in the diagnostic work-up. Mod Pathol 2022;35(3):306–31.

[3] Swerdlow SH, Campo E, Pileri SA, et al. The 2016 revision of the World Health Organization classification of lymphoid neoplasms. Blood 2016;127(20):2375–90.

[4] Jaffe ES. Pathobiology of peripheral T-cell lymphomas. Hematol Am Soc Hematol Educ Program 2006;317–22.

[5] Jaffe ES, Campo E, Harris NL, et al. WHO classification of tumours of haematopoietic and lymphoid tissues. In: Campo E, Harris NL, Jaffe ES, et al, editors. WHO classification of tumors. 4th edition. Lyon, France: World Health Organization; 2017. p. 190–8.

[6] Xie C, Li X, Zeng H, et al. Molecular insights into pathogenesis and targeted therapy of peripheral T cell lymphoma. Exp Hematol Oncol 2020;9(1):30.

[7] Sidorova YV, Sychevskaya KA, Chernova NG, et al. High Incidence of Clonal CD8+ T-cell Proliferation in Non-malignant Conditions May Reduce the Significance of T-cell Clonality Assay for Differential Diagnosis in Onco-hematology. Clin Lymphoma Myeloma Leuk 2020;20(4):203–8.

[8] Sufficool KE, Lockwood CM, Abel HJ, et al. T-cell clonality assessment by next-generation sequencing improves detection sensitivity in mycosis fungoides. J Am Acad Dermatol 2015;73(2):228–36.e2.

[9] Vose J, Armitage J, Weisenburger D. International T-Cell Lymphoma Project. International peripheral T-cell and natural killer/T-cell lymphoma study: pathology findings and clinical outcomes. J Clin Oncol 2008;26(25):4124–30.

[10] Wang T, Feldman AL, Wada DA, et al. GATA-3 expression identifies a high-risk subset of PTCL, NOS with distinct molecular and clinical features. Blood 2014;123(19):3007–15.

[11] Iqbal J, Wright G, Wang C, et al. Lymphoma Leukemia Molecular Profiling Project and the International Peripheral T-cell Lymphoma Project. Gene expression signatures delineate biological and prognostic subgroups in peripheral T-cell lymphoma. Blood 2014;123(19):2915–23.

[12] Amador C, Greiner TC, Heavican TB, et al. Reproducing the molecular subclassification of peripheral T-cell lymphoma-NOS by immunohistochemistry. Blood 2019;134(24):2159–70.

[13] Heavican TB, Bouska A, Yu J, et al. Genetic drivers of oncogenic pathways in molecular subgroups of peripheral T-cell lymphoma. Blood 2019;133(15):1664–76.

[14] Maura F, Dodero A, Carniti C, et al. *CDKN2A* deletion is a frequent event associated with poor outcome in patients with peripheral T-cell lymphoma not otherwise specified (PTCL-NOS). Haematologica 2021;106(11):2918–26.

[15] Watatani Y, Sato Y, Miyoshi H, et al. Molecular heterogeneity in peripheral T-cell lymphoma, not otherwise

specified revealed by comprehensive genetic profiling. Leukemia 2019;33(12):2867–83.
[16] Dobay MP, Lemonnier F, Missiaglia E, et al. Integrative clinicopathological and molecular analyses of angioimmunoblastic T-cell lymphoma and other nodal lymphomas of follicular helper T-cell origin. Haematologica 2017;102(4):e148–51.
[17] Lemonnier F, Couronné L, Parrens M, et al. Recurrent TET2 mutations in peripheral T-cell lymphomas correlate with TFH-like features and adverse clinical parameters. Blood 2012;120(7):1466–9.
[18] Laginestra MA, Cascione L, Motta G, et al. Whole exome sequencing reveals mutations in FAT1 tumor suppressor gene clinically impacting on peripheral T-cell lymphoma not otherwise specified. Mod Pathol 2020;33(2):179–87.
[19] Ji MM, Huang YH, Huang JY, et al. Histone modifier gene mutations in peripheral T-cell lymphoma not otherwise specified. Haematologica 2018;103(4):679–87.
[20] Debackere K, Marcelis L, Demeyer S, et al. Fusion transcripts FYN-TRAF3IP2 and KHDRBS1-LCK hijack T cell receptor signaling in peripheral T-cell lymphoma, not otherwise specified. Nat Commun 2021;12(1):3705.
[21] Abate F, da Silva-Almeida AC, Zairis S, et al. Activating mutations and translocations in the guanine exchange factor VAV1 in peripheral T-cell lymphomas. Proc Natl Acad Sci U S A 2017;114(4):764–9.
[22] Vasmatzis G, Johnson SH, Knudson RA, et al. Genome-wide analysis reveals recurrent structural abnormalities of TP63 and other p53-related genes in peripheral T-cell lymphomas. Blood 2012;120(11):2280–9.
[23] de Leval L, Parrens M, Le Bras F, et al. Angioimmunoblastic T-cell lymphoma is the most common T-cell lymphoma in two distinct French information data sets. Haematologica 2015;100(9):e361–4.
[24] Zhang Y, Lee D, Brimer T, et al. Genomics of Peripheral T-Cell Lymphoma and Its Implications for Personalized Medicine. Front Oncol 2019;10:898.
[25] Yoo HY, Sung MK, Lee SH, et al. A recurrent inactivating mutation in RHOA GTPase in angioimmunoblastic T cell lymphoma. Nat Genet 2014;46(4):371–5.
[26] Sakata-Yanagimoto M, Enami T, Yoshida K, et al. Somatic RHOA mutation in angioimmunoblastic T cell lymphoma. Nat Genet 2014;46(2):171–5.
[27] Ondrejka SL, Grzywacz B, Bodo J, et al. Angioimmunoblastic T-cell Lymphomas With the RHOA p.Gly17Val Mutation Have Classic Clinical and Pathologic Features. Am J Surg Pathol 2016;40(3):335–41.
[28] Nagao R, Kikuti YY, Carreras J, et al. Clinicopathologic Analysis of Angioimmunoblastic T-cell Lymphoma With or Without RHOA G17V Mutation Using Formalin-fixed Paraffin-embedded Sections. Am J Surg Pathol 2016;40(8):1041–50.
[29] Willemsen M, Abdul Hamid M, Winkens B, et al. Mutational heterogeneity of angioimmunoblastic T-cell lymphoma indicates distinct lymphomagenic pathways. Blood Cancer J 2018;8(1):6.
[30] Steinhilber J, Mederake M, Bonzheim I, et al. The pathological features of angioimmunoblastic T-cell lymphomas with $IDH2^{R172}$ mutations. Mod Pathol 2019; 32(8):1123–34.
[31] Lewis NE, Petrova-Drus K, Huet S, et al. Clonal hematopoiesis in angioimmunoblastic T-cell lymphoma with divergent evolution to myeloid neoplasms. Blood Adv 2020;4(10):2261–71.
[32] Quivoron C, Couronné L, Della Valle V, et al. TET2 inactivation results in pleiotropic hematopoietic abnormalities in mouse and is a recurrent event during human lymphomagenesis. Cancer Cell 2011;20(1):25–38.
[33] Nguyen TB, Sakata-Yanagimoto M, Asabe Y, et al. Identification of cell-type-specific mutations in nodal T-cell lymphomas. Blood Cancer J 2017;7(1):e516.
[34] Yoo HY, Kim P, Kim WS, et al. Frequent CTLA4-CD28 gene fusion in diverse types of T-cell lymphoma. Haematologica 2016;101(6):757–63.
[35] Rohr J, Guo S, Huo J, et al. Recurrent activating mutations of CD28 in peripheral T-cell lymphomas. Leukemia 2016;30(5):1062–70.
[36] Zain JM, Hanona P. Aggressive T-cell lymphomas: 2021 Updates on diagnosis, risk stratification and management. Am J Hematol 2021;96(8):1027–46.
[37] Debackere K, van der Krogt JA, Tousseyn T, et al. FER and FES tyrosine kinase fusions in follicular T-cell lymphoma. Blood 2020;135(8):584–8.
[38] Streubel B, Vinatzer U, Willheim M, et al. Novel t(5; 9)(q33;q22) fuses ITK to SYK in unspecified peripheral T-cell lymphoma. Leukemia 2006;20(2):313–8.
[39] Huang Y, Moreau A, Dupuis J, et al. Peripheral T-cell lymphomas with a follicular growth pattern are derived from follicular helper T cells (TFH) and may show overlapping features with angioimmunoblastic T-cell lymphomas. Am J Surg Pathol 2009;33(5):682–90.
[40] Attygalle AD, Feldman AL, Dogan A. ITK/SYK translocation in angioimmunoblastic T-cell lymphoma. Am J Surg Pathol 2013;37(9):1456–7.
[41] Vallois D, Dobay MP, Morin RD, et al. Activating mutations in genes related to TCR signaling in angioimmunoblastic and other follicular helper T-cell-derived lymphomas. Blood 2016;128(11):1490–502.
[42] Falini B, Martelli MP. Anaplastic large cell lymphoma: changes in the World Health Organization classification and perspectives for targeted therapy. Haematologica 2009;94(7):897–900.
[43] Morris SW, Kirstein MN, Valentine MB, et al. Fusion of a kinase gene, ALK, to a nucleolar protein gene, NPM, in non-Hodgkin's lymphoma. Science 1994;263(5151): 1281–4.
[44] Werner MT, Zhao C, Zhang Q, et al. Nucleophosmin-anaplastic lymphoma kinase: the ultimate oncogene and therapeutic target. Blood 2017;129(7):823–31.
[45] Chiarle R, Voena C, Ambrogio C, et al. The anaplastic lymphoma kinase in the pathogenesis of cancer. Nat Rev Cancer 2008;8(1):11–23.

[46] Feldman AL, Vasmatzis G, Asmann YW, et al. Novel TRAF1-ALK fusion identified by deep RNA sequencing of anaplastic large cell lymphoma. Genes Chromosomes Cancer 2013;52(11):1097–102.

[47] Lobello C, Tichy B, Bystry V, et al. STAT3 and TP53 mutations associate with poor prognosis in anaplastic large cell lymphoma. Leukemia 2021;35(5):1500–5.

[48] Larose H, Prokoph N, Matthews JD, et al. Whole Exome Sequencing reveals NOTCH1 mutations in anaplastic large cell lymphoma and points to Notch both as a key pathway and a potential therapeutic target. Haematologica 2021;106(6):1693–704.

[49] Parrilla Castellar ER, Jaffe ES, Said JW, et al. ALK-negative anaplastic large cell lymphoma is a genetically heterogeneous disease with widely disparate clinical outcomes. Blood 2014;124(9):1473–80.

[50] Feldman AL, Dogan A, Smith DI, et al. Discovery of recurrent t(6;7)(p25.3;q32.3) translocations in ALK-negative anaplastic large cell lymphomas by massively parallel genomic sequencing. Blood 2011;117(3):915–9.

[51] Karube K, Feldman AL. Double-hit" of DUSP22 and TP63 rearrangements in anaplastic large cell lymphoma, ALK-negative. Blood 2020;135(9):700.

[52] Crescenzo R, Abate F, Lasorsa E, et al. European T-Cell Lymphoma Study Group, T-Cell Project: Prospective Collection of Data in Patients with Peripheral T-Cell Lymphoma and the AIRC 5xMille Consortium "Genetics-Driven Targeted Management of Lymphoid Malignancies". Convergent mutations and kinase fusions lead to oncogenic STAT3 activation in anaplastic large cell lymphoma. Cancer Cell 2015;27(4):516–32.

[53] Scarfò I, Pellegrino E, Mereu E, et al, European T-Cell Lymphoma Study Group. Identification of a new subclass of ALK-negative ALCL expressing aberrant levels of ERBB4 transcripts. Blood 2016;127(2):221–32.

[54] Boddicker RL, Razidlo GL, Dasari S, et al. Integrated mate-pair and RNA sequencing identifies novel, targetable gene fusions in peripheral T-cell lymphoma. Blood 2016;128(9):1234–45.

[55] Fitzpatrick MJ, Massoth LR, Marcus C, et al. JAK2 Rearrangements Are a Recurrent Alteration in CD30+ Systemic T-Cell Lymphomas with Anaplastic Morphology. Am J Surg Pathol 2021;45(7):895–904.

[56] Luchtel RA, Zimmermann MT, Hu G, et al. Recurrent MSC^{E116K}mutations in ALK-negative anaplastic large cell lymphoma. Blood 2019;133(26):2776–89.

[57] Robb L, Hartley L, Wang CC, et al. musculin: a murine basic helix-loop-helix transcription factor gene expressed in embryonic skeletal muscle. Mech Dev 1998;76(1–2):197–201.

Advances in Molecular Pathology 5 (2022) 59–71
ADVANCES IN MOLECULAR PATHOLOGY

Multiple Myeloma

Loren J. Joseph, MD[a,b,*]
[a]Department of Pathology, Harvard Medical School, Boston, MA, USA; [b]Beth Israel Deaconess Medical Center, 330 Brookline Avenue, Rabb #315, Boston, MA 02215, USA

KEYWORDS
• Myeloma • MGUS (monoclonal gammopathy of uncertain significance) • SMM (smoldering multiple myeloma)
• MRD (minimal residual disease) • NGF (next-generation flow)

KEY POINTS

- Genomic and transcriptomic changes in myeloma have been surveyed in depth but have minimal impact on clinical guidelines.
- Cytogenetic results at diagnosis remain important for management. Complex cytogenetic changes, like chromothripsis, are more common and clinically significant than generally recognized.
- There is a modest genomic heterogeneity among spatially separate myelomatous lesions.
- Detection of minimal residual disease (MRD) in bone marrow aspirates, by flow cytometry or by next-generation sequencing (of the VDJ segments of the IgH locus), is essential to clinical care.
- MRD testing of circulating malignant plasma cells and circulating DNA is a promising research tool.

MULTIPLE MYELOMA OVERVIEW

Malignant myeloma (MM) is the second most common hematologic malignancy in the United States. Malignant plasma cells in multiple myeloma are usually limited to the bone marrow, although circulating malignant cells are detectable in many cases.

Like normal plasma cells, the neoplastic plasma cells in myeloma secrete immunoglobulins. Because the plasma cell expansion is clonal, the malignant plasma cells secrete identical immunoglobulins, all sharing the same sequence and length (the specific sequence is unique and will vary from patient to patient). When the number of malignant plasma cells is high enough, a corresponding paraprotein can be detected as a discrete band on a diffusely stained (polyclonal) background when serum is analyzed by protein electrophoresis (serum protein electrophoresis [SPEP]). Electrophoresis has enabled early detection of monoclonal proteins in asymptomatic people. SPEP is often ordered in the workup of anemia, unexplained proteinuria, and neuropathy. The workup also often includes a bone marrow biopsy, which is examined for the level of plasma cell proliferation and light chain immunotype.

Most people with an incidentally discovered paraprotein and small clonal plasma cell expansion live for years or decades with a slowly increasing monoclonal burden, but without development of overt myeloma. This state is termed monoclonal gammopathy of undetermined significance (MGUS). It is accepted that essentially all MM originates in MGUS, but most MGUS cases do not progress to MM, even after decades. MGUS is found in 5% to 10% of the general population by age 60 years; the subsequent incidence increases 1% per year.

Criteria for diagnosing MGUS, MM, and an intermediate state, "smoldering multiple myeloma" (SMM) have been developed by the International Myeloma Working Group (IMWG) and are set forth in the

*Beth Israel Deaconess Medical Center, 330 Brookline Avenue, Rabb #315, Boston, MA 02215. *E-mail address:* ljjoseph@bidmc.harvard.edu

https://doi.org/10.1016/j.yamp.2022.06.002
2589-4080/22/

National Comprehensive Cancer Network (NCCN) Guidelines for Multiple Myeloma, version 5.2022 (at NCCN.org).

PLASMA CELL BIOLOGY

Quantifying plasma cells morphologically for diagnosis is usually not a diagnostic challenge. Despite a somewhat monotonous appearance, at least 4 human plasma cell subsets are present in normal bone marrow: $CD19^+CD38^{hi}CD138^-$, $CD19^+CD38^{hi}CD138^+$, $CD19^-CD38^{hi}CD138^-$, and $CD19^-CD38^{hi}CD138^+$ [1]. The last subset is primarily limited to bone marrow, and there is evidence that this is a long-lived plasma cell population [2]. The other 3 subsets occur in other tissues. Plasma cells are usually thought of as terminally differentiated cells, which seems problematic for malignant expansion; however, immunohistochemical proliferation assessment does show a modest proliferation index, and apoptosis rates seem to decrease with progression from MGUS to overt MM [2–4].

A panel of antibodies to CD19, CD27, CD38, CD45, CD56, CD81, CD117, CD138, kappa, and lambda (cytoplasmic) will identify most plasma cells. Although such thorough phenotyping is not needed for diagnosis, it is important for subsequent flow cytometric detection of minimal residual disease (MRD). Malignant plasma cells in MGUS and MM frequently show aberrant phenotypes. Next-generation flow (NGF) cytometry can detect at least 1 aberrant plasma cell of 100,000 cells.

CYTOGENETICS

Early cytogenetic studies showed that nearly all MM cases had one of the cytogenetic abnormalities listed in Table 1. Most MGUS cases include one of these cytogenetic changes, with translocations involving the *IGH* gene locus accounting for the majority; this suggests that the altered gene regulation resulting from translocations is necessary but not sufficient for overt malignancy. The translocations involving chromosomes 4, 11, and 14 do not involve fusions; rather, each brings a new gene under the control of the *IGH* gene promoter. The immunoglobulin genes normally undergo significant double-strand DNA (dsDNA) breaks for recombination physiologically, so the increased incidence of pathologic translocation is not surprising. Sequencing shows that the MM-associated translocations show increased Activation-Induced (cytidine) Deaminase (AID) and Apolipoprotein B mRNA Editing enzyme, Catalytic polypeptide (APOBEC) activity at the fusion site [5–7].

TABLE 1
Common Primary Cytogenetic Abnormalities in Multiple Myeloma

Translocation	Incidence	Risk	*IGH* Partner gene
t(11;14)(q13.3;q32)	15%	Standard	*CCND1*
t(4;14)(p16.3;q32)	6%	High	*NSD2*
t(14;16)(q32;q23.2)	4%	High	*MAF*
t(6;14)(p21.1;q32)	<1%	Standard	*CCND3*
t(14;20)(q32;q12)	<1%	High	*MAFB*
IGH (14q32)/ unknown partner	5%	NA	NA
HD without translocation	40%	Standard risk	NA

Abbreviation: HD, hyperdiploidy. NA, Not Applicable
Data is extracted from Laubach JP. Multiple Myeloma:Staging and Prognostic Studies. In:UpToDate, Shefner JM (ed), UpToDate, Waltham, MA. (Accessed August 8, 2022)

Hyperdiploidy denotes an increased chromosome complement that is still in a near-diploid state (typically 47–57 chromosomes), and one or more of the "odd-numbered" chromosomes (3, 5, 7, 9, 11, 15, 19, or 21) are often affected in myeloma. The absence of chromosomes 13 and 17 suggests that the extra dosage of the tumor suppressors *Rb* (chr 13) and *TP53* (chr 17) impedes myeloma development. A biological explanation for this predilection for odd-numbered chromosomes remains elusive (and is most likely "chance").

Traditional karyotyping is limited to dividing cells. Cytogenetic fluorescence in situ hybridization probes can interrogate nondividing and fixed cells. Microarrays, combining both cytogenomicand and single nucleotide polymorphism detection formats can survey the entire genome of bulk samples at a higher genomic resolution than conventional chromosome analysis,(and detect parental disomy) but it cannot achieve cell-level resolution and cannot easily detect balanced chromosomal rearrangements. More recent cytogenetic findings include the following:

1. Subclonal translocations involving *MYC* are present at diagnosis in a small percentage of MGUS cases, in 25% of new cases of MM, and in 50% of advanced MM cases [8].

2. Translocation involving the lambda promoter is associated with especially poor outcome [9].
3. Chromothripsis is present in up to 35% of cases of MM [10,11]; it is a poor prognostic sign, which might, in part, result from an association with biallelic inactivation of *TP53*.
4. Templated insertions are found in about 20% of MM cases [6,10,12]; these are characterized by DNA segments from different areas of the genome, copied, joined, and inserted as one sequence into a chromosome.
5. Copy number aberrations (CNAs) are widespread [13].

GENOMICS

Numerous gene sequence mutations had been reported in multiple myeloma before 2011, all discovered by the traditional single-gene-at-a-time approach [14], but none were dominant or category defining. The Catalogue of Somatic Mutations in Cancer (COSMIC), hosted by the Wellcome Sanger Institute, lists 6962 myeloma cases in its database (as of April 3, 2022). The database is maintained by expert curation of publications and by importing data from other databases, such as The Cancer Genome Atlas (TCGA).

The prevalence of the 20 most frequently mutated genes in the COSMIC database for myeloma is given in Table 2. The genes are ranked by the percentage of positive cases. Until recently most cases were from series that studied only 1 or a few mutations. For example, after the *BRAF* p.V600E mutation was discovered in cancer, hundreds of studies tested for that mutation specifically, and for nothing else. As a consequence COSMIC is a good source for answering the question "Has gene variant X *ever* been reported," but must be used cautiously for quantitative questions like "what is the frequency of variant X in malignancy Y.

TABLE 2
Ten most frequently mutated genes in multiple myeloma

Gene	# samples tested	# with mutation	% mutated
NRAS	1230	238	19
KRAS2	1229	229	19
SYNE1	167	32	19
FAT4	264	34	13
TP53	1021	97	10
CDKN2	436	39	9
TENT5C	576	47	8
BRAF	1947	94	5
ATM	794	41	5

Catalogue of Somatic Mutations in Cancer database

The first genomic study of myeloma was reported in 2011. Chapman and colleagues evaluated 23 myeloma cases with whole genome sequencing (WGS) and 16 additional cases with whole exome sequencing (WES). *NRAS* mutations were present in 9 cases, *KRAS* mutations in 10, *TP53* mutations in 3, and *CCND1* mutations in 2. Chapman and colleagues also identified likely pathogenic variants in 6 other genes, which had not been previously implicated in myeloma.

The TCGA consortium generated its own data and used standardized criteria for accepting, processing, and sequencing samples. The TCGA portal (accessed March 10, 2022) showed a single project for multiple myeloma, which contrasts with 11 for acute myeloid leukemia. The most frequently identified mutations in the MM study are shown in Fig. 1. Another multi-institutional international consortium, the ICGC (International Cancer Genetics Consortium), has no myeloma series.

A comprehensive multiomic myeloma database does exist: the Clinical Outcomes in Multiple Myeloma Personal Assess Study (CoMMpass), an initiative of the Multiple Myeloma Research Foundation. CoMMpass is a longitudinal observation study of 1150 patients with newly diagnosed myeloma at 76 institutions worldwide (accessed April 28, 2022). Each patient's clinical information is collected every 6 months for 8 years. Molecular testing includes WGS, WES, RNA sequencing (RNA-seq), and multicolor flow cytometry. Sera are analyzed for paraproteins. Data are acquired at 8 time points per patient. Both raw and high-level data are stored and available at the Genome Data Commons (https://portal.gdc.cancer.gov/). Fig. 2 shows a typical "oncogrid."

Dutta and colleagues [15] summarize most of the WGS and WES studies through 2021. With high-throughput genomic sequencing (HTGS) the number of genes with probable pathogenic mutations in myeloma reached 80. None of the mutations are present in most cases. These abundant HTGS data are still being mined to address open questions.

1. *Prognosis*. Are any of the mutations or combinations of mutations useful for distinguishing among MGUS, SMM, and MM with respect to the risk of progression?

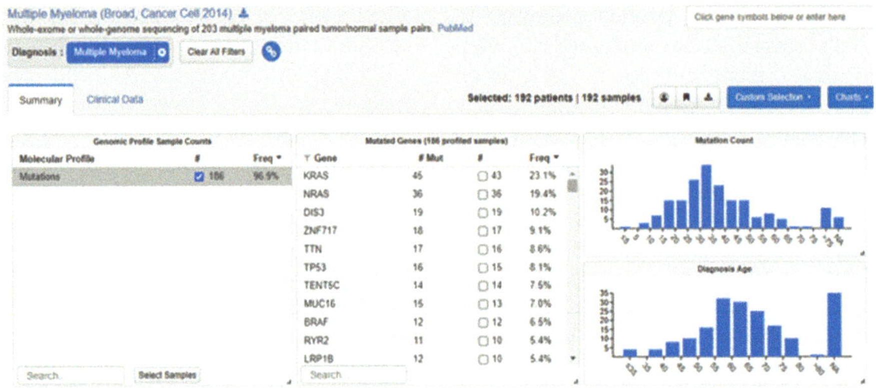

FIG. 1 Most frequently mutated genes in multiple myeloma. The 11 most frequently mutated genes in the TCGA myeloma study are shown. There is modest overlap with the results shown in Figs. 1 and 3. TCGA study viewed at the cBioPortal.

2. *Prediction*. Are any of the mutations or combinations of mutations useful for predicting treatment response or resistance?
   - Methylation of an intronic enhancer leading to decreased *CRBN* [16] expression has been associated with loss of response to lenalidomide
   - Mutations in *PSMB5* (proteasome subunit beta type 5) explains some cases resistant to bortezomib [17].
   - Biallelic loss of *TNFRSF17* (*BCMA*) explains resistance to Chimeric Antigen Receptor T (CAR-T) therapy directed at *TNFRSF17* [18,19].

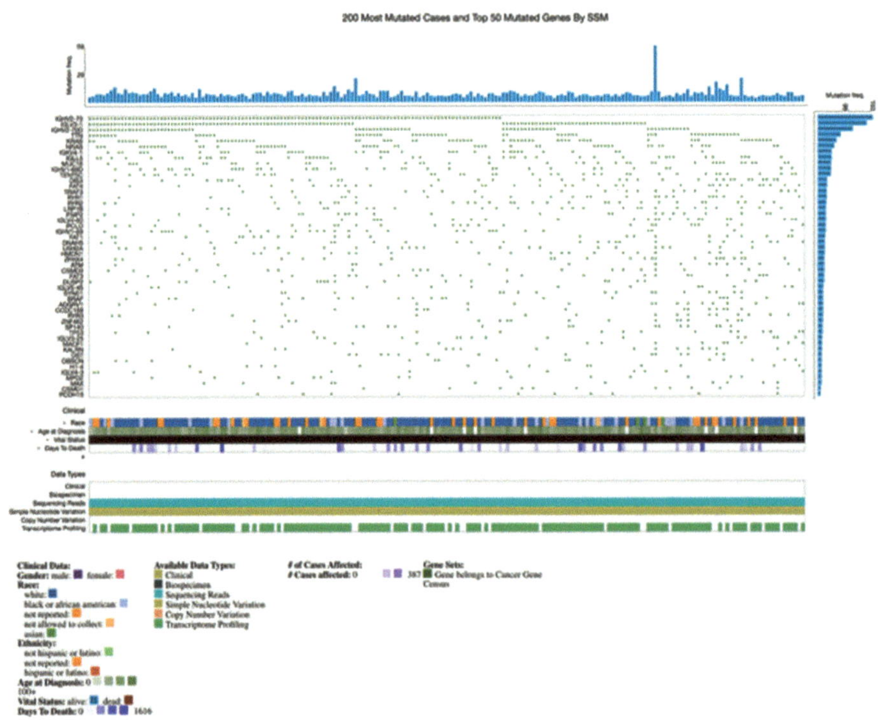

FIG. 2 Representative OncoGrid from the CoMMpass database. Shown is an oncogrid from the CoMMpass database, showing the most frequent mutations in the 200 most mutation-rich samples (of more than 900 cases). Unlike the COSMIC and TCGA databases, this includes the sequences of the immunoglobulin genes.

3. *How does the myeloma genome evolve?* WES or WGS data for 1 sample are enough to permit mathematical modeling, which can enumerate subclones and infer the likely order of acquisition of mutations including the putative initiating mutation [20,21]
4. *Mutation signatures*. On the genomic scale the pattern of alteration in nucleotide sequence, independent of the gene involved, shows characteristic patterns (like dinucleotide frequency) that are characteristic of various mutagenic processes such as exposure to UV light or exposure to melphalan [22–25].

GENE EXPRESSION PROFILES (TRANSCRIPTOMICS)

The international staging system for myeloma developed by the IMWG was based only on beta-2 microglobulin and albumin levels but was updated in 2016 to include several cytogenetic aberrations: del(17p), t(4;14), and t(14;16). Numerous gene expression studies have proposed expression signatures to improve prognostication for MGUS and MM. Initially studies were done using gene expression microarrays, more recently with RNA-seq. Data for many of these studies are housed in the NCBI GEO database. The SKY92 gene expression classifier assay for myeloma risk is among the more recently advocated [26], but none have found widespread acceptance.

SINGLE-CELL ANALYSIS

Single-cell techniques can be used to analyze genomes, transcriptomes, epigenomes, and genome-wide chromatin occupation sites. A few studies have demonstrated combining 2 modalities. The caveat must be kept in mind that single-cell analyses are usually not complete—so statistical imputations are often necessary by looking at multiple similar cells.

With genomic and transcriptomic analysis of several thousand bulk myeloma samples already completed, it is unlikely that single-cell analysis will reveal many novel mutations or transcripts, but several important lines of investigation are opened:

1. *Phylogenetics*: More granular analysis of clonal and subclonal genomic structure, especially determining if mutations co-occur in a cell.
2. *Cell identification*: If the mutation is in an expressed coding region, then RNA-seq can potentially both detect the mutation and identify the cell type, showing how robustly the mutated transcript is expressed. Not all mutations will be in myeloma cells.
3. *Robust detection of low-level mutations*: This is analogous to digital display polymerase chain reaction (PCR). Each cell is like an independent PCR/sequencing reaction chamber. A mutation in a single cell should show a variant allele frequency of 100%, 50%, or 0%.
4. *Determining the transcriptional states of cell types*: For example, do "exhausted" immune cell profiles predict response to immune checkpoint inhibitors.

As with studies of bulk samples, single-cell data have been analyzed for prognostic and predictive factors. A listing of selected single-cell studies on MM is given in Dutta and colleagues [15].

The earliest single-cell study of MM reported an analysis of 6 patients, each carrying t(11;14) [27]. Single-cell analysis was limited to multiplexed real-time PCR, for 5 DNA targets, on CD138$^+$ FACS (fluorescence-activated cell sorting)-sorted cells, ranging from 73 to 243 per case.

Ledergor and colleagues [28] reported a single-cell transcriptomic analysis of 40 subjects spanning the clinical spectrum of MM (11 healthy controls, 7 with MGUS, 6 with SMM, 12 with MM, and 4 with primary light chain amyloidosis). The study analyzed 20,586 CD38$^+$ marrow plasma cells, with samples ranging from 56 to 1821 cells. Among the key findings are the following:

1. Minimal "heterogeneity" among controls.

   Only two cell expression clusters were found among plasma cells in controls. Both clusters were present in all control samples but minimally, if at all, in non-controls. This suggests only two broad physiological states (or plasma cell 'types') are present among the normal plasma cells. This is a little surprising and might only reflect the still small number of cells per sample. This finding depends critically on how "heterogeneity" is measured. The investigators define a "heterogeneity score" based on correlations of the read counts within and between clusters for a given subject.
2. Every myeloma sample showed a unique transcriptional profile. For example, in sample SMM02, one transcriptional state was defined by expression of *DEFB1*, a putative *CCR6* ligand, whereas the other transcriptional state by expression of *FRZB*, a putative member of the Wnt pathway.
3. Several overexpressed genes were identified, not previously noted in MM. Overexpression was confirmed on review of other cases in the CoMMpass database.

a. *LAMP5*: a lysosome-associated membrane protein
b. *WFDC2*: an endopeptidase inhibitor
c. *CDR1*: a short intronless gene on the X chromosome.

4. Most genes overexpressed in multiple myeloma do not change posttreatment. Five subjects were sampled before and after treatment; 2 were complete responders.
5. Circulating malignant plasma cells showed the same transcriptional profiles as the corresponding marrow aspirates.

Cohen and colleagues [29] used single-cell RNA-seq (scRNA-seq) in conjunction with a prospective multicenter single-arm clinical trial to determine safety and efficacy of a 4-drug combination (daratumumab + carfilzomib + lenalidomide + dexamethasone) in patients who had either failed to respond to bortezomib induction or relapsed early (primary refractory MM [PRMM]). The molecular study followed 41 patients longitudinally: at baseline, cycle 4 (month 3), and cycle 10 (month 9). Only 4 subjects had completed the regimen; 15 were ongoing, and 22 discontinued. As controls, samples from 15 patients with "newly" diagnosed MM (NDMM) and 11 healthy controls were used. These controls were from an earlier study (Ledergor and colleagues [28]), which raises some concern over suitability, given the well-known sensitivity of gene expression to preanalytical variables and batch effects, but this seems unlikely to affect the main findings [30,31]. Overall there were 97 samples from 67 subjects. Plasma cells from bone marrow were collected by FACS sorting on CD38. Satisfactory quality was seen in 51,297 cells (@500 cells/sample). The key conclusions are:

1. Every MM case showed a distinctive transcriptional state
2. There was no significant change in expression of driver genes, over time or treatment.
3. Three gene expression signatures (modules) distinguished NDMM from PRMM samples and split PRMM into 2 subsets.
4. Expression of the *PPIA* gene identified a new high-risk MM marker.

The investigators studied the *PPIA* gene, peptidyl-prolyl isomerase A, in detail, deleting it with CRISPr in a human myeloma cell line. The *PPIA* $^{-/-}$ cell line was sensitive to carfilzomib (CFZ). Similarly, fresh MM cells showed synergistic sensitivity to treatment with cyclosporin A and CFZ. Interestingly, cyclosporin was noted to have an effect on myeloma cells in the 1990s but fell out of favor [32].

Several extensive single-cell transcriptome surveys of normal bone marrow, mouse and human, made no mention of plasma cells [33–35]. The single-cell studies of myeloma described earlier were limited to CD38$^+$ plasma cells. The bone marrow has many cell types; several surely influence dormancy or progression of myeloma.

scRNA-seq studies of other bone marrow populations in MM have been reported. Zavidij and colleagues [36] looked at CD45$^+$CD138$^-$ cells, analyzing 19,000 cells from 23 patients (including MGUS, low-risk SMM, high-risk SMM, and MM) and 9 healthy controls. The key findings (some of which could have also been made from flow) are:

1. Significant enrichment in NK, T, and CD16$^+$ cells in MM
2. Decreased plasmacytoid dendritic cells, granzyme K$^+$ lymphocytes, and CD14$^+$ monocytes in MM.
3. These alterations were observed in some MGUS samples

These studies were extended to show that granzyme K (GZMK)$^+$ T cells were associated with significantly longer progression-free survival (PFS) in treated patients with SMM [37].

de Jong and colleagues [38] investigated the nonhematopoietic cell stroma of bone marrow in 13 patients with NDMM and 7 healthy controls. Flow cytometric sorting excluded CD45$^+$ (hematopoietic), CD235$^+$ and CD71$^+$ (erythroid), and CD38$^+$ (plasma) cells. The resulting niche accounted for 0.002% of the total aspirated cells. From this population, they sequenced transcriptomes of 19,983 cells from subjects with MM and 7038 cells from controls. The analysis of MM and control cells together generated 5 mesenchymal stromal cell clusters, MSC1 to MSC5, as well as 1 cluster for endothelial cells, 1 (*SELP*$^+$) for selectin-P-positive cells, and 1 for osteolineage cells. The clusters MSC1 and MSC2 were markedly enriched in the MM cases (Fig. 3), and the gene sets defining these clusters were enriched in genes involved in inflammation, particularly genes mediating tumor necrosis factor-alpha signaling through nuclear factor-κB, well-known MM cell survival factors *IL6* and *LIF*, and multiple chemokines. MSC1 and MSC2 were prominent in all the MM cases, regardless of the cytogenetic abnormalities, and nearly absent in control subjects.

The osteolinage cluster, identified with markers including *RUNX2* and *SP7*, contained few cells. The investigators note an often neglected fact, which is that bone marrow aspirates are often not fully representative of the intact bone marrow.

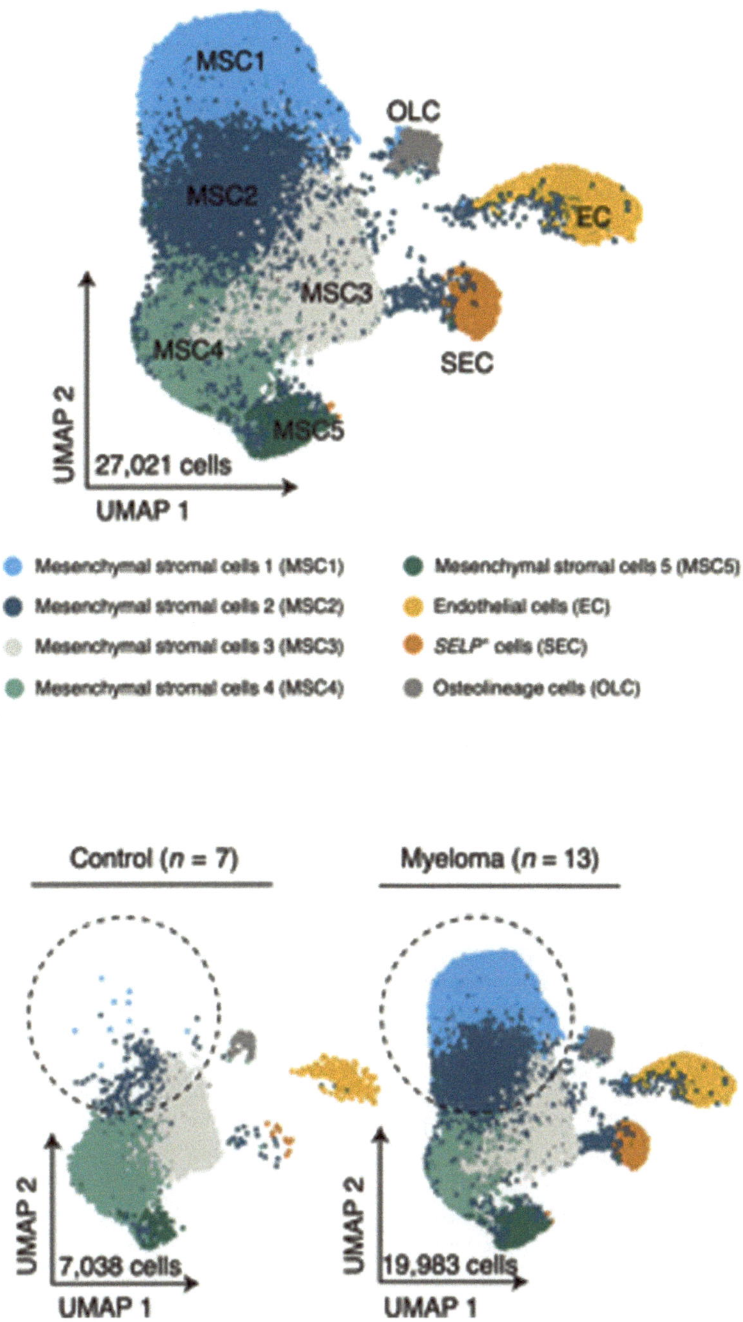

FIG. 3 Cell clustering by UMAP analysis is shown for single-cell transcriptomes of stromal cells in multiple myeloma. (*From* de Jong MME, Kellermayer Z, Papazian N, et al. The multiple myeloma microenvironment is defined by an inflammatory stromal cell landscape. Nat Immunol. 2021;22(6):769-780. doi: https://doi.org/10.1038/s41590-021-00931-3.)

Perhaps the most intriguing finding in this study is that after 4 cycles of therapy, including cases in which MM cells were no longer detected, the MSC population structure remained abnormal.

A commentary by Sklavenitis-Pisotfidis [39] and colleagues compared these results with analysis of MSCs from 2 bulk studies, one showing no effect of successful treatment on the MSC population and the other showing changes.

(MACRO) SPATIAL HETEROGENEITY

Rasche and colleagues (2017) [40] looked at 42 newly diagnosed patients and 11 treated patients with MM. Paired lesions were analyzed—a standard iliac crest biopsy and an image-guided needle core biopsy of a focal lesion elsewhere [40]. Five NDMM cases had 4 to 5 focal lesions biopsied. Cytogenetic microarray studies showed on average 3 different CNAs between the diagnostic and the additional focal lesion (range 1–28 differences). Classic cytogenetic translocations were stable, but in 2 cases hyperdiploid status was not shared. WES showed significant divergences in 75% of the subjects.

Rasche and colleagues [40] relate their findings to theories of cancer evolution. The investigators note that MM primarily grows in the marrow, where free movement among sites through the circulation is assumed, and that their expectation was that when a fitter clone arises, it will sweep to dominance everywhere.

Rasche and colleagues (2022) [41] extended the work by Rasche and colleagues (2017) [40], looking at 144 samples collected over 14 years from 25 patients, each with multiple focal lesions. The investigators describe 3 patterns of evolution: (1) the original dominant clone persists after treatment, (2) preexisting subclones compete after relapse, and (3) distinct subclones persist at different sites. These patterns cover most of the a priori possibilities. More interestingly, they observed that numerically minor subclones can persist for more than 10 years and then expand at relapse.

Merz and colleagues (2022) [42] looked at 24 sites in 10 patients, and did an scRNA-seq analysis, looking at 148,630 cells. Here, too, WES showed limited variation but scRNA-seq showed wide variation.

If 2 sites show divergent genomic or transcriptomic profiles, it could blunt the effectiveness of prognostic/predictive signatures based on the diagnostic bone marrow sample alone. As a practical matter, additional focal lesions are rarely biopsied. Profiling both the standard biopsy and circulating malignant plasma cells could hint at the presence of such a divergence.

SINGLE-CELL SPATIAL GENOMICS

Single-cell genomics and transcriptomics reveal nothing about relationship among cells. In single-cell spatial genomics DNA or RNA is used to construct next-generation sequencing (NGS) libraries on a cell-by-cell basis from all the cells within a tissue section. The geographic location of the cell is registered in an image and correlated with the known unique barcode predeposited at that position of the slide [43–45].

Knowing each transcriptome's location enables exploration of cell-cell interactions. Application to MM might be difficult because the usual sample is a calcified bone core. Ethylenediaminetetraacetic acid incubation can render a bone marrow core susceptible to sectioning, but the effect of incubation on the transcriptome might be substantial.

Treatment

The dismal overall survival (OS) rate began to improve in the 1990s with the introduction of high-dose melphalan, a cytotoxic (and mutagenic) alkylating agent, as an induction agent for subsequent stem cell transplantation [22,46]. When possible, autologous stem cells are used to avoid graft-versus-host disease. Multiple additional novel agents are now available and have demonstrated dramatic improvements in PFS and OS, leaving high-dose therapy with autologous stem cell transplant reserved for refractory cases.

Therapeutic Monoclonal Antibodies (Rx-mAbs)

Ironically, myeloma, the paradigmatic disorder of cells producing monoclonal immunoglobulins, is one of the earliest malignancies to be successfully treated with monoclonal antibodies (mAbs). Most new therapeutic mAbs are IgG1 kappa immunoglobulins, developed in transgenic mice, which have had a human immunoglobulin locus engineered into their genome.

Daratumumab

Daratumumab is directed against CD38, an abundant surface marker on plasma cells. CD38 is also present on many immune cell types and on red blood cells (RBC). CD38 can function as an enzyme, a cyclic ADP ribose hydrolase, but is probably multifunctional. Daratumumab binding to MM cells causes apoptosis by uncertain means. CD38 expression can downregulate, blunting efficacy.

Isatuximab

Isatuximab is directed against CD38, but at an epitope different from that targeted by daratumumab [47].

Elotuzumab

Elotuzumab is directed against the SLAMF7 receptor (CD319), a surface receptor, of uncertain function, at a high level on plasma cells [16].

Laboratory pitfall with therapeutic monoclonals

Therapeutic human monoclonals create a problem for monitoring the response of MM to treatment. Initially the response is monitored by following the patient's endogenous monoclonal level by SPEP. Human therapeutic mAbs can be detected on SPEP as monoclonals; they are "true" false-positives. Each mAb has a characteristic mobility, but this does not always permit distinguishing the therapeutic from the endogenous monoclonal protein on SPEP. Mass spectrometric analysis can distinguish endogenous monoclonal immunoglobulin from multiple Rx-mAbs in a single assay [48,49].

OTHER THERAPIES

Proteasome inhibitors and immunomodulatory drugs have each effected a dramatic improvement in clinical course for myeloma [50–54]. The modes of action, involving proteolysis inhibition and ubiquitination, presage the development of ProTacs, an approach generalizable to multiple cancer types [55–58].

Bortezomib carries a boron molecule that it donates to the 26S complex, shutting down proteolysis. Inhibition of proteolysis affects a wide array of proteins—cyclins, proapoptotic factors, and inhibitors of apoptosis, among them. The net effect seems to be increased apoptosis.

The mechanism of action of immunomodulatory agents such as lenalidomide has been worked out in detail: it interacts with the ubiquitin E3 ligase cereblon and targets this enzyme to degrade the Ikaros transcription factors IKZF1 and IKZF3.

CAR-T cells directed at myeloma are in several clinical trials [59–61]. The most common target is *TNFRSF17*. Examples of resistance, with biallelic deletion of both gene copies, have already been reported. Other targets are *SLAMF7, CD38*, and *CD138* [62].

Other therapies in development include panobinostat, a pan-HDAC inhibitor [52]; selinexor, an exportin inhibitor [63]; venetoclax, a Bcl-2 inhibitor [64]; and immune checkpoint inhibitors.

MINIMAL RESIDUAL DISEASE

With the current 3- and 4-drug regimens and agents for maintenance, a complete remission is attainable in up to 80% of patients; unfortunately the majority are not durable, with a 50% ten-year OS [65,66]. More sensitive assays, to monitor for emergence of malignant plasma cells following completion of treatment, might better distinguish patients who will have durable responses from those who will have relapse. If a patient is identified as MRD positive early in treatment, it raises the possibility of intensifying or changing the treatment, but the merits of such changes in a given setting are usually untested.

It is customary to monitor serum/urine for the diagnostic paraprotein following treatment, but because of the long half-life of immunoglobulins, the level does not decline rapidly; it is also not a sensitive test. For a paraprotein to be detected over background by SPEP typically 5% of plasma cells must be clonal. Serum free light chains show a more rapid decline than do intact monoclonal immunoglobulins, but most myeloma cases do not express a clonal excess of light chains. Nevertheless, moderately sensitive detection of the circulating clonotypic immunoglobulin is feasible by mass spectrometry [67,68].

NGF cytometric and NGS assays of bone marrow are the recommended modalities for sensitive detection of residual malignant plasma cells. Numerous trials have shown that MRD negativity of bone marrow aspirates predicts significantly longer PFS and OS. The IMWG has published criteria for detecting/reporting MRD [69]. It requires a method able to detect a malignant plasma cell with a minimum sensitivity of 1 in 100,000 cells to be designated MRD(−). Because of stochasticity in detecting a single cell, a reliable test cannot assay just 100,000 cells; rather it must assay $10^6$6 cells [66]. Multiple studies show that an MRD cutoff of 1 cell in 1 million leads to even better PFS and OS.

A suitable NGF assay, with validation approved by the IMWG, is the EuroFlow assay. The assay is designed to detect 10 antigens, using 8 fluorophores, in a 2-tube assay: CD138, CD27, CD38, CD56, CD117, CD45, CD19, CD81, c-kappa, c-lambda. It should be noted that this is done on total aspirate, and *not* on $CD138^+$-selected cells. The EuroFlow protocol calls for testing 10^7 cells to detect 2×10^{-6} cells with a 20-cell cutoff [70].

MRD by NGS is designed to detect the myeloma clone-specific rearrangement of the *IGH* gene; this requires a baseline sample from the time of diagnosis. The format is similar to the traditional assay for assessing B-cell clonality. Several primer pools targeting the FR1-3 regions of V_H and J_H portions of *IGH* are used to amplify V-D-J rearrangements by PCR. The NGS assay uses similar primers, but oligonucleotide adapters are ligated to the ends of the target fragments for construction of an NGS library and include unique molecular barcode sequences for pooled sample sequencing. The sensitivity identifying any expanded clone, as in a diagnostic sample, with NGS-based clonality studies is comparable to traditional PCR-based fragment-size analysis methods (eg, EuroClonality/BIOMED-2-based analysis). The sensitivity for detecting a specific sequence (clone) is much higher, and suitable for MRD.

At present (March 30, 2022) the ClonoSeq assay is the only FDA-approved NGS-based assay for detection of MRD in chronic lymphocytic leukemia (CLL), MM, and B-cell acute lymphoblastic leukemia. This assay has been extensively validated and shown to be able to detect 1 malignant plasma cell out of 10^6 cells. Other commercial NGS-based clonality/MRD offerings are available (eg, LymphoTrack, InVivoScribe, Inc., San Diego, CA); Oncomine Clonality Assay, Thermo Fisher Scientific, Waltham , MA) and described in published validations, including one showing comparability to NGF [71]. MRD by NGS has a comparative drawback compared with NGF—it requires analysis of a patient-specific "positive" (baseline) sample, usually from the time of diagnosis. At present this is not routinely provided prospectively. Stored aspirate slides may be acceptable. NGF assays have the comparative drawback that the sample must be analyzed promptly, compounded by the need for many sites to send the sample to a reference laboratory.

IMWG guidelines recommend MRD testing of unfractionated bone marrow aspirates. The optimal time to first test for MRD and optimal interval for monitoring is unsettled. At present, the IMWG guidelines recommend assessing MRD status over the disease course, rather than at a single timepoint after complete response (CR) is achieved, because this may provide a more robust evaluation of disease control [72]. Traditionally the first pull of a bone marrow aspirate is reserved for morphologic analysis, and the last for molecular testing. The trauma of biopsy induces hemorrhage, increasing with every aspiration. MRD testing must be done on the "first pull" [72]. Two other groups have offered informative consensus opinions [72,73].

The clinical utility of monitoring MM by iliac crest biopsy is well established, but for many patients, frail from age or cytopenias, it is not a trivial procedure. MM involvement in the bone marrow can be spotty, complicating reliance on the biopsy. MRD testing has been applied to circulating myeloma cells in blood and circulating free nucleic acids released into blood from myeloma cells. MRD analysis of blood would avoid the problem with single bone marrow aspirates not being representative and could, potentially, also detect mutated genomes shed from other sites of involvement. NGF and NGS assays can detect circulating myeloma cells in a moderate number of putative CR cases but are not as frequently positive as the bone marrow biopsies [74,75]; this could still have a role. Blood can be monitored more frequently; if positive, it might obviate bone marrow biopsy.

SUMMARY

Noncoding RNAs, both long and short, have been relatively underinvestigated, but genomic and transcriptomic analyses of myeloma would seem exhaustive, with more than 80 putative "driver" genes identified. Even so, there has been little clinical impact of genomics on diagnosis, prognosis, or therapy selection. As of 2022 the NCCN guidelines for myeloma (version 5.2022) only takes note of cytogenetics at diagnosis. A modest number of mutations and methylations have been associated with therapy resistance. In MRD, NGS and NGF play a critical role. Meanwhile, novel therapies have continued to markedly improve clinical response including OS.

CLINICS CARE POINTS

- MRD testing must be done on the "first pull" of a bone marrow aspirate.
- Cytogenetic analysis (karyotyping, FISH) remains an essential part of the diagnostic/prognostic workup but the proliferation of effective therapies, often in combination, has made predicting response challenging.
- Minimal Residual Disease (MRD) testing by clone-specific Next Generation Sequencing is the most sensitive approach, but requires availability of a baseline sample from the time of diagnosis.
- At present MRD assessment is only recommended for bone marrow samples, and **must** use the 'first pull' of the aspirate. Testing of circulating cell-free DNA is not yet adequately validated.

REFERENCES

[1] Manakkat Vijay GK, Singh H. Cell fate dynamics and genomic programming of plasma cell precursors. Immunol Rev 2021;303(1):62–71.

[2] Halliley JL, Tipton CM, Liesveld J, et al. Long-lived plasma cells are contained within the CD19(-)CD38(hi)CD138(+) subset in human bone marrow. Immunity 2015;43(1):132–45.

[3] Larsen JT, Chee CE, Lust JA, et al. Reduction in plasma cell proliferation after initial therapy in newly diagnosed multiple myeloma measures treatment response and predicts improved survival. Blood 2011;118(10):2702–7.

[4] Witzig TE, Timm M, Larson D, et al. Measurement of apoptosis and proliferation of bone marrow plasma cells in patients with plasma cell proliferative disorders. Br J Haematol 1999;104(1):131–7.

[5] Samur MK, Aktas Samur A, Fulciniti M, et al. Genome-wide somatic alterations in multiple myeloma reveal a superior outcome group. J Clin Oncol 2020;38(27):3107–18.

[6] Oben B, Froyen G, Maclachlan KH, et al. Whole-genome sequencing reveals progressive versus stable myeloma precursor conditions as two distinct entities. Nat Commun 2021;12(1):1861.

[7] Maura F, Petljak M, Lionetti M, et al. Biological and prognostic impact of APOBEC-induced mutations in the spectrum of plasma cell dyscrasias and multiple myeloma cell lines. Leukemia 2018;32(4):1044–8.

[8] Affer M, Chesi M, Chen WDG, et al. Promiscuous MYC locus rearrangements hijack enhancers but mostly super-enhancers to dysregulate MYC expression in multiple myeloma. Leukemia 2014;28(8):1725–35.

[9] Barwick BG, Neri P, Bahlis NJ, et al. Multiple myeloma immunoglobulin lambda translocations portend poor prognosis. Nat Commun 2019;10(1):1911.

[10] Rustad EH, Yellapantula VD, Glodzik D, et al. Revealing the impact of structural variants in multiple myeloma. Blood Cancer Discov 2020;1(3):258–73.

[11] Maura F, Boyle EM, Rustad EH, et al. Chromothripsis as a pathogenic driver of multiple myeloma. Semin Cell Dev Biol 2022;123:115–23.

[12] Aktas Samur A, Minvielle S, Shammas M, et al. Deciphering the chronology of copy number alterations in multiple myeloma. Blood Cancer J 2019;9(4):39.

[13] Bergsagel PL, Kuehl WM. Molecular pathogenesis and a consequent classification of multiple myeloma. J Clin Oncol 2005;23(26):6333–8.

[14] Chapman MA, Lawrence MS, Keats JJ, et al. Initial genome sequencing and analysis of multiple myeloma. Nature 2011;471(7339):467–72.

[15] Dutta AK, Alberge JB, Sklavenitis-Pistofidis R, et al. Single-cell profiling of tumour evolution in multiple myeloma - opportunities for precision medicine. Nat Rev Clin Oncol 2022;1–14.

[16] Haertle L, Barrio S, Munawar U, et al. Cereblon enhancer methylation and IMiD resistance in multiple myeloma. Blood 2021;138(18):1721–6.

[17] Allmeroth K, Horn M, Kroef V, et al. Bortezomib resistance mutations in PSMB5 determine response to second-generation proteasome inhibitors in multiple myeloma. Leukemia 2021;35(3):887–92.

[18] Samur MK, Fulciniti M, Aktas Samur A, et al. Biallelic loss of BCMA as a resistance mechanism to CAR T cell therapy in a patient with multiple myeloma. Nat Commun 2021;12(1):868.

[19] Da Vià MC, Dietrich O, Truger M, et al. Homozygous BCMA gene deletion in response to anti-BCMA CAR T cells in a patient with multiple myeloma. Nat Med 2021;27(4):616–9.

[20] Rustad EH, Yellapantula V, Leongamornlert D, et al. Timing the initiation of multiple myeloma. Nat Commun 2020;11(1):1917.

[21] Maura F, Rustad EH, Boyle EM, et al. Reconstructing the evolutionary history of multiple myeloma. Best Pract Res Clin Haematol 2020;33(1):101145.

[22] Maura F, Weinhold N, Diamond B, et al. The mutagenic impact of melphalan in multiple myeloma. Leukemia 2021;35(8):2145–50.

[23] Walker BA, Boyle EM, Wardell CP, et al. Mutational spectrum, copy number changes, and outcome: results of a sequencing study of patients with newly diagnosed myeloma. J Clin Oncol 2015;33(33):3911–20.

[24] Walker BA, Wardell CP, Murison A, et al. APOBEC family mutational signatures are associated with poor prognosis translocations in multiple myeloma. Nat Commun 2015;6:6997.

[25] Maura F, Rustad EH, Yellapantula V, et al. Role of AID in the temporal pattern of acquisition of driver mutations in multiple myeloma. Leukemia 2020;34(5):1476–80.

[26] van Beers EH, Huigh D, Bosman L, et al. Analytical validation of SKY92 for the identification of high-risk multiple myeloma. J Mol Diagn 2021;23(1):120–9.

[27] Melchor L, Brioli A, Wardell CP, et al. Single-cell genetic analysis reveals the composition of initiating clones and phylogenetic patterns of branching and parallel evolution in myeloma. Leukemia 2014;28(8):1705–15.

[28] Ledergor G, Weiner A, Zada M, et al. Single cell dissection of plasma cell heterogeneity in symptomatic and asymptomatic myeloma. Nat Med 2018;24(12):1867–76.

[29] Cohen YC, Zada M, Wang SY, et al. Identification of resistance pathways and therapeutic targets in relapsed multiple myeloma patients through single-cell sequencing. Nat Med 2021;27(3):491–503.

[30] Meißner T, Seckinger A, Hemminki K, et al. Profound impact of sample processing delay on gene expression of multiple myeloma plasma cells. BMC Med Genomics 2015;8:85.

[31] Ahmann GJ, Chng WJ, Henderson KJ, et al. Effect of tissue shipping on plasma cell isolation, viability, and RNA integrity in the context of a centralized good laboratory practice-certified tissue banking facility. Cancer Epidemiol Biomarkers Prev 2008;17(3):666–73.

[32] Sonneveld P, Durie BG, Lokhorst HM, et al. Modulation of multidrug-resistant multiple myeloma by cyclosporin. Lancet 1992;340(8814):255–9.

[33] Baccin C, Al-Sabah J, Velten L, et al. Combined single-cell and spatial transcriptomics reveal the molecular, cellular

and spatial bone marrow niche organization. Nat Cell Biol 2020;22(1):38–48.
[34] Tikhonova AN, Dolgalev I, Hu H, et al. The bone marrow microenvironment at single-cell resolution. Nature 2019. https://doi.org/10.1038/s41586-019-1104-8.
[35] Coutu DL, Kokkaliaris KD, Kunz L, et al. Three-dimensional map of nonhematopoietic bone and bone-marrow cells and molecules. Nat Biotechnol 2017; 35(12):1202–10.
[36] Zavidij O, Haradhvala NJ, Mouhieddine TH, et al. Single-cell RNA sequencing reveals compromised immune microenvironment in precursor stages of multiple myeloma. Nat Cancer 2020;1(5):493–506.
[37] Sklavenitis-Pistofidis R, Dutta AK, Ujwary S, et al. Single-cell RNA-sequencing identifies immune biomarkers of response to immunotherapy in patients with high-risk smoldering myeloma. Blood 2021;138(Supplement 1): 330.
[38] de Jong MME, Kellermayer Z, Papazian N, et al. The multiple myeloma microenvironment is defined by an inflammatory stromal cell landscape. Nat Immunol 2021; 22(6):769–80.
[39] Sklavenitis-Pistofidis R, Getz G, Ghobrial I. Single-cell RNA sequencing: one step closer to the clinic. Nat Med. Published online March 2021;4. https://doi.org/10.1038/s41591-021-01276-y.
[40] Rasche L, Chavan SS, Stephens OW, et al. Spatial genomic heterogeneity in multiple myeloma revealed by multi-region sequencing. Nat Commun 2017;8(1):268.
[41] Rasche L, Schinke C, Maura F, et al. The spatio-temporal evolution of multiple myeloma from baseline to relapse-refractory states. Nat Commun 2022;13:4517.
[42] Merz M, Merz AMA, Wang J, et al. Deciphering spatial genomic heterogeneity at a single cell resolution in multiple myeloma. Nat Commun 2022;13(1):807.
[43] Cho CS, Xi J, Si Y, et al. Microscopic examination of spatial transcriptome using Seq-Scope. Cell 2021; 184(13):3559–72.e22.
[44] Lewis SM, Asselin-Labat ML, Nguyen Q, et al. Spatial omics and multiplexed imaging to explore cancer biology. Nat Methods 2021. https://doi.org/10.1038/s41592-021-01203-6.
[45] Merritt CR, Ong GT, Church SE, et al. Multiplex digital spatial profiling of proteins and RNA in fixed tissue. Nat Biotechnol 2020;38(5):586–99.
[46] Kazandjian D, Dew A, Hill E. The changing role of high dose melphalan with stem cell rescue in the treatment of newly diagnosed multiple myeloma in the era of modern therapies-back to the future. Best Pract Res Clin Haematol 2020;33(1):101150.
[47] Frampton JE. Isatuximab: a review of its use in multiple myeloma. Target Oncol 2021;16(5):675–86.
[48] Murray DL, Puig N, Kristinsson S, et al. Mass spectrometry for the evaluation of monoclonal proteins in multiple myeloma and related disorders: an International Myeloma Working Group Mass Spectrometry Committee Report. Blood Cancer J 2021;11(2):24.
[49] Dasari S, Kohlhagen MC, Dispenzieri A, et al. Detection of plasma cell disorders by mass spectrometry: a comprehensive review of 19,523 cases. Mayo Clin Proc 2022; 97(2):294–307.
[50] Attal M, Lauwers-Cances V, Hulin C, et al. Lenalidomide, bortezomib, and dexamethasone with transplantation for myeloma. N Engl J Med 2017;376(14):1311–20.
[51] Rosiñol L, Oriol A, Teruel AI, et al. Bortezomib and thalidomide maintenance after stem cell transplantation for multiple myeloma: a PETHEMA/GEM trial. Leukemia 2017. https://doi.org/10.1038/leu.2017.35.
[52] Laubach JP, Schjesvold F, Mariz M, et al. Efficacy and safety of oral panobinostat plus subcutaneous bortezomib and oral dexamethasone in patients with relapsed or relapsed and refractory multiple myeloma (PANORAMA 3): an open-label, randomised, phase 2 study. Lancet Oncol 2021;22(1):142–54.
[53] Grosicki S, Simonova M, Spicka I, et al. Once-per-week selinexor, bortezomib, and dexamethasone versus twice-per-week bortezomib and dexamethasone in patients with multiple myeloma (BOSTON): a randomised, open-label, phase 3 trial. Lancet 2020;396(10262):1563–73.
[54] Goldschmidt H, Mai EK, Dürig J, et al. Response-adapted lenalidomide maintenance in newly diagnosed myeloma: results from the phase III GMMG-MM5 trial. Leukemia 2020;34(7):1853–65.
[55] Lim S, Khoo R, Peh KM, et al. bioPROTACs as versatile modulators of intracellular therapeutic targets including proliferating cell nuclear antigen (PCNA). Proc Natl Acad Sci U S A 2020;117(11):5791–800.
[56] Burslem GM, Crews CM. Proteolysis-targeting chimeras as therapeutics and tools for biological discovery. Cell 2020;181(1):102–14.
[57] Pfaff P, Samarasinghe KTG, Crews CM, et al. Reversible spatiotemporal control of induced protein degradation by bistable PhotoPROTACs. ACS Cent Sci 2019;5(10): 1682–90.
[58] Dale B, Cheng M, Park KS, et al. Advancing targeted protein degradation for cancer therapy. Nat Rev Cancer 2021;21(10):638–54.
[59] Berdeja JG, Madduri D, Usmani SZ, et al. Ciltacabtagene autoleucel, a B-cell maturation antigen-directed chimeric antigen receptor T-cell therapy in patients with relapsed or refractory multiple myeloma (CARTITUDE-1): a phase 1b/2 open-label study. Lancet 2021;398(10297):314–24.
[60] Munshi NC, Anderson LD Jr, Shah N, et al. Idecabtagene vicleucel in relapsed and refractory multiple myeloma. N Engl J Med 2021;384(8):705–16.
[61] Mikkilineni L, Kochenderfer JN. CAR T cell therapies for patients with multiple myeloma. Nat Rev Clin Oncol 2021;18(2):71–84.
[62] Teoh PJ, Chng WJ. CAR T-cell therapy in multiple myeloma: more room for improvement. Blood Cancer J 2021;11(4):84.
[63] Chari A, Vogl DT, Gavriatopoulou M, et al. Oral selinexor-dexamethasone for triple-class refractory multiple myeloma. N Engl J Med 2019;381(8):727–38.

[64] Neri P, Maity R, Alberge JB, et al. Mutations and copy number gains of the BCL2 family members mediate resistance to venetoclax in multiple myeloma (MM) patients. Blood 2019;134(Supplement_1):572.

[65] Diamond BT, Rustad E, Maclachlan K, et al. Defining the undetectable: the current landscape of minimal residual disease assessment in multiple myeloma and goals for future clarity. Blood Rev 2021;46:100732.

[66] Maclachlan KH, Came N, Diamond B, et al. Minimal residual disease in multiple myeloma: defining the role of next generation sequencing and flow cytometry in routine diagnostic use. Pathology 2021;53(3):385–99.

[67] Eveillard M, Rustad E, Roshal M, et al. Comparison of MALDI-TOF mass spectrometry analysis of peripheral blood and bone marrow-based flow cytometry for tracking measurable residual disease in patients with multiple myeloma. Br J Haematol 2020;189(5):904–7.

[68] Dispenzieri A, Krishnan A, Arendt B, et al. Mass-fix better predicts for PFS and OS than standard methods among multiple myeloma patients participating on the STAMINA trial (BMT CTN 0702 /07LT). Blood Cancer J 2022;12(2):27.

[69] Kumar S, Paiva B, Anderson KC, et al. International Myeloma Working Group consensus criteria for response and minimal residual disease assessment in multiple myeloma. Lancet Oncol 2016;17(8):e328–46.

[70] Roshal M. Minimal residual disease detection by flow cytometry in multiple myeloma: why and how? Semin Hematol 2018;55(1):4–12.

[71] Ho C, Syed M, Roshal M, et al. Routine evaluation of minimal residual disease in myeloma using next-generation sequencing clonality testing: feasibility, challenges, and direct comparison with high-sensitivity flow cytometry. J Mol Diagn 2021;23(2):181–99.

[72] Costa LJ, Derman BA, Bal S, et al. International harmonization in performing and reporting minimal residual disease assessment in multiple myeloma trials. Leukemia 2021;35(1):18–30.

[73] Yee AJ, Raje N. Minimal residual disease in multiple myeloma: why, when, where. Hematol Am. Soc Hematol Educ Program 2021;2021:37–45.

[74] Lohr JG, Kim S, Gould J, et al. Genetic interrogation of circulating multiple myeloma cells at single-cell resolution. Sci Transl Med. 8:363ra147.

[75] Waldschmidt JM, Vijaykumar T, Knoechel B, et al. Tracking myeloma tumor DNA in peripheral blood. Best Pract Res Clin Haematol 2020;33(1):101146.

Infectious Disease

Advances in Molecular Pathology 5 (2022) 73–84
ADVANCES IN MOLECULAR PATHOLOGY

Prevalence and Clinical Disease Severity of Respiratory Coinfections During the Coronavirus Disease 2019 Pandemic

Maxwell D. Weidmann, MD, PhD, Gregory J. Berry, PhD, Daniel A. Green, MD, Fann Wu, MD, PhD*
Department of Pathology & Cell Biology, Columbia University Irving Medical Center, 622 West 168th Street, New York NY 10032, USA

KEYWORDS
• Coinfection • Superinfection • COVID-19 • Respiratory virus • SARS-CoV-2 • Influenza

KEY POINTS

- An increased use of multiplex polymerase chain reaction–based assays has challenged the notion of a single respiratory pathogen always being responsible for a given disease.
- Rates of coinfection between severe acute respiratory syndrome coronavirus 2 and other respiratory viruses is highly variable based on etiology and patient population.
- Rates of coinfection or superinfection with bacteria are generally lower in patients with coronavirus disease 2019 than for those with influenza or respiratory syncytial virus.
- Higher rates of bacterial and fungal pneumonia in ventilated patients with coronavirus disease 2019 in the intensive care unit warrants increased diagnostic testing and empirical antibiotic therapy.
- Low rates of community-acquired respiratory coinfections, and higher rates of antimicrobial resistance, warrant greater antibiotic stewardship for patients with nonsevere coronavirus disease 2019.

INTRODUCTION

Respiratory tract infections represent a major global health concern. Coronavirus disease 2019 (COVID-19), which is caused by severe acute respiratory syndrome coronavirus 2 (SARS-CoV-2), has resulted in more than 470 million confirmed cases and approximately 6 million deaths worldwide [1]. Since the beginning of COVID-19 pandemic, the presence of more than 1 pathogenic organism in the respiratory tract of patients with COVID-19 has been widely recognized owing to the availability of advanced molecular detection technologies, such as multiplex polymerase chain reaction (PCR) and next-generation sequencing. However, the association between the occurrence of multiple pathogen infections and clinical disease severity remains unclear. In the study of disease evolution, multiple infections fall into 2 broad categories: coinfection and superinfection. Coinfection occurs when a person is found to be infected by two or more micro-organisms, but which infection was established first cannot be clearly determined, while superinfection is an infection arising when one or more infections is already present. A substantial number of patients with COVID-19 were also coinfected with various pathogens, including other respiratory viruses, bacteria, and fungi, which can influence infectious disease dynamics. This

*Corresponding author. Children's Hospital Central (CHC) 3-308, 622 West 168th Street, New York, NY 10032. *E-mail address:* fw108@cumc.columbia.edu

https://doi.org/10.1016/j.yamp.2022.07.003
2589-4080/22/

review presents an overview of the prevalence and clinical disease severity of respiratory coinfections and superinfections (Table 1) and discusses possible mechanisms of the interactions between viral infections, including SARS-CoV-2, and bacterial infections during the COVID-19 pandemic.

RESPIRATORY VIRAL COINFECTIONS

In late 2019, an acute respiratory disease, COVID-19, emerged in humans caused by a novel coronavirus, SARS-CoV-2. Unlike previously known coronaviruses, SARS-CoV-2 combines greater pathogenicity with high transmissibility during the presymptomatic or asymptomatic period [2]. COVID-19 has spread rapidly across the globe and has become a major pandemic disease. The increasing number of infections prompt the need to use rapid antigen-based assays and real-time reverse transcription PCR technology to rapidly detect SARS-CoV-2 RNA and confirm the clinical diagnosis of COVID-19 [3].

Respiratory virus infections are associated with a wide spectrum of clinical symptoms. This classical thinking that a single virus is associated with clinical symptoms has been challenged by the more advanced multiplexed PCR-based assays, which may simultaneously identify multiple pathogens associated with one clinical syndrome [4]. Broad respiratory syndromic testing is widely used to identify viral pathogens that cocirculate with SARS-CoV-2. Coinfections involving viruses are recognized to influence the disease dynamics that occur relative to a single infection [5].

Prevalence of respiratory viral coinfections

Respiratory viral coinfection with SARS-CoV-2 refers to the simultaneous infection of other respiratory viruses at the time of COVID-19 diagnosis. Previous reports have shown viral coinfection and superinfection are rare [6]. This article focuses on the prevalence and outcome of viral coinfection.

Viral coinfection in adults

The overall rate of coinfection of SARS-CoV-2 and other respiratory viruses in adults is considerably variable as reported. The rate of viral coinfection depends on the cocirculation of respiratory viruses in the specific time of the year and the geographic region where the study was conducted. In the beginning of COVID-19 pandemic, Yue and colleagues [7] carried out an epidemiologic study in Wuhan, China, between January 12 and February 21, 2020, and reported that the prevalence of SARS-CoV-2 and influenza coinfections was as high as 57.3% (176/307 cases), although the diagnosis of influenza was based on IgM serologic testing alone. From March 3 through 25, 2020, Kim and colleagues [8] conducted a study to assess the prevalence of coinfections in Northern California.. A total of 1217 nasopharyngeal swabs of symptomatic adult patients were tested by multiplex real-time reverse transcription PCR assays for SARS-CoV-2 and other respiratory pathogens. Of the 116 specimens positive for SARS-CoV-2, 24 were positive for 1 or more additional pathogens including influenza, rhinovirus, enterovirus, respiratory syncytial virus (RSV), and non–SARS-CoV-2 coronaviridae. The rates of coinfection between SARS-CoV-2 and other respiratory pathogens were 20.7%.

When the California Department of Public Health assessed influenza activity in California during the 2020 to 2021 influenza season, their analyses revealed that, among the 255 positive influenza cases, 58 persons were coinfected with SARS-CoV-2. The occurrence of influenza and SARS-CoV-2 coinfections was 23%, with influenza B being the predominant type (39/58 [67%]) [9]. The report indicated that SARS-CoV-2 testing was prioritized over influenza virus testing and infrequent influenza testing might have contributed to underestimates of influenza transmission [9]. Since the highly transmissible SARS-CoV-2 virus became the predominant circulating respiratory virus in humans, its impact on the circulation of other respiratory viruses has been evaluated [10]. The majority of cocirculating respiratory viruses seem to be less prevalent since the onset of the COVID-19 pandemic. This finding might be attributable to both intrinsic viral characteristics and viral interference [10].

Viral coinfection in children

The prevalence of viral coinfections is significantly higher in children than adults. A study from 6 US children's hospitals located in areas with high COVID-19 incidence during July and August 2021 found viral coinfections with SARS-COV-2 was common (113/713 [16%]) in pediatric patients aged less than 18 years. The coinfection rate was even higher among infants (32.4%) and young children aged 1 to 4 years (36.1%). The predominant (>65%) viral coinfections were caused by RSV [11].

Children with COVID-19 present with distinct epidemiologic and clinical characteristics that differ from adults. They may be asymptomatic or symptomatic with generalized clinical manifestations, like fever, cough, and nasal congestion. This pattern of symptoms makes it difficult to distinguish children with COVID-19 from those with infection of other common

TABLE 1
Prevalence of common coinfections in patients with COVID-19

Coinfections	Geography	Patient Population	Diagnostic Method for Coinfected Agents	No. of Patients	No. of Coinfected Case	Coinfection Rate	Reference[a]
Viral coinfection							
SARS-CoV-2 coinfected with influenza A/B	China	Aged ≥ 50 y	IgM serology	213	97	45.5%	Cheng et al,[25] 2021
	Spain	Adults	NAAT	255	7	2%–8%	Garcia-Vidal et al,[13] 2021
	Japan	Adults	NAAT	298	28	9.4%	Ishiguro et al,[14] 2021
	USA	Adults	NAAT	116	1	0.9%	Kim et al,[8] 2020
	Turkey	Adults	Direct fluorescent antibody	1103	6	0.5%	Ozaras et al,[17] 2020
	USA	Adults	NAAT	255	58	22.8%	Rizzo et al,[9] 2021
	China	Children	NAAT	34	1	2.9%	Wu et al,[12] 2020
	China	Adults	NAAT	145	2	1.4%	Xiang et al,[26] 2021
	China	Adults	IgM serology	307	176	57.3%	Yue et al,[7] 2020
SARS-CoV-2 coinfected with RSV	Spain	Adults	NAAT	256	1	0.4%	Garcia-Vidal et al,[13] 2021
	USA	Adults	NAAT	116	6	5.2%	Kim et al,[8] 2020
	USA	Children	NAAT	713	75	10.5%	Wanga et al,[11] 2021
	China	Children	NAAT	34	3	8.8%	Wu et al,[12] 2020
Bacterial coinfection							
Community-acquired coinfections	Spain	Adults	Culture	989	25	2.5%	Garcia-Vidal et al,[13] 2021
	Sweden	Adults	Culture, NAAT antigen	1243	46	4.0%	Hedberg et al,[58] 2022
	USA	Adults	Culture, NAAT antigen	1705	59	3.5%	Vaughn et al,[63] 2021
Community-acquired coinfections (72 h)	USA	Adults	Culture	3028	183	6.0%	Kubin et al,[64] 2021

(continued on next page)

TABLE 1
(continued)

Coinfections	Geography	Patient Population	Diagnostic Method for Coinfected Agents	No. of Patients	No. of Coinfected Case	Coinfection Rate	Reference[a]
Community-acquired pneumonia	USA	Adults	Culture, NAAT antigen	1705	26	1.7%	Vaughn et al,[63] 2021
	USA	Adults	Culture	3796	35	0.9%	Weidmann et al,[60] 2022
Health care–associated superinfections (>72 h)	USA	Adults	Culture	3028	350	11.6%	Kubin et al,[64] 2021
Hospital-acquired superinfections	Spain	Adults	Culture	989	38	3.8%	Garcia-Vidal et al,[13] 2021
Ventilator-associated lower respiratory tract superinfections	Sweden	Intubated Adults	Culture	426	129	29.4%	Hedberg et al,[61] 2022
Ventilator-associated pneumonia	USA	Intubated Adults	Culture	631	246	39.0%	Weidmann et al,[60] 2022

Abbreviation: NAAT, nucleic acid amplification test.
[a] References included in the review are arranged alphabetiacally within each type of coinfection.

respiratory viruses. A retrospective study of previous healthy children exposed to SARS-COV-2 in their household, who subsequently tested positive for SARS-COV-2, reported 19 of 34 children (51%) coinfected with other respiratory pathogens [12].

Clinical outcomes of respiratory viral coinfections

The COVID-19 pandemic has caused great challenges for health care systems globally. Viral coinfections are commonly seen in hospitalized patients [13]. A retrospective study found that, even though viral coinfection was common at 30.5% in patients hospitalized with COVID, coinfection was not an independent risk factor for the severity of hospital admission, need for high-flow oxygen therapy or mechanical ventilation, or mortality [14]. Another study analyzed inpatient data and revealed that patients positive for SARS-CoV-2 had a lower rate of coinfection with other respiratory viruses compared with those positive for other respiratory viruses (1.4% vs 4.8%). Patients with COVID-19 testing positive for other viruses including rhinovirus, parainfluenza, and seasonal coronavirus presented with mild disease and did not progress to pneumonia [15]. The proportion of SARS-COV-2 coinfected patients requiring care in the intensive care unit (ICU) (4/21 [19%]) was significantly lower than the proportion of those infected with SARS-CoV-2 alone (113/280 [47%]), indicating that coinfection with other respiratory viruses might not worsen the outcome of SARS-CoV-2–associated respiratory disease [16].

The clinical disease severity of respiratory viral coinfections in patients with COVID-19 could be impacted by the specific organism(s) causing of coinfection.

Coinfection with influenza

Influenza virus is a frequent cause of community-acquired pneumonia (CAP). Coinfection with SARS-CoV-2 may worsen COVID-19 symptoms and increase mortality, especially for the elderly [9]. Patients coinfected with SARS-CoV-2 and influenza B virus have presented with symptoms of fatigue (13%), abnormalities on a computed tomography scan of the chest (100%) or decreased lymphocytes and poor prognosis compared with SARS-CoV-2 single positive patients [7]. Ozaras and colleagues [17] reported 6 patients with COVID-19 who were coinfected with influenza and suffered from pneumonia. A thoracic computed tomography scan showed multiple lesions in the lung in 2 cases, bilateral lung lesions in 3 cases, and a single central lesion in 1 case [17]. A recent research study using an animal model for SARS-CoV-2 infection demonstrated that coinfection with influenza A virus causes more severe and prolonged pneumonia in SARS-CoV-2–infected hamsters [18]. The research team examined the respiratory organs of coinfected hamsters using immunohistochemical stain and found the infected regions were clearly divided into SARS-CoV-2–patterned and influenza-patterned areas and both viruses never coexisted at the same site in these organs, indicating that each virus may have distinct cell tropism and can efficiently spread in the respiratory organ without interference with the other [18].

Coinfection with Respiratory Syncytial Virus

RSV is the most common cause of bronchiolitis and pneumonia in children younger than 1 year of age. Patients coinfected with SARS-Cov-2 have been reported and hospitalized [11]. A retrospectively study found that 6 of 32 hospitalized children (18.7%) less than 24 months of age coinfected with SARS-CoV-2 and RSV, and had a significantly longer length of stay (7 days vs 3 days) than those without [19]. However, there was no difference in the need for intensive care or mechanical ventilation or mortality [19]. Similar findings were presented by Giannattasio and colleagues [20] among 6 infants aged 18 days to 9 months coinfected with both SARS-CoV-2 and RSV. The infants experienced mild fever and respiratory symptoms with an uncomplicated resolution [20]. RSV, which can cause more severe disease in infants, caused relatively mild disease in coinfected infants in this study of limited size. The authors speculate that this finding could be due to increased infectivity and replication of SARS-CoV-2, which may suppress RSV replication and clinical expression [20].

Virological mechanisms that determine viral persistence or exclusion during coinfections

Viral competition for resources in the respiratory tract

Molecular methods of viral detection and their increased sensitivity over culture have led to increased diagnoses of viral respiratory infections. This increase has also led to a greater frequency of viral coinfections being detected. When looking at the interactions between individual viruses during viral–viral respiratory coinfections, there seem to be both cases of inhibition and enhancement of one virus over another.

In the case of inhibition, it has been demonstrated through mathematical modeling that one virus can block infection with another virus by being the first to infect a cell [21]. In addition, the replication speed of the virus played a role with a rapidly replicating virus, such as rhinovirus, decreasing the replication of other viruses and a slow-growing virus, such as parainfluenza virus, being out-competed and subsequently suppressed in a viral–viral coinfection model [21]. This pattern is consistent with reports of viral coinfections seen during the pandemic, with 1 study reporting 8% of cases as coinfected, with rhinovirus comprising 6% and influenza virus comprising 2% of SARS-CoV-2 coinfections [22].

Ferret models of SARS-CoV-2 and influenza A virus coinfection showed that influenza A outcompeted SAR-CoV-2 in both viral titers and infectivity when coinfected ferrets were cohoused with uninfected ferrets [23]. Additional animal studies in murine models also showed increased influenza viral loads in coinfections and increased mortality, which could be ameliorated by prior immunity to influenza [24].

Studies in humans have been more ambiguous, with some studies showing similar clinical outcomes in patients infected with SARS-CoV-2 alone versus with a viral coinfection [25] and others showing higher rates of viral–viral coinfections in patients with severe cases of COVID-19 [7,26,27] or who had died [28]. Data published before the pandemic looking at influenza viral coinfections suggested that detection of more than 1 virus correlated with less severe disease [29] or had no difference in clinical disease severity [30]. This finding will need to be investigated in the context of SARS-CoV-2 coinfections. One large observational study in more than 21,000 positive specimens found that, although viral coinfection was not associated with an increase in viral load when compared with single-virus infections, there was evidence of viral competition that decreased the viral load [31].

Epithelial and organ damage

Although the significance of viral coinfection is unknown, the mechanisms of coinfection include virus-induced airway damage, decreased mucociliary clearance, and damage to the immune system [32].

Animal models of SARS-CoV-2 and influenza A virus coinfection led to significantly more weight loss and more severe inflammation in both the nose and lungs when compared with animals singly infected with each virus [23,33]. In addition, influenza A virus preinfection led to an increase in SARS-CoV-2 infectivity in cell-based models and also led to more lung damage and higher viral loads in mouse models [34]. Other models of epithelial, endothelial, and mononuclear cells have also shown infectivity with high viral loads, leading to cell damage and deterioration of barrier function [35].

Impact on the pattern of immune responsiveness

Because of the damage to the immune system caused by the coinfection, the presentation of patients who are positive for both SARS-CoV-2 and other viruses may be more severe [36]. It has been shown that SARS-CoV-2 infection leads to epithelial cell damage and the release of interferon [35]. Increases in proinflammatory cytokine levels early in infections have been linked to worse outcomes, with severe COVID-19 being linked with an increased cytokine response throughout disease progression [37].

When looking at influenza A and SARS-CoV-2 coinfection, one study showed an increase in serum cytokines (interleukin-2R [IL-2R], IL-6, IL-8, and tumor necrosis factor-α), cardiac troponin I, and a higher incidence of lymphadenopathy in patients solely infected with SARS-CoV-2 [25]. A hamster model of SARS-CoV-2 and influenza coinfection also showed a higher histology score for pulmonary edema, vasculitis, and inflammatory cell infiltration than single-virus infected animals [33]. Additionally, looking at the impact of influenza A and SARS-CoV-2 coinfections in adult inpatients showed that coinfection led to an increased odds of acute heart failure, multilobar infiltrates, acute kidney injury, secondary bacterial infection, and ICU admission. Coinfected patients also had a relatively higher SARS-CoV-2 viral load based on relative cycle threshold values than patients singly infected with SARS-CoV-2, which significantly correlated with acute kidney injury and acute respiratory distress syndrome [38].

BACTERIAL COINFECTION IN THE SETTING OF RESPIRATORY VIRAL ILLNESS

Respiratory viral infection may predispose hosts to bacterial pneumonia, but the degree to which this occurs varies widely based on the viral pathogen. We will examine 3 commonly occurring respiratory viral pathogens—influenza virus, RSV, and SARS-CoV-2—to understand how each affects risk for bacterial coinfection, outcomes associated with coinfection, and the mechanisms underlying these associations.

Influenza-associated bacterial coinfection

As a long-known cause of seasonal epidemics and occasional pandemics, the association of influenza with bacterial superinfection has long been established, with review of autopsy findings from the 1918 Spanish Flu pandemic displaying that bacterial superinfection was likely a central risk factor for mortality [39]. A variety of studies have attempted to characterize the rates of bacterial coinfection or superinfection in the setting of influenza, yet many of these have been limited to a single influenza season [40,41]. A metanalysis found rates varying from 2% to 65%; however, when the studies contributing the majority of heterogeneity were removed the range was 11% to 35% [42]. More recently, a prospective multicenter study from Spain has assessed rates of bacterial pneumonia from 2009 to 2015, including years of both pandemic and seasonal epidemic influenza [43]. These authors found lower rates of bacterial coinfection during 2009 (11.4%), associated with the H1N1 pandemic during that year, relative to increased rates in subsequent years (17.3%–23.4%) [43]. A metanalysis focusing on pandemic H1N1 influenza during 2009 found that 19% of hospitalized patients were found to have secondary bacterial pneumonia and that this rate increased to 23% when looking at autopsy specimens from fatal influenza cases [41].

Outcomes in patients with influenza have been found to be consistently worse in the setting of bacterial coinfection. Authors of the 2009 to 2015 Spanish study finding an adjusted odds ratio (OR) of 1.9 (95% CI, 1.5–2.5) for hospital mortality, whereas another retrospective study of 209 patients hospitalized with influenza from the Netherlands, 41 of whom had community-acquired bacterial coinfection (19.6%), found an adjusted hazard ratio of 2.6 (95% confidence interval [CI], 1.252–5.480) for mortality associated with bacterial coinfection [44]. Of note, this latter study found a large difference in mortality by bacterial species responsible for coinfection, with *Staphylococcus aureus* producing a mortality (adjusted hazard ratio) of 6.267 (95% CI, 2.679–14.662). A smaller study comparing mortality rates in patients with bacterial pneumonia in the setting of influenza (VI; n = 57) or other types of respiratory viral illness (NI; n = 77), they found that VI patients had lower rates of bacterial pneumonia than NI patients (23% vs 44%), as well as overall lower length of hospital and ICU stay, but no significant trends associated with bacterial pneumonia status [45].

A large portion of bacterial pneumonia in the setting of influenza has been found to be community acquired. One study involving 4313 patients with influenza hospitalized between 2010 and 2015 at 179 US hospitals found a CAP rate of 10.6%, with *S aureus* presenting as the most common etiology, and a mortality adjusted OR of 3.00 (95% CI, 2.17–4.16) [46]. Bacterial isolates identified were also more consistent with CAP, with the largest study of all types of bacterial pneumonia in patients with influenza identifying *Streptococcus pneumoniae* as the most common etiology (51.0%) by a large margin [43], and the most comprehensive meta-analysis of this subject has also found *S pneumoniae* as the most common etiology (35%), although *S aureus* made a more significant contribution (28%) [42].

There are a number of pathways by which influenza has been identified in both animal and human studies to increase susceptibility to bacterial pneumonia, including (1) depletion of alveolar macrophages by 90% during the first week of influenza infection in mice [47], (2) inhibition of the phagocytic activity of macrophages and neutrophils through induction of type 1 IFN responses [48,49], (3) inhibition of Th17 T cells that modulate the immune surveillance of pathogenic bacteria via type 1 IFN signaling, as well as (4) an increase in bacterial binding sites in the upper and lower respiratory tract produced by neuraminidase cleavage of sialic acid [50], and upregulation of surface receptors recognized by bacteria from the host inflammatory response and wound healing [51,52]. Interestingly, the mortality rates for influenza with bacterial pneumonia have been found to be highest in animal studies when bacterial infection occurs during the first week of viral infection [53], which in conjunction with high rates of CAP and the mechanisms listed elsewhere in this article, suggest that viral and bacterial infection act synergistically to decrease pulmonary function and inhibit host responses.

RSV-associated bacterial coinfection

Before the COVID-19 pandemic, RSV represented the leading cause of lower respiratory tract infection in children, with an estimated 2.7 to 3.8 million cases in 2015, causing higher rates of hospitalization and mortality relative to influenza in children under 5 years [54]. A wide range of bacterial coinfection rates is associated with RSV. One study of children with bronchopulmonary RSV found that 43.6% had a concurrent respiratory culture positive for pathogenic bacteria [55], with the most common pathogens being *Haemophilus influenzae* (43.9%), *S pneumoniae* (36.6%), and *Moraxella catarrhalis* (29.3%). A larger study of children with RSV pneumonia between 2010 and 2019 found that 32.4% had a concurrent respiratory bacterial infection, the most common etiologies of which were *S pneumonia* (40.8%), *S aureus* (40.8%), and *H influenzae* (25.4%) [56]. This study also assessed the effect of bacterial coinfection on clinical outcomes in children with bacterial coinfection compared with RSV alone, finding significantly higher rates of invasive ventilation (3.0% vs 0.0%) and ICU care (11.9% vs 6.4%), although mortality was not reported. One study focusing on 165 patients with RSV who were intubated and treated in the ICU found similarly high rates of respiratory culture positivity (42.6%); however, they used quantitative culture to separate bacterial coinfection (21.8%) and low bacterial growth or possible coinfection (20.8%) based on whether their cultures grew greater or less than 10^5 CFU/mL, respectively [57]. Although there was no significant difference in mortality rates, this study found a small but significant increase in length of mechanical ventilation in the bacterial coinfection group (6 days vs 4 days).

Interestingly, a retrospective cohort study concluding within the past year has directly compared rates of CAP in admitted adult patients testing positive for Influenza, RSV, or SARS-CoV-2 [58]. Hedberg and colleagues (2022) [58] found that roughly similar proportions of adults with influenza or RSV had concurrent CAP, 27% and 29% respectively, whereas only 4% of patients with SARS-CoV-2 had CAP. For all 3 viral infections, no significant differences in length of stay, ICU admission, or 30-day mortality between patients with or without CAP were seen, except a lower adjusted hazard ratio of being discharged alive for patients with influenza and CAP relative to those without CAP (0.76; 95% CI, 0.64–0.90). Of note, this study assessed only adult patients, whereas most studies of coinfection in the setting of RSV have focused on pediatric patients. Therefore, in adults, RSV infection involves high rates of bacterial pneumonia, similar to or increased in prevalence compared with influenza coinfection; however, exacerbation of outcomes by coinfection in pediatric populations is modest in comparison with that of influenza.

SARS-CoV-2–associated bacterial coinfection

The literature to date on bacterial coinfection in the setting of SARS-CoV-2 has shown significant differences from influenza or RSV coinfection. One study of 4267 patients hospitalized with COVID-19 in New York City found that only 2.1% had positive respiratory cultures and 1.9% had positive blood cultures, although 71% received at least 1 dose of an antibiotic [59]. Whereas Hedberg, Johansson, and colleagues [58] reported a CAP coinfection rate of 4% with SARS-CoV-2, other studies assessing CAP have found significantly lower rates. A multicenter study of 1705 patients hospitalized with COVID-19 in Michigan found that only 1.5% qualified as having CAP (defined as positive culture <3 days from admission). Another study of 3796 hospitalized patients with COVID-19 in New York City found that only 0.9% of patients with COVID-19 had CAP (defined as positive culture <2 days from admission), which only represented 12.2% of bacterial pneumonia cases in patients with COVID-19, whereas the large majority of cases were due to ventilator-associated pneumonia (VAP, 85.7%) [60]. This study also found that a significantly higher proportion of bacterial pneumonia in patients with COVID-19 was ventilator-associated relative to patients who did not have COVID. Rates of bacterial pneumonia among ventilated patients were also found to be significantly higher for those testing positive for SARS-CoV-2, was also seen in an independent study of a large cohort in Sweden [61]. Although meta-analyses have only looked at overall rates of bacterial coinfection in the setting of SARS-CoV-2, the largest of these found considerable heterogeneity between studies, with subgroup analyses showing rates of 4% in all hospitalized patients and 14% for ICU patients alone, consistent with the largest individual studies described elsewhere in this article [59,62,63].

Although Hedberg and colleagues did not report significant differences in the risk of ICU admission or 30-day mortality for patients with COVID-19 with CAP relative to those without, another large observational study looking specifically at clinically confirmed CAP found significantly increased rates of ICU admission (rate ratio = 4.45), mechanical ventilation (rate ratio = 6.74), higher rates of septic shock (rate ratio = 4.60), longer length of stay (mean 7 vs 5 days) and greater mortality (47.5% vs 18.0%) for patients with CAP [63]. A study specifically assessing hospital-acquired respiratory coinfections with bacterial or fungal pathogens found that that they occurred in 6.8% of patients with COVID-19, and more than 10-fold as many positive respiratory cultures relative to community-acquired infections [64]. For both hospital- and community-acquired infections, the vast majority were associated with bacterial etiologies, with only 4% of community-acquired and 2% of health care–associated pathogens involving fungal isolates (*Aspergillus*). Few other studies have directly assessed the rate of fungal respiratory infection in the setting of hospitalized patients with COVID-19. Of these, Nori and colleagues [59] represents the largest and also found low rates of coinfection with fungal pathogens, with 3 of 112 (2.7%) positive respiratory isolates of fungal etiology (*Candida* and *Aspergillus* spp). However, high rates of pulmonary aspergillosis have been demonstrated among patients with COVID-19 admitted to an ICU, with 1 meta-analysis of 30 studies covering 3441 patients demonstrating a pooled incidence rate of 14%

(95% CI, 11%–17%) with a case fatality rate of 52% (95% CI, 47%–56%) [65].

The etiologies of bacterial respiratory infections also reflect a relatively high proportion of health care–associated and/or ventilator-associated pathogens in patients with COVID-19, relative to pathogens found in patients with influenza. Although *S pneumoniae* represented the most common bacterial pneumonia pathogen for patients with influenza, *Staphylococcus, Pseudomonas,* and Enterobacterales spp (such as *Klebsiella*) represented the most common etiologies in patients with COVID-19 found by studies looking at both community-acquired and health care–associated pneumonia [59,60,64]. In a large observational study looking specifically at CAP in patients with COVID-19, bacterial pathogen profiles were more similar to that of patients with influenza, with the most common pathogen being *S pneumoniae* (28%), albeit far lower than coinfection in patients with influenza (56%), and with patients with COVID-19 with CAP having a higher proportion of *S aureus* as the second-most common pathogen (26% vs 19%) [58].

Despite the lower rates of bacterial respiratory coinfection in patients with COVID-19 relative to patients with influenza and RSV, high rates of early antibiotic therapy have been observed in these patient populations. The 3 largest such studies, including 4267, 3028, and 1705 patients with COVID-19 from Spring 2020, respectively, found that 71%, 67%, and 57% of patients received some form of antibiotic therapy during their treatment [59,63,64]. Interestingly, the smallest of these studies found that 54% of those patients with COVID-19 started on early antimicrobial therapy had it discontinued within 1 day after SARS-CoV-2 tests returned positive, but of those remaining on antimicrobial therapy, only 7.4% had a community-onset bacterial infection confirmed [63]. Another meta-analysis of 24 studies including 3338 patients also found that 72% of patients received antibiotics (95% CI, 56%–88%). However, most of the studies have looked at cases dating from the first or second wave of the COVID-19 pandemic in 2020, when effective antivirals were not available, and it remains to be seen whether such high rates of antibiotic therapy have continued into 2021 to 2022.

Nori and colleagues (2021) [59] also assessed antibiotic use in health care–associated infections, finding that 79% of patients who had a positive bacterial culture (blood or respiratory) had received antibiotics in the 30 days before positive culture, and all 21 patients with multi-drug resistant pathogens were in this group. Kubin and colleagues (2021) [64] found increasing rates of antimicrobial resistance in isolates recovered later in patients' hospital stay, 33% of *S aureus* isolates were methicillin resistant, 76% of which were respiratory isolates, 42% of Enterobacterales were cephalosporin resistant and 7% were carbapenem resistant (the majority of which were respiratory isolates). However, a study from the same institution comparing rates of antimicrobial resistance for bacterial respiratory isolates in patients with and without COVID-19 found no significant increase in any of these categories except for patients with COVID-19 with methicillin-resistant *S aureus* and overall resistance to penicillin class antibiotics [60]. Thus, antimicrobial resistance rates seemed comparable for COVID-19 and patient populations without COVID-19, with the exception of methicillin-resistant *S aureus*, but increasing risk of resistance with hospital stay further highlights the need for stewardship in early antibiotic treatment, particularly for nonintubated patients. This finding is corroborated by health care–associated infection risk factors assessed in Kubin and colleagues (2021), the leading of which were invasive mechanical ventilation (OR, 6.0; 95% CI, 3.7–10.0), ICU care (OR, 4.1; 95% CI, 2.5–6.8), and steroid treatment (OR, 1.9; 95% CI, 1.4–2.6).

Although there are a host of mechanisms by which influenza has been found to predispose human epithelia to bacterial coinfection, with high rates of CAP to support the manifestation of these mechanisms in real-world settings, there is a paucity of research into which of these mechanisms may also operate in the setting of SARS-CoV-2 infection. However, observational studies have found far lower rates of CAP in SARS-CoV-2 relative to patients with influenza, and instead prolonged exposure to health care settings and particularly mechanical ventilation seem to be driving the majority of bacterial and fungal pneumonia cases seen in patients with COVID-19. Respiratory culture ordering and antibiotic use should, therefore, be primarily considered in severe COVID-19 disease requiring ICU-level care and invasive mechanical ventilation.

DISCLOSURE

The authors have nothing to disclose.

REFERENCES

[1] World Health Organization Coronavirus. COVID-19) Dashboard. Available at: https://covid19.who.int/. Accessed on March 22, 2022.

[2] Tan J, Liu S, Zhuang L, et al. Transmission and clinical characteristics of asymptomatic patients with SARS-

CoV-2 infection. Future Virol 2020. https://doi.org/10.2217/fvl-2020-0087.
[3] Wang W, Xu Y, Gao R, et al. Detection of SARS-CoV-2 in Different Types of Clinical Specimens. JAMA 2020; 323(18):1843–4.
[4] Ramanan P, Bryson AL, Binnicker MJ, et al. Syndromic Panel-Based Testing in Clinical Microbiology. Clin Microbiol Rev 2017;31(1):e00024-17.
[5] Kumar N, Sharma S, Barua S, et al. Virological and Immunological Outcomes of Coinfections. Clin Microbiol Rev 2018;31(4):e00111-7.
[6] Musuuza JS, Watson L, Parmasad V, et al. Prevalence and outcomes of co-infection and superinfection with SARS-CoV-2 and other pathogens: a systematic review and meta-analysis. PLoS One 2021;16(5):e0251170.
[7] Yue H, Zhang M, Xing L, et al. The epidemiology and clinical characteristics of co-infection of SARS-CoV-2 and influenza viruses in patients during COVID-19 outbreak. J Med Virol 2020;92(11):2870–3.
[8] Kim D, Quinn J, Pinsky B, et al. Rates of Co-infection Between SARS-CoV-2 and Other Respiratory Pathogens. JAMA 2020;323(20):2085–6.
[9] Rizzo KR, Hoover C, Jain S, et al. Influenza and SARS-CoV-2 Co-infections in California, USA, September 2020-April 2021. Emerg Infect Dis 2021;27(11): 2923–6.
[10] Uhteg K, Amadi A, Forman M, et al. Circulation of Non-SARS-CoV-2 Respiratory Pathogens and Coinfection with SARS-CoV-2 Amid the COVID-19 Pandemic. Open Forum Infect Dis 2021;9(3):ofab618.
[11] Wanga V, Gerdes ME, Shi DS, et al. Characteristics and clinical outcomes of children and adolescents aged <18 years hospitalized with COVID-19 - six hospitals, United States, July-August 2021 [published correction appears in MMWR Morb Mortal Wkly Rep. 2022 Feb 04;71(5):185]. MMWR Morb Mortal Wkly Rep 2021;70(5152): 1766–72.
[12] Wu Q, Xing Y, Shi L, et al. Coinfection and Other Clinical Characteristics of COVID-19 in Children. Pediatrics 2020;146(1):e20200961.
[13] Garcia-Vidal C, Sanjuan G, Moreno-García E, et al. Incidence of co-infections and superinfections in hospitalized patients with COVID-19: a retrospective cohort study. Clin Microbiol Infect 2021;27(1):83–8.
[14] Ishiguro T, Kobayashi Y, Shimizu Y, et al. Frequency and Significance of Coinfection in Patients with COVID-19 at Hospital Admission. Intern Med 2021;60(23):3709–19.
[15] Wee LE, Ko KKK, Ho WQ, et al. Community-acquired viral respiratory infections amongst hospitalized inpatients during a COVID-19 outbreak in Singapore: co-infection and clinical outcomes. J Clin Virol 2020;128: 104436.
[16] Burrel S, Hausfater P, Dres M, et al. Co-infection of SARS-CoV-2 with other respiratory viruses and performance of lower respiratory tract samples for the diagnosis of COVID-19. Int J Infect Dis 2021;102:10–3.
[17] Ozaras R, Cirpin R, Duran A, et al. Influenza and COVID-19 coinfection: report of six cases and review of the literature. J Med Virol 2020;92(11):2657–65.
[18] Kinoshita T, Watanabe K, Sakurai Y, et al. Co-infection of SARS-CoV-2 and influenza virus causes more severe and prolonged pneumonia in hamsters. Sci Rep 2021;11: 21259.
[19] Alvares PA. SARS-CoV-2 and respiratory syncytial virus coinfection in hospitalized pediatric patients. Pediatr Infect Dis J 2021;40(4):e164–6.
[20] Giannattasio A, Maglione M, D'Anna C, et al. Silent RSV in infants with SARS-CoV-2 infection: a case series. Pediatr Pulmonol 2021;56(9):3044–6.
[21] Pinky L, Dobrovolny HM. Coinfections of the respiratory tract: viral competition for resources. PLoS One 2016; 11(5):e0155589.
[22] Kim KW, Deveson IW, Pang CNI, et al. Respiratory viral co-infections among SARS-CoV-2 cases confirmed by virome capture sequencing. Sci Rep 2021;11:3934.
[23] Huang Y, Skarlupka AL, Jang H, et al. SARS-CoV-2 and Influenza A Virus Coinfections in Ferrets. J Virol 2022; 96(5):e0179121.
[24] Achdout H, Vitner EB, Politi B, et al. Increased lethality in influenza and SARS-CoV-2 coinfection is prevented by influenza immunity but not SARS-CoV-2 immunity. Nat Commun 2021;12:5819.
[25] Cheng Y, Ma J, Wang H, et al. Co-infection of influenza A virus and SARS-CoV-2: a retrospective cohort study. J Med Virol 2021;93(5):2947–54.
[26] Xiang X, Wang ZH, Ye LL, et al. Co-infection of SARS-COV-2 and influenza A virus: a case series and fast review. Curr Med Sci 2021;41(1):51–7.
[27] Stowe J, Tessier E, Zhao H, et al. Interactions between SARS-CoV-2 and influenza, and the impact of coinfection on disease severity: a test-negative design. Int J Epidemiol 2021;50(4):1124–33.
[28] Hashemi SA, Safamanesh S, Ghasemzadeh-Moghaddam H, et al. High prevalence of SARS-CoV-2 and influenza A virus (H1N1) coinfection in dead patients in Northeastern Iran. J Med Virol 2021;93(2): 1008–12.
[29] Martin ET, Kuypers J, Wald A, et al. Multiple versus single virus respiratory infections: viral load and clinical disease severity in hospitalized children. Influenza Other Respir Viruses 2012;6(1):71–7.
[30] Asner SA, Science ME, Tran D, et al. Clinical disease severity of respiratory viral co-infection versus single viral infection: a systematic review and meta-analysis. PLoS One 2014;9(6):e99392.
[31] Burstein R, Althouse BM, Adler A, et al. Interactions among 17 respiratory pathogens: a cross-sectional study using clinical and community surveillance data. Preprint Medrxiv 2022 22270474.
[32] Vareille M, Kieninger E, Edwards MR, et al. The airway epithelium: soldier in the fight against respiratory viruses. Clin Microbiol Rev 2011;24:210–29.

[33] Zhang AJ, Lee AC, Chan JF, et al. Coinfection by Severe Acute Respiratory Syndrome Coronavirus 2 and Influenza A(H1N1)pdm09 Virus Enhances the Severity of Pneumonia in Golden Syrian Hamsters. Clin Infect Dis 2021;72(12):e978–92.

[34] Bai L, Zhao Y, Dong J, et al. Coinfection with influenza A virus enhances SARS-CoV-2 infectivity. Cell Res 2021;31: 395–403.

[35] Deinhardt-Emmer S, Böttcher S, Häring C, et al. SARS-CoV-2 causes severe epithelial inflammation and barrier dysfunction [published online ahead of print, 2021 Feb 26]. J Virol 2021;95(10):e00110–21.

[36] Tay MZ, Poh CM, Rénia L, et al. The trinity of COVID-19: immunity, inflammation and intervention. Nat Rev Immunol 2020;20(6):363–74.

[37] Lucas C, Wong P, Klein J, et al. Longitudinal analyses reveal immunological misfiring in severe COVID-19. Nature 2020;584(7821):463–9.

[38] Zheng J, Chen F, Wu K, et al. Clinical and virological impact of single and dual infections with influenza A (H1N1) and SARS-CoV-2 in adult inpatients. Plos Negl Trop Dis 2021;15(11):e0009997.

[39] Morens DM, Taubenberger JK, Fauci AS. Predominant role of bacterial pneumonia as a cause of death in pandemic influenza: implications for pandemic influenza preparedness. J Infect Dis 2008;198(7):962–70.

[40] Shah NS, Greenberg JA, McNulty MC, et al. Bacterial and viral co-infections complicating severe influenza: incidence and impact among 507 U.S. patients, 2013-14. J Clin Virol 2016;80:12–9.

[41] MacIntyre CR, Chughtai AA, Barnes M, et al. The role of pneumonia and secondary bacterial infection in fatal and serious outcomes of pandemic influenza a(H1N1) pdm09. BMC Infect Dis 2018;18(1):637.

[42] Klein EY, Monteforte B, Gupta A, et al. The frequency of influenza and bacterial coinfection: a systematic review and meta-analysis. Influenza Other Respir Viruses 2016;10(5):394–403.

[43] Martin-Loeches I, JS M, Vincent JL, et al. Increased incidence of co-infection in critically ill patients with influenza. Intensive Care Med 2017;43(1):48–58.

[44] Teng F, Liu X, Guo SB, et al. Community-acquired bacterial co-infection predicts severity and mortality in influenza-associated pneumonia admitted patients. J Infect Chemother 2019;25(2):129–36.

[45] Manna S, Baindara P, Mandal SM. Molecular pathogenesis of secondary bacterial infection associated to viral infections including SARS-CoV-2. J Infect Public Health 2020;13(10):1397–404.

[46] Bartley PS, Deshpande A, Yu PC, et al. Bacterial coinfection in influenza pneumonia: rates, pathogens, and outcomes. Infect Control Hosp Epidemiol 2022;43(2): 212–7.

[47] Ghoneim HE, Thomas PG, McCullers JA. Depletion of alveolar macrophages during influenza infection facilitates bacterial superinfections. J Immunol 2013;191(3): 1250–9.

[48] Sun K, Metzger DW. Inhibition of pulmonary antibacterial defense by interferon-gamma during recovery from influenza infection. Nat Med 2008;14(5):558–64.

[49] Tian X, Xu F, Lung WY, et al. Poly I:C enhances susceptibility to secondary pulmonary infections by gram-positive bacteria. PLoS One 2012;7(9):e41879.

[50] Foster TJ, Hook M. Surface protein adhesins of Staphylococcus aureus. Trends Microbiol 1998;6(12):484–8.

[51] Bucior I, Pielage JF, Engel JN. Pseudomonas aeruginosa Pili and Flagella Mediate Distinct Binding and Signaling Events at the Apical and Basolateral Surface of Airway Epithelium. Plos Pathog 2012;8(4).

[52] Davison VE, Sanford BA. Adherence of Staphylococcus-Aureus to Influenza-a Virus-Infected Madin-Darby Canine Kidney-Cell-Cultures. Infect Immun 1981; 32(1):118–26.

[53] Jamieson AM, Pasman L, Yu S, et al. Role of tissue protection in lethal respiratory viral-bacterial coinfection. Science 2013;340(6137):1230–4.

[54] Shi T, McAllister DA, O'Brien KL, et al. Global, regional, and national disease burden estimates of acute lower respiratory infections due to respiratory syncytial virus in young children in 2015: a systematic review and modelling study. Lancet 2017;390(10098):946–58.

[55] Hishiki H, Ishiwada N, Fukasawa C, et al. Incidence of bacterial coinfection with respiratory syncytial virus bronchopulmonary infection in pediatric inpatients. J Infect Chemother 2011;17(1):87–90.

[56] Lin HC, Liu YC, Hsing TY, et al. RSV pneumonia with or without bacterial co-infection among healthy children. J Formos Med Assoc 2022;121(3):687–93.

[57] Thorburn K, Harigopal S, Reddy V, et al. High incidence of pulmonary bacterial co-infection in children with severe respiratory syncytial virus (RSV) bronchiolitis. Thorax 2006;61(7):611–5.

[58] Hedberg P, Johansson N, Ternhag A, et al. Bacterial co-infections in community-acquired pneumonia caused by SARS-CoV-2, influenza virus and respiratory syncytial virus. BMC Infect Dis 2022;22(1):108.

[59] Nori P, Cowman K, Chen V, et al. Bacterial and fungal coinfections in COVID-19 patients hospitalized during the New York City pandemic surge. Infect Control Hosp Epidemiol 2021;42(1):84–8.

[60] Weidmann MD, Berry GJ, Zucker JE, et al. Bacterial Pneumonia and Respiratory Culture Utilization among Hospitalized Patients with and without COVID-19 in New York City. J Clin Microbiol 2022; 60(7):e0017422.

[61] Hedberg P, Ternhag A, Giske CG, et al. Ventilator-Associated Lower Respiratory Tract Bacterial Infections in COVID-19 Compared With Non-COVID-19 Patients. Crit Care Med 2022;50(5):825–36.

[62] Lansbury L, Lim B, Baskaran V, et al. Co-infections in people with COVID-19: a systematic review and meta-analysis. J Infect 2020;81(2):266–75.

[63] Vaughn VM, Gandhi TN, Petty LA, et al. Empiric antibacterial therapy and community-onset bacterial coinfection

in patients hospitalized with coronavirus disease 2019 (COVID-19): a multi-hospital cohort study. Clin Infect Dis 2021;72(10):e533–41.

[64] Kubin CJ, McConville TH, Dietz D, et al. Characterization of Bacterial and Fungal Infections in Hospitalized Patients With Coronavirus Disease 2019 and Factors Associated With Health Care-Associated Infections. Open Forum Infect Dis 2021;8(6):ofab201.

[65] Chen W, Yin C, Zhong M, et al. Incidence and outcomes of patients with COVID-19 associated pulmonary aspergillosis (CAPA) in intensive care units: a systematic review and meta-analysis of 31 cohort studies. Ann Palliat Med 2022;11(7):2202–9.

Advances in Molecular Pathology 5 (2022) 85–108
ADVANCES IN MOLECULAR PATHOLOGY

Applications of Long-Read Sequencing Technology in Clinical Genomics

Shivaprasad H. Sathyanarayana, PhD, Sophie J. Deharvengt, PhD, Guohong Huang, PhD, Rachael E. Barney, BS, Parth S. Shah, MD, Joel A. Lefferts, PhD*

Department of Pathology and Laboratory Medicine, Clinical Genomics and Advanced Technology Laboratory, Geisel School of Medicine at Dartmouth, Dartmouth-Hitchcock Medical Center, Lebanon, NH 03756, USA

KEYWORDS

• Long-read sequencing • PacBio • Oxford Nanopore Technology • Short-read sequencing • Infectious disease • Cancer genomics • Structural variants

KEY POINTS

- Long-read sequencing (LRS) technologies with improving accuracy and high throughput capabilities have multiple applications in genetics and clinical genomics.
- Long-read technologies can generate reads of thousands of kilobases (kb) to megabases (Mb) in length.
- LRS has successfully shown its potential to resolve complicated structural variants in the most challenging regions of the human genome.
- LRS, also known as third-generation sequencing technology, has revolutionized genomics by revealing the full spectrum of human genome variation responsibile for hereditary conditions and novel disease mechanisms.
- Diverse LRS technologies will soon permit the routine assembly of diploid genomes and telomere-to-telomere assemblies.

INTRODUCTION

Genetics and genomics research has constantly been guided by state-of-the-art sequencing technologies, which initially emerged from Sanger sequencing and were later followed by next-generation sequencing (NGS) [1]. NGS technology has transformed modern genetics and genomics research, including clinical genetics applications. For over a decade, NGS has an integral to genetic research in academia and the health care industry by discovering novel disease-causing genes and variants [2]. In addition, clinical gene panels and whole-exome sequencing (WES) have primarily replaced, single-gene testing for improved clinical investigation due to high performance and low pricing compared with traditional Sanger sequencing approaches [2,3]. The Illumina sequencing platforms have dominated both genomic research and clinical genomic testing (Fig. 1A). Illumina sequencing chemistry is based on the short-read sequence by synthesis methods to resolve the order of nucleotides in deoxyribonucleic acid (DNA) sequences [1] (Fig. 1B). With massive scalability and cost-effectiveness, this technology provides greater than 99.9% sequencing accuracy, and currently, it is a benchmark in research and clinical

Conflict of Interest Statement: The authors declare no commercial or financial relationships that could be construed as a potential conflict of interest.

*Corresponding author, *E-mail address:* Joel.A.Lefferts@hitchcock.org

https://doi.org/10.1016/j.yamp.2022.07.004
2589-4080/22/

ABBREVIATIONS

ARFGEF9	ADP ribosylation factor guanine nucleotide exchange factor 9
BLAST	Basic local alignment search tool
CAMPHOR	Comprehensive analysis method for polymorphic and somatic structural variations
CDKN2A	Cyclin-dependent kinase inhibitor 2A
CHEK2	Checkpoint kinase 2
CLN6	Ceroid-lipofuscinosis neuronal 6
CRISPR	Clustered regularly interspaced short palindromic repeats
CX26	Connexin 26
CYP21A2	Cytochrome P450 family 21 subfamily A member 2
CYP2D6	Cytochrome P450 family 2 subfamily D member 6
ERBB2	Erb-B2 receptor tyrosine kinase
FMLRC	FM-index long read corrector
LR-WGS	Long-read whole genome sequencing
PDCL3P4	Phosducin-like 3 pseudogene 4
PKD1	Polycystic kidney disease 1
PMS2	PMS1 homolog 2, mismatch repair system component
PRKAR1A	Protein kinase cAMP-dependent type I regulatory subunit alpha
PTPN11	Protein tyrosine phosphatase non-receptor type 11
RASSF2	Ras association domain family member 2
RET	RET proto-oncogene
SLC23A2	Solute carrier family 23 member 2
SMAD4	SMA- and MAD-related 4
SMN1	Survivor of motor neuron 1
SR-NGS	Short-read next generation sequencing
TCOF1	Treacle ribosome biogenesis factor 1

settings (Table 1). Over the past several years, short-read sequencing (SRS) has led to valuable novel discoveries that have advanced our understanding of genomics. This discovery includes a growing knowledge of genetic diseases and their associated pathogenic variants that consist of single-nucleotide variants (SNVs), copy number variants (CNVs), insertions, and deletions [4–9].

However, the increased complexity of repetitive sequences in the human genome could be technically challenging for SRS [10,11]. Inherent challenges with SRS include the inability to precisely map or assemble the short reads (SRs) coming from repetitive sequences, detecting complex structural variation (SV), and sequencing through regions of high GC content within the genome [11]. These technical limitations might lead to errors or failure to detect genetic variants in certain complex regions in the genome [12]. With the recent accomplishment in finding the most challenging genome regions and completing the human genome sequence, long-read sequencing (LRS) is assured to bypass the limitations of short-read NGS-based research for human diseases [13–17]. Compared to SRS, the advantage of LRS is the ability to read 10 kilobases (kb) or even longer derived from a single DNA molecule [18]. Also, library preparation can be conducted without polymerase chain reaction (PCR) amplification or relatively low cycle numbers, with sequencing progress appearing in real-time [19]. Having unique technological features, LRS can generate high-quality genome assembly with clinical significance [20,21].

In addition, LRS can provide clinical information related to infectious diseases and its management, monitoring of emerging infectious diseases outbreak, identification of pathogen drug resistance, and epidemiologic data [22,23]. With numerous examples, LRS

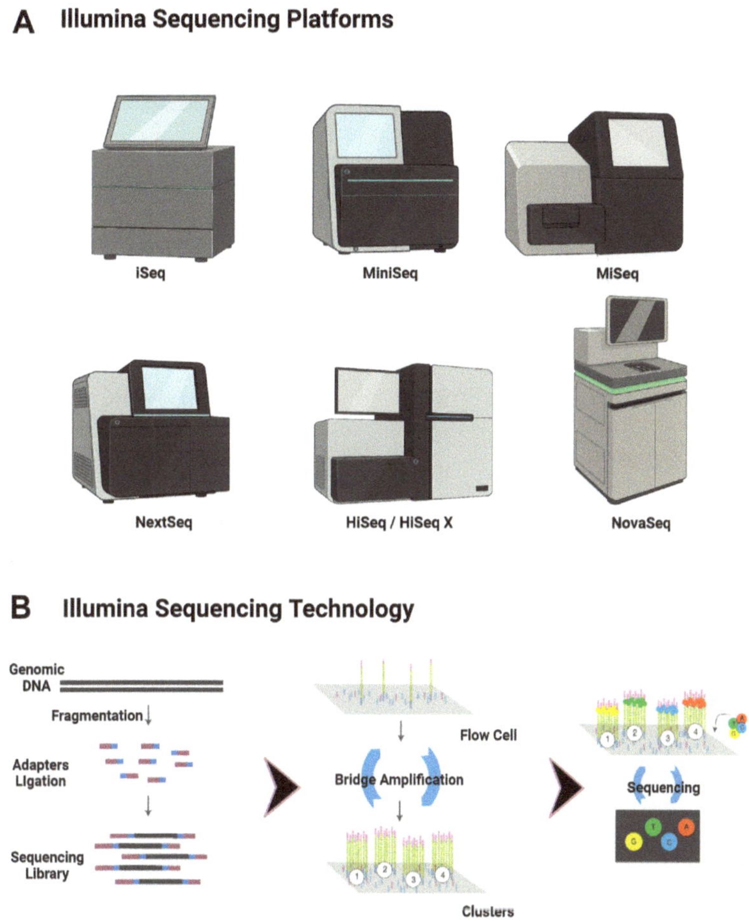

FIG. 1 *Overview of short-read sequencing technologies by Illumina.* (*A*) Representation of different SRS platforms by Illumina (*B*) SRS chemistry by Illumina. The sequencing library is made by fragmenting genomic DNA (gray) molecules and ligating specific adapters (pink and blue) to both the fragment ends. The ligated adapters carry unique molecular barcodes and sequences complementary to the oligonucleotides attached to the surface of a flow cell. Adapter-tagged DNA library is loaded into a flow cell, and the fragments are hybridized to the flow cell surface. Once these DNA library fragments have been attached, cluster generation initiates. Each bound fragment is amplified into a clonal cluster in thousands of copies generated through the bridge amplification. After this process, the reverse DNA strands are cleaved and washed away, resulting in only the forward strands. Then, sequencing by synthesis begins as the sequencing reagents, and fluorescently labeled nucleotides are incorporated into newly synthesized DNA strands at each cycle. After that, a laser excites the fluorophore on the strand, imaged, and the signal emission recorded are used to identify the specific nucleotide base. (*Created with* Biorender.com)

has successfully identified disease-causing SVs, resolved phasing issues, differentiated genes from pseudogenes, captured repeat sequence expansions, identified infectious disease pathogens and novel pathogenic variants [24–26]. In this comprehensive review, we emphasize two LRS platforms: Pacific Biosciences (PacBio) with its single-molecule real-time (SMRT) sequencing technology and Oxford Nanopore Technologies (ONT) with its nanopore-based sequencing. These two LRS technologies are rapidly advancing in genetics and clinical genomics research.

PacBio. The PacBio launched its first commercial long-read sequencer in 2011. After that, numerous technological advances have been made to their sequencing

TABLE 1
The difference between short-read and long-read technologies and its platform based on the type of data, read length, and throughput

Sequencing technology	Platform	Data Type	Read Length in kb		Read Accuracy in %	Throughput Per Flow Cell in Gb	
			N50	Maximum		Mean	Maximum
Illumina	NovaSeq 6000	Single End	0.05–0.25	0.25	>99.9%	65–3000	>3000
		Paired-end	0.10–0.5	0.50			
	NextSeq 550	Single End	0.075–0.15	0.15		16–30	>30
		Paired-end	0.15–0.30	0.30		32–120	>120
Oxford Nanopore Technologies (ONT)	PromethION	Long read	10–60	>1000	87%–98%	50–100	180
	MinION/ GridION	Long read	10–60	>1000		2–20	30
		Ultra-long read	100–200	>1500		0.5–2	2.5
Pacific Biosciences (Pac Bio)	Sequel II	Hi-Fi Read	10–20	>20	>99%	15–30	35
		CLR	30–60	>200	87%–92%	50–100	160
	Sequel	CLR	25–50	>100		5–10	20

Data from Logsdon GA, Vollger MR, Eichler EE. Long-read human genome sequencing and its applications. *Nature Reviews Genetics*. 2020;21(10). https://doi.org/10.1038/s41576-020-0236-x.

platforms [27,28] (Fig. 2A). The foundation of the PacBio systems is single-molecule realtime (SMRT) sequencing, which happens within SMRT cells and consists of zero-mode waveguides (ZMW), which are chambers that carry inactive polymerase [29]. This specific technology uses a circular DNA template called SMRTbell by supplementing hairpin adaptors at both ends of double-stranded DNA [30]. Once the SMRTbell is ready, DNA polymerase is attached and loaded onto a SMRT cell containing up to 8 million ZMWs, for sequencing (see Fig. 2A). The polymerase synthesizes new complementary strands as fluorescently labeled nucleotides are added to the sequencing reaction. A laser excites the fluorophores as fluorescence pulses and is recorded into real-time data after each inclusion. This process is continuously repeated to identify each base in the SMRTbell template. Thus, the released signals are converted into a nucleotide sequence called a continuous long-read (CLR) [29].

The PacBio CLR is the most common form of data generated with DNA inserts exceeding 30 Kb in length [29]. CLR data comes from Sequel platforms with a range of 20 Gb up to 160 Gb of data per flow cell with 99.9% accuracy [31,32] (see Table 1). In addition, PacBio high-fidelity (HiFi) reads are the newest data type improved by PacBio, using 10 to 30 Kb DNA inserts with an accuracy of greater than 99% with circular consensus sequencing (CCS) [29]. Thus, with greater than 99% accuracy, PacBio reads have significantly advanced variant detection, improved time efficiency in genome assembly, and identified complex regions in the genome [32–34].

ONT. ONT-LRS uses linear DNA molecules instead of circular ones. In 1995, the plan of sequencing a single molecule using biological nanopores was first proposed [29], In 2012, ONT officially introduced the MinION as their new generation nanopore sequencer that may require a low cycle number amplification or fluorescence labels [35,36]. The DNA inserts used in ONT are typically several hundred kb to Mb in length [37–40]. In the ONT platform, with the aid of motor protein, sequencing commences within a double-stranded DNA molecule ligated connecting to a sequencing adaptor preloaded with a motor protein on one or both ends. Later, DNA samples are loaded onto a flow cell that consists of thousands of protein nanopores that are effectively inserted into a solid phase conductive membrane [29]. Thus, the sequencing is initiated via a motor protein unwinding the double-stranded DNA. At a controlled rate, negatively charged DNA drives through the pore with an electric current, leading to distinct changes in the current captured in real-time

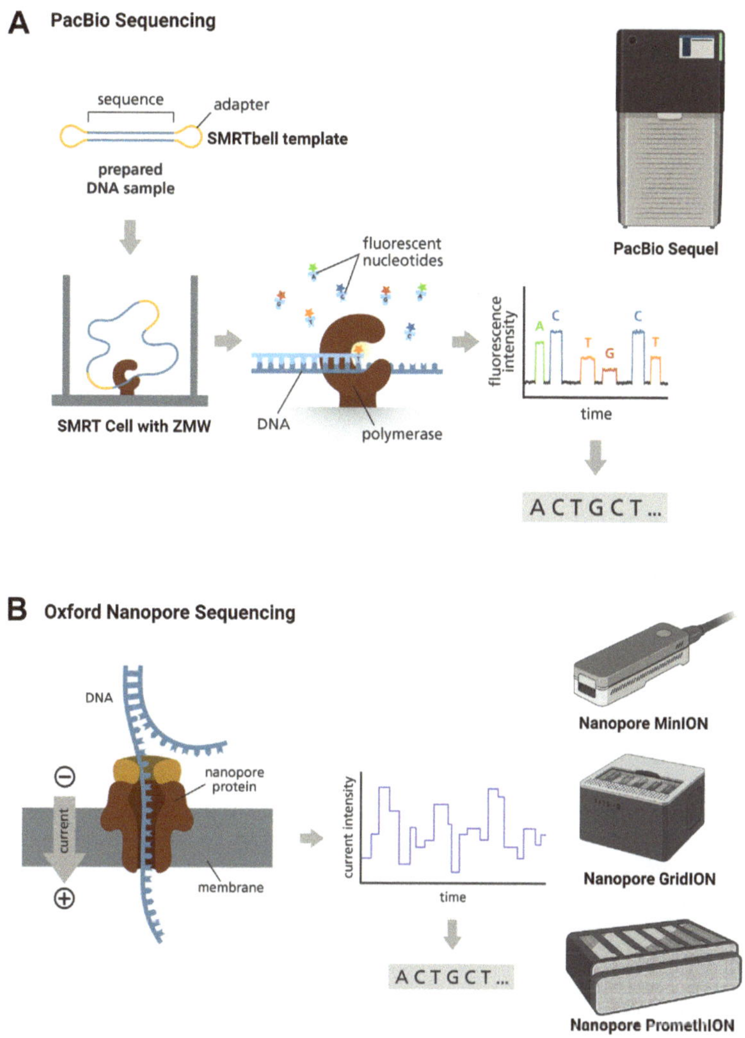

FIG. 2 *Overview of long-read sequencing technologies by PacBio and ONT* (*A*) PacBio long-read sequencing platform and chemistry with PacBio Sequel II LRS system. In PacBio SMRT sequencing, fragmented DNA (blue) is ligated with hairpin adapters (yellow) that form a circular molecule called an SMRT bell template. Once the SMRTbell is made, those are loaded onto an SMRT Cell for sequencing tagged with DNA polymerase in an inactive state. Each SMRT Cell contains up to 8 million zero-mode waveguides (ZMWs), holding a small sample volume. As the DNA samples are loaded into this SMRT Cell with ZMWs, the SMRTbell template and the polymerase become restrained, and fluorescently labeled nucleotides (dNTPs) are incorporated to initiate the sequencing reaction. As the polymerase synthesizes the new strand, fluorescently labeled dNTPs are excited by the light emission. The excited fluorophores will be captured by a real-time camera that records fluorescence intensity over time, corresponding to an individual nucleotide base representation. (*B*) Overview of Oxford Nanopore Sequencing Technologies (ONT). Presentation of different sequencing platforms by ONT. Long DNA (blue) is tagged with sequencing adapters with one or both ends in the ONT platform. The DNA is combined with Nanopore proteins embedded inside the sequencing flow cell into an artificial membrane. The sequencing adapters insert into the opening of the nanopore, and the motor protein starts to unwind the DNA. An electric current is applied across the membrane forcing the negatively charged DNA to pass through the nanopores at 450 bases per second. As the DNA moves through the pores, the obstruction of a nanopore by a DNA fragment causes a change in the current measured continuously within the flow cell used to identify the DNA sequence. (*Created with* Biorender.com)

to reveal the specific bases in the DNA strand [40] (see Fig. 2B).

Compared with PacBio, ONT can exceed read lengths by spawning continuous sequences up to hundreds or thousands of kb. The standard ONT long read is the most commonly produced, typically 10 to 100 kb in length with 87% to 98% accuracy [37,39,40]. In addition to the MinION sequencer (which can hold one flow cell), ONT LRS is also available with the GridION (which can hold up to 5 flow cells) and PromethION (which can hold up to 48 flow cells) [29] (see Fig. 2B). Each of these three ONT sequencers varies significantly in size, flow cell capacity, and data output. MinION and GridION share a similar flow cell type, with 2048 nanopores split into 512 channels generating up to 2 to 20 Gb long-read data per flow cell. Meanwhile, PromethION uses higher capacity flow cells with 12,000 nanopores split into 3000 channels to generate 50 to 100 Gb data per flow cell [37,39,40] (see Table 1). Another type of data produced with the ONT platform is ONT ultra-long-reads longer than 100 Kb, typically in the Mb range, with 87% to 98% accuracy [37,38,40]. Using MinION or GridION, only 500 Mb to 2 Gb ultra-long-read data can be produced per flow cell [39,40] (see Table 1). Further, ONT's long and ultra-long-read have substantially impacted several areas of genomic research, including variant discovery, de-novo assembly, disease correlation, and genome complexity [14,15,20,31,34,37,39–47].

Here, we discuss the comprehensive applications of the LRS technology in different thrust areas of clinical genomics and how they facilitate new biological insights with significant progress in genomic research. In addition, we have also briefly discussed the data analytics associated with these systems, and the detailed evaluation of the various LRS genome informatics pipelines and software has been illustrated elsewhere [48].

LONG-READ TECHNOLOGY IN GENETICS AND GENOMICS RESEARCH

Genetic research in clinical laboratories is always robust and powered by new sequencing technologies. Efforts toward updating sequencing technologies continued to pave the way for more accurate and complete genome assembly, which was initiated with Sanger sequencing and gradually advanced by different NGS platforms [1]. However, the LRS technology can overcome most of the drawbacks of the traditional NGS approach to human diseases by distinguishing the complex DNA sequences and filling gaps in the human genome assemblies [14,15,20,37]. In clinical lab tests, the WES platform by Illumina is frequently used to examine genetic diseases as a primary testing option. The popularity of Illumina has taken clinical genetic testing and diagnostics to a different level [2]. Remarkably, the individual human genome consists of more than 20,000 structural variants (that are >50 base pairs (bp)) and thousands of indels (<50 bp), spanning dozens of megabases (Mbs). Long-read-whole-genome sequencing (WGS) uncovers these structural variants, often missed with conventional SR-NGS [13–15,44,49,50]. Moreover, such unknown structural variants or indels might interfere with relevant genes causing dosage sensitivity among individuals with common inherited diseases or disorders.

STRUCTURAL VARIANTS DETECTION AND CANCER

SVs are substantial modifications in the genome that often occur in repetitive genomic locations. The variants include inversions, translocations, deletions, duplications, and CNVs of various sizes and magnitudes. These SVs alter genome architecture and are associated with both genetic diseases and cancer [51,52] (Fig. 3). SRS-based methods can detect SVs but may be limited in their ability to identify or accurately characterize large or complex deletions, duplications, and rearrangements [12,44,53,54]. However, LRS platforms like ONT and PacBio provide much more reliable and accurate SV detection, a feature that often overshadows its lower - quality reads. The power and utility of LRS for detecting CNVs and other SVs have been shown in several genetic diseases, including cancers [55–59].

The detection of SVs from LRS is performed using two comprehensive methods: (1) the mapping-based approach and (2) *the de-novo* assembly-based approach. In the mapping-based approach, the sequence data is split into two or more subreads, and those reads will be mapped to a reference genome (hg19 or hg38) [60]. However, in the *de-novo* assembly type, regions of overlap between reads are used to construct a whole genome without considering the reference genome. However, considering the availability of the reference genome and the cost, the alignment-based method is more efficient and is generally used in SV detection. Moreover, given the complexity and heterozygosity of the cancer genome, the *de novo* assembly-based approach won't successfully assemble accurate genomic contigs [60].

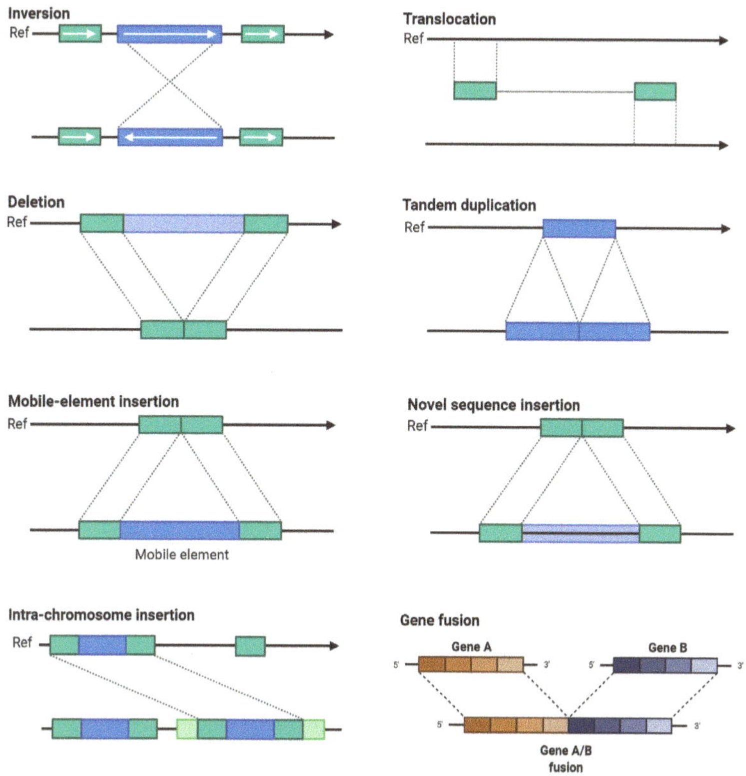

FIG. 3 Different types of structural variants that observed in several cancer types and genetic disorders. (*Created with* Biorender.com)

There are multiple examples of studies using LRS for SV detection. Sakamoto and colleagues [60] used ONT-based MinION to study the transcripts of fusion genes in lung adenocarcinoma cell lines via full-length cDNA sequencing and identified the fusion gene junction between *coiled-coil domain-containing 6 (CCDC6)* and *RET* accurately. In addition, the group also studied five non-small-cell lung cancer (NSCLC) cell lines and 20 clinical samples with lung cancer. Utilizing ONT-MinION and PromethION WGS platform, and the group identified complex SVs including local tandem inversion, duplication, and microdeletions. In another study, using ONT MinION, Fujimoto and colleagues [61] evaluated 11 Japanese liver cancer samples previously sequenced by the International Cancer Genome Consortium (ICGC). The study group assembled germline and somatic SVs from LRS data advancing a new analytical pipeline (CAMPHOR). Valle-Inclan and colleagues [62] used ONT LRS and quantitative real-time PCR to establish a low sequence depth approach. The study identified SVs from circulating tumor (Ct) DNA to track tumor burden (TB) using somatic SVs as biomarkers from liquid biopsies.

Using the combination of targeted LRS and adaptive sequencing on the ONT, Miller and colleagues [63] detected all genomic aberrations, including SNVs, CNVs, repeat expansions, methylation change, and complex structural rearrangements in 10 patients who required complete molecular diagnosis. Further, this study also captured precise resolution of the genetic variants, guiding amendments in clinical management. Aganezov and colleagues[64] evaluated multiplatform (ONT, PacBio, 10X Genomics, and Illumina sequencing) for WGS of cancer cell line (SKBR3) and normal organoids from two breast cancer clinical samples. The authors showed that LRS permits significantly more accurate and sensitive SV detection even at relatively low coverage. In addition, 90% to 95% of variants identified via different long-read technology platforms were intercomparable [64,65]. With ONT MinION and PromethION, Sakamoto and colleagues [66] conducted WGS of the LC2/ad lung cancer cell line and revealed unique structural aberrations consisting of complex local duplications, inversions, and microdeletions.

In 2018, using a PacBio sequencer, Nattestad and coworkers studied SVs in a breast cancer cell line. The study emphasized the *ERBB2*, considered the most significant gene involved in tumorigenesis and diagnosis of breast cancer. In addition, the study group recorded complex SVs associated with *the ERBB2* gene and nested duplications, with five translocations [67]. In another study on the application of SVs, Norris, and colleagues [58] used the ONT-LRS platform to sequence pancreatic cancer cell lines to uncover SVs by focusing on well-characterized *CDKN2A and SMAD4* genes. The authors could detect SVs, including translocations, inversions, and large deletions, suggesting an ideal platform for the low-level finding of cancer-associated SVs essential for molecular relapse early discovery and suitable therapeutic supervision.

In one of the studies, combining Cas9-Assisted Targeting of CHromosome segments (CATCH), a CRISPR-Cas9-based method, and ONT-LRS, the study group successfully sequenced the *breast cancer 1 gene (BRCA1)* region with 70X coverage [68,69]. Thus, these study results significantly show new directions about cancer initiation's driver events and advancement. With the available evidence, we are aware that several complex SVs (deletions, duplications, inversions, and translocations) hold critical roles in tumorigenesis and cancer progression [60]. Therefore, finding those important SVs and indels has the potential to unravel the causative factor for different cancer types and its event that can be accurately investigated using specific LRS platforms.

STRUCTURAL VARIATIONS AND GENETIC DISORDERS

Deep sequencing by NGS is a reliable and cost-effective method for detecting SNVs, indels, and other structural rearrangements [3,12] Although chromosomal microarrays and karyotyping have been used extensively to detect CNVs or other SVs, these technologies are often unable to resolve complex SVs (see Fig. 3) and incapable of providing in-depth resolution of such alterations [51]. Moreover, the SRS-based approach often fails in sensitivity, shows an excess of false positives, and misinterprets complex SVs that include larger genomic deletions, duplications, and rearrangements [12,53,54]. On the contrary, LRS generates reads spanning SV breakpoints or the whole SVs [44,50,54]. Thus, LRS platforms can offer better resolution and substantially increase the uniformity of capturing and mapping SVs. In one of the diagnostic case investigations, a female patient with intellectual disability and seizure presented with a balanced reciprocal translocation between chromosomes X and 20. Using the ONT-WGS, the investigators identified the breakpoints in Xp11.1 (*ARFGEF9* gene) and 20p13 (*RASSF2* and *SLC23A2*) [70] (Table 2). Similarly, a patient with a negative WES report for progressive myoclonic epilepsy was found to have a 12 kb homozygous deletion in *CLN6* after testing via PacBio-WGS [71].

Merker and colleagues,[72] using PacBio SMRT-WGS, managed to detect a pathogenic 2-kb heterozygous deletion of a patient's first coding exon of the *PRKAR1A* gene who had received an unremarkable report from a clinical NGS panel (see Table 2). Similarly, using a PacBio LRS in a patient with autosomal recessive Bardet–Biedl syndrome, a 72-kb homozygous deletion in chromosome 7q14.3 was revealed [73]. In another instance, ONT-based LRS confirmed the presence of pathogenic SV with ~7.1kb deletion within *glucose 6-phosphatase catalytic (G6PC)* in a patient with a recessive glycogen storage disease undetected in a traditional NGS-WES method [74] (see Table 2). Sanchis-Juan and colleagues [75] analyzed a patient with neonatal hypoxic-ischemic encephalopathy and reported duplication-inversion-duplication overlap in *cyclin-dependent kinase-like 5 (CDKL5)* using the ONT-LRS platform. Overall, the above examples suggest clinically significant SVs that may be undetected with current clinical tests can be effectively identified using LRS and a suitable bioinformatics approach.

TRANSPOSABLE ELEMENTS

Transposable elements (TEs) facilitate forming the structure and function of the human genome [76]. TE insertions are also a significant source of genomic variation leading to human genetic disease [5,77]. Few studies have shown that TEs influence human development and health (i.e. placental development and innate immunity) [78,79]. In addition, more than a hundred TE insertions have been associated with hereditary cancers and Mendelian disorders. TE affects gene regulation via different means, including insertional mutagenesis, premature polyadenylation, and alteration of RNA expression and splicing [77,80].

The application of LRS is also used to distinguish such genetic alteration. For example, Gonçalves and colleagues [81] described an intronic long-interspersed element 1 (*LINE-1*) insertion within the *duchenne muscular dystrophy (DMD)* gene in a patient with Becker muscular dystrophy by using the PacBio and

TABLE 2
Different human genetic diseases and disorders examined with long-read sequencing technology.

Clinical Phenotype	Platform	Variant Type	Gene/Loci	References
Tandem repeat expansion				
Fragile X syndrome	PacBio	CGG expansion	*FMR1*	Ardui et al. [27], 2018
Huntington's disease	PacBio	CAG expansion	*HTT*	Hoijer et al., [120], 2018
Myotonic dystrophy	PacBio	CTG expansion	*DMPK*	Cumming et al., [219], 2017
Parkinson's disease	PacBio	Repeat expansion	*ATXN10*	Schule et al., [144], 2017
Spinocerebellar ataxia type 10	PacBio	ATTCT expansion	*ATXN10*	McFarland et al. [121], 2013
Structural Variation				
Bardet-Biedl Syndrome	PacBio	7q14.3 deletion	7q14.3	Reiner et al. [73], 2018
Carney complex	PacBio	2 kb deletion	*PRKAR1A*	Merker et al. [72], 2018
Congenital abnormalities	Nanopore	Complex rearrangements	-	Cretu Stancu et al., [220], 2017
Glycogen storage disease IA	Nanopore	7.1 kb deletion	*G6PC*	Miao et al. [74], 2018
Intellectual Disability	Nanopore	Translocation	*ARFGEF9*	Dutta et al. [70], 2019
Neonatal hypoxic-ischemic encephalopathy	Nanopore	Duplication – inversion	*CDKL5*	Sanchis-Juan et al. [75], 2018
Progressive myoclonic epilepsy	PacBio	12 kb deletion	*CLN6*	Mizuguchi et al. [71], 2019
Transposable Elements				
Becker muscular dystrophy	PacBio	L1 insertion	*DMD*	Goncalves et al., [81], 2017
X –linked Parkinsonism	PacBio	SVA Insertion	*TAF1*	Aneichyk et al. [24], 2018
Resolving Allele Phasing				
Keratitis-ichthyosis-deafness	PacBio	Revertant mosaicism	*CX26*	Gudmundsson et al. [98], 2017
Treacher Collins and Noonan syndrome	PacBio	de novo mutations	*TCOF, PTPN11*	Wilbe et al. [96], 2017
Pseudogenes discrimination				
Autosomal dominant polycystic kidney disease	PacBio	Pseudogene discrimination	*PKD1*	Borras et al., [108], 2017
Drug metabolism	PacBio/ONT	Pseudogene discrimination	*CYP2D6*	Buermans et al., [109], 2017

transcriptome analysis (see Table 2). In another investigation, a combination of PacBio, Illumina, and 10X Genomics approaches was used for an unbiased *de-novo* assembly to unfold the SINE-VNTR-Alu insertion in the *TAF1*, the prime source of X-linked dystonia-parkinsonism [24]. Ewing and colleagues [82] used ONT-LRS and new computational tools to directly infer CpG methylation of novel and extant TE insertions. The samples for this study included hippocampus, heart, liver, paired tumor and nontumor liver samples from one post-mortem individual and another from a patient who underwent surgical resection. Thus, these examples illustrate that TE insertions are accountable for certain genetic diseases and not be ignored. Further, a detailed study on the broad applications of LRS in especially WES or WGS false-negative cases allows the detection of these TE insertions that could interrupt different genes depending on germline or somatic mutations.

HAPLOTYPE RESOLUTION

The process of reforming individual haplotypes is called "haplotyping" or "haplotype phasing" and has significant implications for elucidating the disease risks. A cluster of genetic variants inherited on a paternal or maternal chromosome describes a haplotype due to its genetic linkage [83]. Several studies have classified haplotype as protecting or threatening several ailments, such as breast cancer, Alzheimer's disease, and thrombosis [84–87]. In addition to simply identifying individual sequence variants, there is an increasing need to establish the haplotype or phasing of multiple variants between the two homologous pairs of a given chromosome (maternal and paternal). Distinguishing between two variants that co-occur on a single chromosome or copy of a gene, and two variants present within different copies of that chromosome or gene can be critical. For example, haplotyping is crucial in linkage analysis, association studies, population genetics, and clinical genetics and cannot be performed by conventional genotyping or sequencing approaches [88–92]. From the clinical point of view, phasing is essential to understanding the inheritance patterns, allele-specific expression, mosaicism, disease risk-haplotypes, and the parental origin of de novo mutations [93].

In the conventional SR-NGS approach, despite using paired-end reads, only a limited number of variants (~30% substitutions) can be captured [94]. Currently, the benefit of LRS platforms facilitates directly phasing the variants greater than 10 kb apart in the complicated genomic regions [95]. Especially for compound heterozygosity, identifying whether two genetic variations in the same gene are cis (same chromosome) or trans (on different homologous chromosomes) can be necessary for clinical diagnostic purposes [93]. Using the ONT and PacBio LRS platform with long-range PCR, Laver and colleagues [95] identified two SNVs within the *RET* gene that were 9 kb apart. By direct phasing, the study group excluded the need to examine the parents as it is necessary to predict phasing when traditional SRS or other genotyping methods are in use. Interestingly, using LRS in preimplantation genetic diagnosis (PGD) provides the upper hand in studying haplotype ancestry, gonadal mosaicism, and investigating the parental source of pathogenic *de-novo* mutations. For example, a study employed PacBio SMRT sequencing and ddPCR to investigate the parental origin of genetic variants in *TCOF1* and *PTPN11*. In addition, the study also estimated recurrence risk in families who have undergone assisted reproduction [96].

Zhang and colleagues [97] characterized the exact positions of inversion breakpoints using the ONT LRS approach in four patients undergoing assisted reproduction. Further, the study group validated the breakpoints using the Sangers sequencing method and a genome-wide haplotype linkage analysis based on SNP microarray. In another example, using the PacBio SMRT approach, Gudmundsson and colleagues [98] allele phased in a case of severe hearing impairment and a rare, genetic, multisystem disease (keratitis–ichthyosis–deafness). Maestri and colleagues [83] investigated a clinically significant 12 kb region of the *Apolipoprotein E (APOE)* locus, a hotspot for mutations and haplotypes associated with aging-related ailments and longevity. The study showed an efficient workflow model for haplotype and phasing based on ONT MinION sequencing data. Further, haplotype phasing made possible by LRS delivers a unique possibility to advance investigations to identify the relationship between phenotypes and unique haplotype combinations [93].

IDENTIFYING PSEUDOGENES

Pseudogenes are functionless gene copies due to acquired deleterious mutations or transcriptional silencing. These carry sequences that are highly like known functional genes but fail to make functional proteins [99–101]. At least 14,000 pseudogenes are present in the human genome [102]. Clinically significant genes, *PMS2*, *CYP2D6*, *CHEK2*, *SMN1*, *PKD1*, and others have corresponding pseudogenes with high sequence homology that can interfere in sequencing efforts due to pseudogene reads aligning to the protein-coding gene and vice versa [103]. These pseudogenes can lead to inaccurate variant calling, classification, and interpretation [104,105]. Functional genes may acquire reads from the pseudogenes in conventional SRS methods and trigger reading errors, artificially low variant allele fractions, and high false-positives rates [105]. Thus, SRS-based NGS assays are not always consistent for examining genes with high pseudogenes homology.

Several studies have used the LRS approach to explore essential clinical genes with pseudogenes homology [106–110]. Most studies have implemented long-range PCR, with specific primers to determine the rare mismatch positions that differentiate the gene of interest from its pseudogenes [110]. However, the main advantage of the LRS platform is covering the complete long-range-PCR amplicon, by preserving the phase details [109]. For instance, owing to its extreme size, and pseudogene homology, Polycystin 1 (*PKD1*) is involved in autosomal dominant polycystic kidney disease it is challenging to analyze with SR-NGS or standard Sanger sequencing [111]. However, the combination of long-range PCR and PacBio–SMRT platforms omitted the *PKD1* pseudogene amplification and other alignment uncertainty by identifying only SVs [108] (see Table 2). Stephens and colleagues [112] studied *PMS2* and *CYP21A2* characterizing in clinical samples as a part of a diagnostic assay for congenital adrenal hyperplasia. Similarly, Troskie and colleagues [113] investigated *PDCL3P4* deletion and its biological impact on other genes using PacBio sequencing. Moreover, several groups have studied the *CYP2D6* genotyping and phasing using the LRS platform, considered one of the vital genes required in drug metabolism that was quite challenging to explore via traditional approach [14,106,107,109]. Hence, including consistent pseudogene differentiation to generate accurate reference datasets and interpretations for complex genes, LRS platforms are considered more reliable and allow advances in variant classification.

TANDEM REPEAT EXPANSION DISEASES

Short tandem repeats (STRs) consist of multiple tandem copies of a short-repeated sequence (~ 1–6 bp) within genomic DNA. According to the University of California Santa Cruz (UCSC) annotation, approximately 1 million tandem-repeat sequences are present within the human genome [114]. Owing to errors in replication, the lengths of these repeats have become highly variable within the human population, making them useful in forensics and other DNA identity testing applications. In addition, over thirty different human genetic diseases are known to be caused by increased STR repeat units or expansions [115]. These disease-causing repeats are lengthier than conventional SRS reads, making them undetectable by most clinical NGS tests [54,116,117]. Several research groups have investigated whether LRS technologies can sequence these clinically significant long repeat expansions [118–121]. For example, myotonic dystrophy is caused by CTG repeat expansion in the 3′ untranslated regions of the *myotonic dystrophy protein kinase (DMPK)* gene with pathogenic repeat expansions varying between several hundred to thousands of copies (see Table 2).

The size and repetitive nature of these expanded *DMPK* alleles cause them to evade detection by traditional NGS. Few studies have shown that the ONT platform could be appropriate for investigating these kinds of large repeat expansions over 4 Mb [122]. Likewise, using PacBio sequencing, Cumming and colleagues [119] studied the repeat expansion in the *DMPK* gene. The above examples suggest that using different LRS platforms can identify undiscovered repeat diseases within the range of repeat expansion. In addition, in the subsequent section, we have discussed neurologic-related tandem repeat expansion diseases such as fragile X syndrome (FXS), spinocerebellar ataxia (SCA), and Huntington's disease.

APPLICATIONS OF LONG-READ TECHNOLOGY IN NEUROGENOMICS

Neurodevelopmental and neurodegenerative diseases are a class of neurologic issues differentiated by various groups of conditions that lead cognitive decline, motor disturbance, physical and intellectual disabilities [123,124]. However, several of these neurologic diseases are consequences due to significant genetic variations with several genes known to associate with the disorder, which is *de-novo* in nature [125]. Considering the cause, WES or WGS sequencing has proven to be the most robust approach for both clinical and research on the genetic causes of neurodevelopmental or neurodegenerative issues. Even after WES or WGS, several reasons state that most the neurodevelopmental and neurodegenerative diseases cannot be traced to an underlying genetic variant [126]. Owing to read error, false positives, or false negatives, it is likely that detection of several such variants is simply invisible to short-read analysis. The possible methodology to overcome variant detection limitations is to adopt robust sequencing platforms that provide longer reads, allowing for more comprehensive and accurate read alignment to the reference assembly [127,128].

FRAGILE X SYNDROME

The human fragile X messenger ribonucleoprotein 1 (*FMR1*) gene consists of CGG trinucleotide repeats in the 5′-untranslated region of the gene which is located on the X chromosome [129–132]. Expansion of this trinucleotide repeat region results in hypermethylation and transcriptional silencing. Thus the hypermethylation of *FMR1* result in the loss of *fragile X messenger ribonucleoprotein (FMRP)* expression (the protein encoded by *FMR1*) causing FXS which is considered the most common cause of heritable intellectual disability [132–136]. The mutation range of 55 to 200 CGG repeats is known as pre-mutation, whereas 200 repeats or greater are classified as full mutations, leading to FXS. The *FMR1* pre-mutation range of CGG trinucleotide repeats is susceptible to expanding into a full mutation in the next generation on maternal transmission (see Table 2). However, the inserted occurrence of AGG interruptions in each 9 or 10 CGG repeats can reduce the instability [137]. Hence, to tackle the challenging detection and position of AGG interruptions in female pre-mutation carriers, PacBio SMRT sequencing delivered a straight demonstration of AGG interruptions within the CGG repeat expansions by separating a large number of reads containing AGG repeats [27]. Moreover, the beneficial information offered by this technique estimates the CGG repeats expansion risk in female pre-mutation carriers, and can further aid them to consider prenatal genetic testing or PGD, to investigate the fragile X status of the fetus [138,139].

SPINOCEREBELLAR ATAXIAS

SCA indicates a group of hereditary conditions characterized by heterogeneous neurodegenerative changes in the part of the brain and sometimes in the spinal cord, with a core symptom of progressive cerebellar ataxia and oculomotor abnormalities [124]. CAG repeat expansions lead to SCA in coding regions, instigating a long abnormal chain of polyglutamine or PolyQ disorders [140]. So far, approximately 50 genetically distinct SCAs (i.e. SCA1–SCA48) have been cataloged, emphasizing the importance of genetic testing with high sensitivity and specificity to confirm the clinical diagnosis and the family history [141]. In addition, the other aspect is the presence of clinical anticipation due to the tendency for repeat expansions to change the size mainly by expanding further when it is transmitted to the subsequent generation [141]. Thus, the generations carrying larger repeats would show more severe clinical symptoms. For instance, SCA10, a subtype of the SCA family, is described by significant cerebellar symptoms, seizures, and generalized motor seizures [142]. The pentanucleotide ATTCT is a large noncoding repeat expansion and is a significant cause for SCA10 in intron 9 of *Ataxin10 (ATXN10)* gene on chromosome 22 [142] (see Table 2). Generally, the standard length of ATTCT is 10 to 32 repeats, and intermediate alleles with 280 to 850 repeats show reduced penetrance, whereas the pathogenic alleles ranging from 850 to 4500 repeats trigger complete penetrance [143].

Further, it is well proven that interruptions in the expanded ATTCT repeat strongly correlate with an increased prevalence of epileptic attacks [142]. Despite the prominent lengths of the SCA10 expansion, PacBio SMRT sequencing successfully sequenced the whole span of the expansion, varying from 2.5 to 4.4 kb in size, from three SCA10 patients with different clinical manifestations [121]. Moreover, the genetic architecture of the SCA10 repeat expansion may serve as a phenotypic modifier in combination with the LRS technology, uncovering novel and various assemblies of interruption motifs and establishing a genotype-phenotype relationship between Parkinson's disease and *ATXN10* [121,144]. Further, these similar discoveries using suitable LRS platforms may shed light on investigating several other patterns of SCA.

HUNTINGTON'S DISEASE

Huntington's disease is an adult-onset rare, inherited neurodegenerative disorder with an autosomal dominant inheritance that is clinically characterized by progressive neuronal degeneration in the brain, including cognitive dysfunction, and personality disorders [145]. The prime contributing factor to Huntington's disease is the CAG repeat expansions in the *HTT* (huntingtin gene) on chromosome 4 [146] (see Table 2). In the general population, CAG repeat is up to 26. In contrast, the intermediate alleles contain 27 to 35 repeats and are likely to cause disease in the subsequent generation [147]. In addition, individuals with 36 to 39 CAG repeats are presented with reduced penetrance, whereas full penetrance patients represent 40 or more CAG repeats [147].

Fragment analysis of the PCR products is performed in the clinical setting to determine repeat sizes based on the distinct PCR product sizes correlating to the disease phenotypes [120]. However, owing to the concern of PCR false-negative and excessive GC content, there is a demand for more advanced and robust approaches. With the CRISPR/Cas9 system and SMRT sequencing applications, CAG repeats in clinically relevant Huntington's disease samples can be analyzed [120]. Moreover, several studies have valued the multiplexing efficacy of additional target genes including *FMR1*, *ATXN10*, and others causing FXS and SCA10, [120]. In summary, LRS generates an accurate estimation of the repeat count to confidently examine repeat alterations and provide more comprehensive information on the exact location of interruption motifs.

LONG-READ TECHNOLOGY IN INFECTIOUS DISEASE AND RESEARCH

Most clinical labs depend on microbial culture for pathogen identification. Moreover, the causative diagnosis of infectious diseases is extremely challenging due to the high heterogeneity of pathogens that can cause contagious infections [22]. However, fast, and precise detection of deadly pathogenic microorganisms is a fundamental to diagnosing clinical infectious diseases [148]. High throughput platforms, like Illumina NGS-based assay, have recently been introduced in clinical setup to trace contagious diseases and their complexity. Moreover, a significant limiting factor of sequencing clinical samples for a viral genome is the low viral copies within specimens. In addition, ample sequencing coverage and precise agreement are also crucial and challenging factors [23]. However, WGS has not been introduced for routine clinical testing due to the high-cost estimation. Few studies have shown the utility of PacBio sequencers for WGS of different pathogenic human viruses and their efficiency in identifying other viral species [149,150]. For instance, despite a long turnaround time, PacBio managed to sequence complete Norovirus GII, the most common cause of gastroenteritis infection, with 99.11% high coverage [150].

Moreover, to study the evolution of the severe acute respiratory syndrome coronavirus 2 (*SARS-CoV-2*) and its progression, the PacBio sequencing platform was introduced [151]. Likewise, nanopore sequencing has been widely used to identify viral pathogens in disease diagnostics and its assessment. In a conventional NGS approach, one of the drawbacks is the incapability to characterize on-site field testing and analysis. However, the ONT-based nanopore sequencing technology addresses this issue by identifying pathogenic viruses on-site and is also appropriate for analyzing a broad range of clinical samples [152,153]. Further, studies have reported the high uniformity in nanopore sequencing results versus microbial culture results, including culture-negative samples [154–156].

Most importantly, the ONT platforms can deliver the run results for patients with severe illnesses within a fast turnaround time [154,157] (Fig. 4). Also, ONT sequencing platforms have played a critical role in exposing viral pathogens during major disease epidemics. For example, from 2014 to 2016, the Ebola epidemic in West Africa [153,158,159], the Zika virus epidemic, the Yellow fever virus, and the Lassa fever outbreak in Nigeria [160–162]. Similarly, WGS of clinical samples, which includes human metapneumovirus influenza, chikungunya, dengue, and hepatitis C virus, have also been investigated [162–165]. In less than 24 h of sample collection, Meredith and colleagues [166] successfully generated 747 *SARS-CoV-2* genomes from coronavirus disease-2019 (COVID-19)-positive samples using the Nanopore sequencing. In 2020, with the COVID-19 outburst, Wang and colleagues [157] established *SARS-COV-2* genome sequencing using Nanopore targeted sequencing, which helped identify infected patients. In another example, to facilitate further action and control over COVID-19 infection, epidemiologic data on increase in the *SARS-CoV-2* variant was generated using the ONT sequencing platform [166,167].

In addition, excluding cDNA conversion, direct ribonucleic acid (RNA) sequencing can also be performed using an ONT platform. In 2015, a rough influenza genome was created using the ONT platform, sequencing the RNA virus for the first time [168]. However, nanopore technology is more suitable than the conventional NGS approach for direct RNA sequencing by eliminating reverse transcription and PCR amplification steps, facilitating epigenetic RNA alteration investigations and the source of pathogen resistance [16,169]. Thus, LRS technology can handle deadly infectious disease outbreaks and offer precise and suitable support for outbreak management, prevention, and control of infectious disease and its evolutional research.

LONG-READ SEQUENCING IN METAGENOMICS APPLICATION

With the help of LRS, the identification and classification of the bacterial and viral species within a clinical setting are more evolved than that for fungal infections [23]. By adapting the no target amplification sequencing method, the smaller size of bacterial and viral genomes enables to explore the whole-genome sequencing. The study by Earl and colleagues [170] using a PacBio sequencer showed the capability to detect 20 different bacteria identified to the species level in a given sample. Using the ONT metagenomics platform, Bialasiewicz and colleagues [171] reported the fast and precise diagnosis of illness due to *Capnocytophaga canimorsus* infection in a 62-year-old woman in less than 19 h. Similarly, several other studies have also revealed rapid processing times of 6 to 8 h from starting the sample preparation to pathogen identification [155,172–174]. Interestingly, Gu and colleagues identified pathogenic bacterial species accurately from various clinical samples including cultured bacteria, PCR-positive and PCR-negative samples. Employing ONT metagenomics and Illumina platforms for the study comparision, the turnaround time was 6 h for nanopore sequencing versus 24 h for Illumina sequencing [175–177].

The combination of LRS and SRS approaches, assembled whole genomes of major fungal pathogens, also known as "hybrid assemblies" [178–185] In another

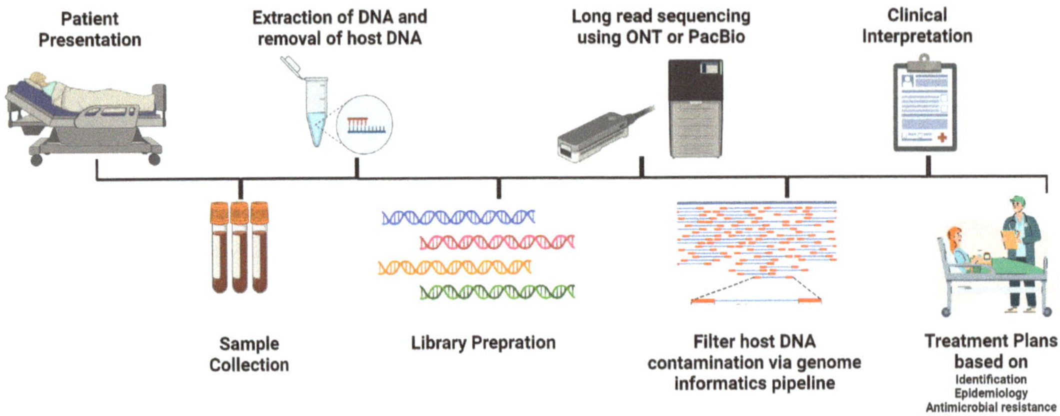

FIG. 4 Possible workflow for long-read sequencing-based approach for clinical diagnosis in metagenomics application. (*Created with* Biorender.com)

example, PacBio LRS distinguished the fungal constitution of fecal samples from 14 healthy individuals characterizing various fungal species [186]. In one of the studies, using ONT's MinION platform, three patient samples, positive for *Pneumocystis jirovecii* fungal disease and three samples with no infection, underwent metagenomic sequencing. The sequencing reads were defined and evaluated using two different analysis tools, designed by ONT and the general nucleotide BLAST approach. All three positive patient samples produced *P jirovecii* reads, while surprisingly, *P jirovecii* reads were also detected in culture-negative samples when ONT-specific tools were used [187]. This observation flagged that using ONT had several technical constraints, not limited to the minimal host to pathogen ratio, deficiency of broad reference sequence databases, and inadequacy of specific bioinformatics tools [187].

A study by Gu and colleagues [177] assessed the diagnostic sensitivity and specificity of Illumina and ONT sequencing on body fluid samples from 87 patients. For the fungal pathogen detection, ONT showed a sensitivity of 90.9% and specificity of 100%, matched to 90.6% and 89.0% for the Illumina platform. Although the above studies could detect pathogens through LRS, the study also emphasized concerns presently related to practical applications in routine diagnostics. The complications include i) the importance of the quality of the input DNA, ii) the ratio of a pathogen to host DNA, and iii) the availability of comprehensive reference databases for analysis [177] which have been discussed in the following section.

CHALLENGES AND ISSUES IN LONG-READ TECHNOLOGY

The rapid improvement in LRS technologies will be beneficial and become the next base of high throughput sequencing. Thus, these advancement permit access to the most complicated regions of the genome, bringing value to clinical applications in diagnosis, prediction, and personalized medicine. However, on the contrary, compared with SRS, the comprehensive usage of LRS platforms in clinical settings have several limitations, such as higher error rate, lower throughput, and higher cost per base [41]. Moreover, sequencing accuracy varies from 87% to 99% in PacBio, whereas 87% to 98% in ONT platforms which could be problematic and cause difficulties in accurately detecting point mutations. Moreover, achieving significant high-molecular-weight DNA and full-length RNA in clinical samples is always challenging [188]. Also, for histopathological staining and long-term storage purpose, most clinical specimens and biopsies generally undergo a formalin-fixed paraffin-embedded (FFPE) procedure [188]. The DNA or RNAs extracted from FFPE samples experience severe damage and fragmentation that could impact sequencing reads. Further, good library preparation for high yield and sequencing workflow for samples with low volume are still an issue for LRS [188]. Although LRS is extremely promising for identifying variants in inherited diseases, it is not ideal for sequencing when looking for somatic variants in small and compromised biopsies.

On the other hand, LRS has effectively identified different bacteria and fungi species and sub-species

TABLE 3
Basic genome informatics tools specific to ONT and PacBio used for long-read sequencing analysis

Application	ONT	PacBio
Base-calling	Albacore, Guppy	Unanimity
Quality control	NanoQC, NanoStat, Nanofilt, NanoLyse	Isoseq3, DALIGNER
Read error correction (Non-hybrid method)	Canu, FLAS. LoRMA, wtdbg2	ToFU, LoRMA
Read error correction (Hybrid method)	Nanocorr, FMLRC	LORDEC, LSC, proovread, Jabba
Read polishing	Nanopolish, Racon, ntEdit	Arrow, Pilon, Racon
Read alignment	Pbmm2	Pbmm2, BLAS, minimap2

with the metagenomics and metabarcoding approaches [23]. Moreover, pathogens typically exist at low loads at the point of infection. Therefore, both the sample's quality and are critical for the sequencing success [23]. Hence, samples with high DNA concentrations are ideal for confirming sufficient sequencing coverage of the pathogen and its proper identification. Moreover, specifically for ONT and PacBio, several DNA isolation protocols are already described but not used in clinical settings [189–191]. Meanwhile, improving extraction procedures is essential to progress the application of LRS to precise clinical diagnosis platforms [23]. Another critical issue in metagenomics is the high host DNA in the sample that interfere with the pathogen DNA detection. Balancing the ratio of pathogen DNA versus human DNA in the clinical samples could resolve the above issue [155,192–194]. However, alternatively using the nanopore adaptive sequencing method, by substituting the voltage across the membrane, specific DNA fragments are designated by recognizing unwanted sequences, thereby blocking the sequencing [195,196]. Thus, more work is needed to improve and balance the host and pathogen DNA ratio that would significantly provide the essential information and benefit the clinical diagnosis and its further implementation.

DATA ANALYTICS

In the area of genome informatics, LRS technologies have unlocked exciting paths. Recent improvements in bioinformatics pipelines could greatly benefit LRS. However, there is still a need for adavancement and scalability in analytical tools used in LRS data analysis [48]. In addition, to capture various genome alterations, there are currently numerous informatics tools for base calling, genome assembly, error correction, base polishing, mapping, and phasing for the data which comes from LRS [197–205] (Table 3). One of the biggest challenges in long-read technology is scalability and benchmarking [48].

Similarly, Peregrine, Flye, TULIP, Ra, wtdbg2, and Shasta are de novo long-read assemblers and rapidly implemented in handling large amounts of long-read genome data [201,206–210]. In addition, minimap2, a versatile sequence alignment program for long mapping reads, has gained popularity for its speed and accuracy [211]. The ONT-developed Nanopolish, a software platform, is well known for assembly correction and base alteration detection, but it is time-consuming while handling more extensive data [212]. Hence, rapid processing is crucial for routine clinical applications to enable faster and more accurate clinical diagnoses. Regardless of the growing accuracy of both ONT and PacBio platforms, substantial improvement in fixing the error rate should be a top priority in the LRS pipelines. Also, advancements in SRS compel low input sample volume to combine both SRS and LRS.

Moreover, combining hybrid methods and using other technologies such as optical genome mapping by Bionano Genomics and Hi-C deep sequencing from Illumina will be beneficial [21]. However, one should also consider genomic project cost and its analytical complexity. Thus, LRS technologies surpass initial drawbacks in terms of accuracy and high throughput by slowly broadening their applications in clinical genetics.

SUMMARY AND FUTURE PROSPECTS

LRS is increasingly used across multiple genomic scale sequencing domains due to its rapid advancement. Compared with SRS, the wide application of LRS is yet to be realized, and issues such as low throughput, error rate corrections, and higher cost per base also matter [21]. However, on a positive note, SVs, nucleotide repeat expansion, TEs, pseudogenes, and complex genomic regions that are impossible to track using a conventional approach can currently be captured with LRS [41]. The present two major LRS platforms, ONT and PacBio, have produced the most exemplary results. The best example is the first telomere to telomere assembly of the human genome using PacBio CLR and ONT ultra-long read to navigate the centromeric region [17]. One of the most portable sequencing platforms, ONT makes the sequencing reads long and continues. On the other hand, PacBio generates highly accurate LRS data [29]. Both PacBio and ONT technologies will significantly impact clinical genetics in the long run. However, ONT's main challenge is decreasing the error rate and increasing the accuracy. On the contrary, PacBio has to reduce its high cost per base. Once these limitations are addressed, these platforms could perform routine clinical runs. Also, to examine all genetic modifications present in an individual genome, there is an excellent potential that long-read WGS could aid as a standard test. In addition, LRS technology has always had the upper hand regarding tandem repeat expansion diseases and complex chromosomal rearrangements. Combining SRS and LRS approaches (hybrid sequencing) can also be efficient for highly accurate variant calling and assembly [31]. Although excitement in the medical genetics community and clinical labs for LRS has been significantly growing, a few technical aspects have to be overcome timely for LRS platforms for recognition as a mainstream tool in clinical laboratories [41]. The current sequencing and technological advancement could capture all genetic variation in an individual sooner. Further, this could open the door to producing a few hundred to thousands of new human reference genomes specific to different ethnicities. Thus, such technological advancement will considerably expand our interpretation of genetic inheritance, population diversity, and the origin of genetic diseases.

Moreover, in parallel, other commercial technologies or platforms are under active development and hopefully might soon be accessible. These novel technologies include nanopore-based sequencing from Roche [213,214] (formerly Genia and Stratos genomics) and Roswell Biotechnologies electronic nanodevice sequencing [215]. In addition, other similar technologies, for example, Strand-Seq, a single-cell sequencing method that determines individual homologs within a cell [216,217]. Hyb & Seq, a library-free, amplification-free single-molecule sequencing technique from Nanostring, and high-resolution genome mapping from Bionano Genomics might align with the LRS technology vision [14,218].

Thus, we are at the next level of the sequencing technological revolution. As soon as we overcome the accuracy, analysis pipelines, error correction, and cost challenges, that moment would be accurate to shift into individual complete phased LRS and its de novo genome assembly. Further, this enables tracking of all genetic variants irrespective of their form and status. Finally, using such technologies from the clinical laboratory standpoint will aid us in advancing our information on cancer genomics, the genetic basis of complex disorders, infectious diseases and their evolution, which carry significant associations for clinical diagnosis.

CLINICS CARE POINTS

- Long-read seqeuncing (LRS) is an emerging technology that has multiple possible uses in the clinical setting.
- LRS will only become a routine technology in clincal molecular laboratories with additional studies to confirm its clinical utility.
- Individual clinical laboratories can only introduce LRS as a clinical test with rigorous validations of specific tests in accordance with local regulations and laws concerning clinical laboratory testing.

ACKNOWLEDGMENTS

The authors would like to thank Dr. Wahab Khan, director of clinical cytogenetics and assistant director of molecular genetics, Dartmouth Hitchcock Medical Center, and Shrey S. Sukhadia, assistant director of bioinformatics, Dartmouth Hitchcock Medical Center, for their suggestions and edits.

REFERENCES

[1] Shendure J, Balasubramanian S, Church GM, et al. DNA sequencing at 40: Past, present and future. Nature 2017; 550(7676). https://doi.org/10.1038/nature24286.

[2] Gilissen C, Hoischen A, Brunner HG, et al. Unlocking Mendelian disease using exome sequencing. Genome Biol 2011;12(9). https://doi.org/10.1186/gb-2011-12-9-228.

[3] Goodwin S, McPherson JD, McCombie WR. Coming of age: Ten years of next-generation sequencing

technologies. Nat Rev Genet 2016;17(6). https://doi.org/10.1038/nrg.2016.49.
[4] Sudmant PH, Rausch T, Gardner EJ, et al. An integrated map of structural variation in 2,504 human genomes. Nature 2015;526(7571). https://doi.org/10.1038/nature15394.
[5] Sudmant PH, Mallick S, Nelson BJ, et al. Global diversity, population stratification, and selection of human copy-number variation. Science (1979) 2015;(6253):349. https://doi.org/10.1126/science.aab3761.
[6] Ng SB, Bigham AW, Buckingham KJ, et al. Exome sequencing identifies MLL2 mutations as a cause of Kabuki syndrome. Nat Genet 2010;42(9). https://doi.org/10.1038/ng.646.
[7] Kircher M, Witten DM, Jain P, et al. A general framework for estimating the relative pathogenicity of human genetic variants. Nat Genet 2014;46(3). https://doi.org/10.1038/ng.2892.
[8] Simonson TS, Yang Y, Huff CD, et al. Genetic evidence for high-altitude adaptation in Tibet. Science (1979) 2010;(5987):329. https://doi.org/10.1126/science.1189406.
[9] Sudmant PH, Kitzman JO, Antonacci F, et al. Diversity of human copy number variation and multicopy genes. Science (1979). 2010;330(6004). doi:10.1126/science.1197005
[10] de Koning APJ, Gu W, Castoe TA, et al. Repetitive elements may comprise over Two-Thirds of the human genome. PLoS Genet 2011;7(12). https://doi.org/10.1371/journal.pgen.1002384.
[11] Treangen TJ, Salzberg SL. Repetitive DNA and next-generation sequencing: Computational challenges and solutions. Nat Rev Genet 2012;13(1). https://doi.org/10.1038/nrg3117.
[12] Ashley EA. Towards precision medicine. Nat Rev Genet 2016;17(9). https://doi.org/10.1038/nrg.2016.86.
[13] Chaisson MJP, Wilson RK, Eichler EE. Genetic variation and the de novo assembly of human genomes. Nat Rev Genet 2015;16(11). https://doi.org/10.1038/nrg3933.
[14] Seo JS, Rhie A, Kim J, et al. De novo assembly and phasing of a Korean human genome. Nature 2016;538(7624). https://doi.org/10.1038/nature20098.
[15] Shi L, Guo Y, Dong C, et al. Long-read sequencing and de novo assembly of a Chinese genome. Nat Commun 2016;7. https://doi.org/10.1038/ncomms12065.
[16] Smith AM, Jain M, Mulroney L, et al. Reading canonical and modified nucleobases in 16S ribosomal RNA using nanopore native RNA sequencing. PLoS One 2019;14(5). https://doi.org/10.1371/journal.pone.0216709.
[17] Nurk S, Koren S, Rhie A, et al. The complete sequence of a human genome. Science (1979) 2022;2376(6588).
[18] van Dijk EL, Jaszczyszyn Y, Naquin D, et al. The Third Revolution in Sequencing Technology. Trends Genet 2018;34(9). https://doi.org/10.1016/j.tig.2018.05.008.
[19] Schadt EE, Turner S, Kasarskis A. A window into third-generation sequencing. Hum Mol Genet 2010;19(R2). https://doi.org/10.1093/hmg/ddq416.
[20] Chaisson MJP, Huddleston J, Dennis MY, et al. Resolving the complexity of the human genome using single-molecule sequencing. Nature 2015;517(7536). https://doi.org/10.1038/nature13907.
[21] Pollard MO, Gurdasani D, Mentzer AJ, et al. Long reads: Their purpose and place. Hum Mol Genet 2018;27(R2). https://doi.org/10.1093/hmg/ddy177.
[22] Zhu X, Yan S, Yuan F, et al. The Applications of Nanopore Sequencing Technology in Pathogenic Microorganism Detection. Can J Infect Dis Med Microbiol 2020;2020:1–8.
[23] Hoang MTV, Irinyi L, Hu Y, et al. Long-Reads-Based Metagenomics in Clinical Diagnosis With a Special Focus on Fungal Infections. Front Microbiol 2022;12. https://doi.org/10.3389/fmicb.2021.708550.
[24] Aneichyk T, Hendriks WT, Yadav R, et al. Dissecting the Causal Mechanism of X-Linked Dystonia-Parkinsonism by Integrating Genome and Transcriptome Assembly. Cell 2018;172(5). https://doi.org/10.1016/j.cell.2018.02.011.
[25] Ishiura H, Doi K, Mitsui J, et al. Expansions of intronic TTTCA and TTTTA repeats in benign adult familial myoclonic epilepsy. Nat Genet 2018;50(4). https://doi.org/10.1038/s41588-018-0067-2.
[26] Zeng S, Zhang MY, Wang XJ, et al. Long-read sequencing identified intronic repeat expansions in SAMD12 from Chinese pedigrees affected with familial cortical myoclonic tremor with epilepsy. J Med Genet 2019;56(4). https://doi.org/10.1136/jmedgenet-2018-105484.
[27] Ardui S, Ameur A, Vermeesch JR, et al. Single molecule real-time (SMRT) sequencing comes of age: Applications and utilities for medical diagnostics. Nucleic Acids Res 2018;46(5). https://doi.org/10.1093/nar/gky066.
[28] Tedersoo L, Albertsen M, Anslan S, et al. Perspectives and Benefits of High-Throughput Long-Read Sequencing in Microbial Ecology. Appl Environ Microbiol 2021;87(17). https://doi.org/10.1128/AEM.00626-21.
[29] Logsdon GA, Vollger MR, Eichler EE. Long-read human genome sequencing and its applications. Nat Rev Genet 2020;21(10). https://doi.org/10.1038/s41576-020-0236-x.
[30] Eid J, Fehr A, Gray J, et al. Real-time DNA sequencing from single polymerase molecules. Science (1979) 2009;323(5910). https://doi.org/10.1126/science.1162986.
[31] Chaisson MJP, Sanders AD, Zhao X, et al. Multi-platform discovery of haplotype-resolved structural variation in human genomes. Nat Commun 2019;10(1). https://doi.org/10.1038/s41467-018-08148-z.
[32] Vollger MR, Logsdon GA, Audano PA, et al. Improved assembly and variant detection of a haploid human genome using single-molecule, high-fidelity long reads. Ann Hum Genet 2020;84(2). https://doi.org/10.1111/ahg.12364.
[33] Wenger AM, Peluso P, Rowell WJ, et al. Accurate circular consensus long-read sequencing improves variant detection and assembly of a human genome. Nat

Biotechnol 2019;37(10). https://doi.org/10.1038/s41587-019-0217-9.
[34] Vollger MR, Dishuck PC, Sorensen M, et al. Long-read sequence and assembly of segmental duplications. Nat Methods 2019;16(1). https://doi.org/10.1038/s41592-018-0236-3.
[35] Eisenstein M. Oxford Nanopore announcement sets sequencing sector abuzz. Nat Biotechnol 2012;30(4). https://doi.org/10.1038/nbt0412-295.
[36] Deamer D, Akeson M, Branton D. Three decades of nanopore sequencing. Nat Biotechnol 2016;34(5). https://doi.org/10.1038/nbt.3423.
[37] Jain M, Koren S, Miga KH, et al. Nanopore sequencing and assembly of a human genome with ultra-long reads. Nat Biotechnol 2018;36(4). https://doi.org/10.1038/nbt.4060.
[38] Payne A, Holmes N, Rakyan V, et al. Bulkvis: A graphical viewer for Oxford nanopore bulk FAST5 files. Bioinformatics 2019;35(13). https://doi.org/10.1093/bioinformatics/bty841.
[39] Shafin K, Pesout T, Lorig-Roach R, et al. Nanopore sequencing and the Shasta toolkit enable efficient de novo assembly of eleven human genomes. Nat Biotechnol 2020;38(9). https://doi.org/10.1038/s41587-020-0503-6.
[40] Miga KH, Koren S, Rhie A, et al. Telomere-to-telomere assembly of a complete human X chromosome. Nature 2020;585(7823). https://doi.org/10.1038/s41586-020-2547-7.
[41] Mantere T, Kersten S, Hoischen A. Long-read sequencing emerging in medical genetics. Front Genet 2019;10(MAY). https://doi.org/10.3389/fgene.2019.00426.
[42] Kronenberg ZN, Fiddes IT, Gordon D, et al. High-resolution comparative analysis of great ape genomes. Science (1979) 2018;(6393):360. https://doi.org/10.1126/science.aar6343.
[43] Audano PA, Sulovari A, Graves-Lindsay TA, et al. Characterizing the Major Structural Variant Alleles of the Human Genome. Cell 2019;176(3). https://doi.org/10.1016/j.cell.2018.12.019.
[44] Huddleston J, Chaisson MJP, Steinberg KM, et al. Discovery and genotyping of structural variation from long-read haploid genome sequence data. Genome Res 2017; 27(5). https://doi.org/10.1101/gr.214007.116.
[45] Okubo M, Doi H, Fukai R, et al. GGC Repeat Expansion of NOTCH2NLC in Adult Patients with Leukoencephalopathy. Ann Neurol 2019;86(6). https://doi.org/10.1002/ana.25586.
[46] Sone J, Mitsuhashi S, Fujita A, et al. Long-read sequencing identifies GGC repeat expansions in NOTCH2NLC associated with neuronal intranuclear inclusion disease. Nat Genet 2019;51(8). https://doi.org/10.1038/s41588-019-0459-y.
[47] Hsieh PH, Vollger MR, Dang V, et al. Adaptive archaic introgression of copy number variants and the discovery of previously unknown human genes. Science (1979) 2019;(6463):366. https://doi.org/10.1126/science.aax2083.
[48] Amarasinghe SL, Su S, Dong X, et al. Opportunities and challenges in long-read sequencing data analysis. Genome Biol 2020;21(1). https://doi.org/10.1186/s13059-020-1935-5.
[49] Pendleton M, Sebra R, Pang AWC, et al. Assembly and diploid architecture of an individual human genome via single-molecule technologies. Nat Methods 2015; 12(8). https://doi.org/10.1038/nmeth.3454.
[50] de Coster W, de Rijk P, de Roeck A, et al. Structural variants identified by Oxford Nanopore PromethION sequencing of the human genome. Genome Res 2019; 29(7). https://doi.org/10.1101/gr.244939.118.
[51] Alkan C, Coe BP, Eichler EE. Genome structural variation discovery and genotyping. Nat Rev Genet 2011; 12(5):363–76.
[52] Kloosterman WP, Hochstenbach R. Deciphering the pathogenic consequences of chromosomal aberrations in human genetic disease. Mol Cytogenet 2014;7(1). https://doi.org/10.1186/s13039-014-0100-9.
[53] Tattini L, D'Aurizio R, Magi A. Detection of genomic structural variants from next-generation sequencing data. Front Bioeng Biotechnol 2015;3(JUN). https://doi.org/10.3389/fbioe.2015.00092.
[54] Sedlazeck FJ, Lee H, Darby CA, et al. Piercing the dark matter: Bioinformatics of long-range sequencing and mapping. Nat Rev Genet 2018;19(6). https://doi.org/10.1038/s41576-018-0003-4.
[55] Leija-Salazar M, Sedlazeck FJ, Toffoli M, et al. Evaluation of the detection of GBA missense mutations and other variants using the Oxford Nanopore MinION. Mol Genet Genomic Med 2019;7(3). https://doi.org/10.1002/mgg3.564.
[56] Euskirchen P, Bielle F, Labreche K, et al. Same-day genomic and epigenomic diagnosis of brain tumors using real-time nanopore sequencing. Acta Neuropathol 2017;134(5). https://doi.org/10.1007/s00401-017-1743-5.
[57] Suzuki A, Suzuki M, Mizushima-Sugano J, et al. Sequencing and phasing cancer mutations in lung cancers using a long-read portable sequencer. DNA Res 2017;24(6). https://doi.org/10.1093/dnares/dsx027.
[58] Norris AL, Workman RE, Fan Y, et al. Nanopore sequencing detects structural variants in cancer. Cancer Biol Ther 2016;17(3). https://doi.org/10.1080/15384047.2016.1139236.
[59] Minervini CF, Cumbo C, Orsini P, et al. TP53 gene mutation analysis in chronic lymphocytic leukemia by nanopore MinION sequencing. Diagn Pathol 2016; 11(1). https://doi.org/10.1186/s13000-016-0550-y.
[60] Sakamoto Y, Zaha S, Suzuki Y, et al. Application of long-read sequencing to the detection of structural variants in human cancer genomes. Comput Struct Biotechnol J 2021;19. https://doi.org/10.1016/j.csbj.2021.07.030.
[61] Fujimoto A, Wong JH, Yoshii Y, et al. Whole-genome sequencing with long reads reveals complex structure and origin of structural variation in human genetic variations

and somatic mutations in cancer. Genome Med 2021; 13(1). https://doi.org/10.1186/s13073-021-00883-1.

[62] Valle-Inclan JE, Stangl C, de Jong AC, et al. Optimizing Nanopore sequencing-based detection of structural variants enables individualized circulating tumor DNA-based disease monitoring in cancer patients. Genome Med 2021;13(1). https://doi.org/10.1186/s13073-021-00899-7.

[63] Miller DE, Sulovari A, Wang T, et al. Targeted long-read sequencing identifies missing disease-causing variation. Am J Hum Genet 2021;108(8). https://doi.org/10.1016/j.ajhg.2021.06.006.

[64] Aganezov S, Goodwin S, Sherman RM, et al. Comprehensive analysis of structural variants in breast cancer genomes using single-molecule sequencing. Genome Res 2020;30(9). https://doi.org/10.1101/GR.260497.119.

[65] Aganezov S, Raphael BJ. Reconstruction of clone- And haplotype-specific cancer genome karyotypes from bulk tumor samples. Genome Res 2020;30(9). https://doi.org/10.1101/GR.256701.119.

[66] Sakamoto Y, Xu L, Seki M, et al. Long read sequencing reveals a novel class of structural aberrations in cancers: Identification and characterization of cancerous local amplifications. bioRxiv 2019. https://doi.org/10.1101/620047.

[67] Nattestad M, Goodwin S, Ng K, et al. Complex rearrangements and oncogene amplifications revealed by long-read DNA and RNA sequencing of a breast cancer cell line. Genome Res 2018;28(8). https://doi.org/10.1101/gr.231100.117.

[68] Jiang W, Zhao X, Gabrieli T, et al. Cas9-Assisted Targeting of CHromosome segments CATCH enables one-step targeted cloning of large gene clusters. Nat Commun 2015; 6. https://doi.org/10.1038/ncomms9101.

[69] Gabrieli T, Sharim H, Fridman D, et al. Selective nanopore sequencing of human BRCA1 by Cas9-assisted targeting of chromosome segments (CATCH). Nucleic Acids Res 2018; 46(14). https://doi.org/10.1093/nar/gky411.

[70] Dutta UR, Rao SN, Pidugu VK, et al. Breakpoint mapping of a novel de novo translocation t(X;20)(q11.1; p13) by positional cloning and long read sequencing. Genomics 2019;111(5). https://doi.org/10.1016/j.ygeno.2018.07.005.

[71] Mizuguchi T, Suzuki T, Abe C, et al. A 12-kb structural variation in progressive myoclonic epilepsy was newly identified by long-read whole-genome sequencing. J Hum Genet 2019;64(5). https://doi.org/10.1038/s10038-019-0569-5.

[72] Merker JD, Wenger AM, Sneddon T, et al. Long-read genome sequencing identifies causal structural variation in a Mendelian disease. Genet Med 2018;20(1). https://doi.org/10.1038/gim.2017.86.

[73] Reiner J, Pisani L, Qiao W, et al. Cytogenomic identification and long-read single molecule real-time (SMRT) sequencing of a Bardet-Biedl Syndrome 9 (BBS9) deletion. npj Genomic Med 2018;3(1). https://doi.org/10.1038/s41525-017-0042-3.

[74] Miao H, Zhou J, Yang Q, et al. Long-read sequencing identified a causal structural variant in an exome-negative case and enabled preimplantation genetic diagnosis. Hereditas 2018;155. https://doi.org/10.1186/s41065-018-0069-1.

[75] Sanchis-Juan A, Stephens J, French CE, et al. Complex structural variants in Mendelian disorders: identification and breakpoint resolution using short- and long-read genome sequencing. Genome Med 2018;10(1). https://doi.org/10.1186/s13073-018-0606-6.

[76] Chu C, Borges-Monroy R, Viswanadham Vv, et al. Comprehensive identification of transposable element insertions using multiple sequencing technologies. Nat Commun 2021;12(1). https://doi.org/10.1038/s41467-021-24041-8.

[77] Hancks DC, Kazazian HH. Active human retrotransposons: Variation and disease. Curr Opin Genet Dev 2012;22(3). https://doi.org/10.1016/j.gde.2012.02.006.

[78] Dupressoir A, Lavialle C, Heidmann T. From ancestral infectious retroviruses to bona fide cellular genes: Role of the captured syncytins in placentation. Placenta 2012;33(9). https://doi.org/10.1016/j.placenta.2012.05.005.

[79] Chuong EB, Elde NC, Feschotte C. Regulatory evolution of innate immunity through co-option of endogenous retroviruses. Science (1979) 2016;(6277):351. https://doi.org/10.1126/science.aad5497.

[80] Cordaux R, Batzer MA. The impact of retrotransposons on human genome evolution. Nat Rev Genet 2009; 10(10). https://doi.org/10.1038/nrg2640.

[81] Gonçalves A, Oliveira J, Coelho T, et al. Exonization of an intronic LINE-1 element causing becker muscular dystrophy as a novel mutational mechanism in dystrophin gene. Genes (Basel) 2017;8(10). https://doi.org/10.3390/genes8100253.

[82] Ewing AD, Smits N, Sanchez-Luque FJ, et al. Nanopore Sequencing Enables Comprehensive Transposable Element Epigenomic Profiling. Mol Cell 2020;80(5). https://doi.org/10.1016/j.molcel.2020.10.024.

[83] Maestri S, Maturo MG, Cosentino E, et al. A long-read sequencing approach for direct haplotype phasing in clinical settings. Int J Mol Sci 2020;21(23). https://doi.org/10.3390/ijms21239177.

[84] Lescai F, Chiamenti AM, Codemo A, et al. An APOE haplotype associated with decreased 4 expression increases the risk of late onset alzheimer's disease. J Alzheimer's Dis 2011;24(2). https://doi.org/10.3233/JAD-2011-101764.

[85] Clipperton-Allen AE, Page DT. Pten haploinsufficient mice show broad brain overgrowth but selective impairments in autism-relevant behavioral tests. Hum Mol Genet 2014; 23(13):3490–505. https://doi.org/10.1093/hmg/ddu057.

[86] Vymetalkova V, Soucek P, Kunicka T, et al. Genotype and haplotype analyses of TP53 gene in breast cancer patients: Association with risk and clinical outcomes. PLoS One 2015;10(7). https://doi.org/10.1371/journal.pone.0134463.

[87] Williams MA, McKay GJ, Carson R, et al. Age-Related Macular Degeneration-Associated Genes in Alzheimer Disease. Am J Geriatr Psychiatry 2015;23(12). https://doi.org/10.1016/j.jagp.2015.06.005.
[88] Pasaniuc B, Rohland N, McLaren PJ, et al. Extremely low-coverage sequencing and imputation increases power for genome-wide association studies. Nat Genet 2012;44(6). https://doi.org/10.1038/ng.2283.
[89] Ripke S, O'Dushlaine C, Chambert K, et al. Genome-wide association analysis identifies 13 new risk loci for schizophrenia. Nat Genet 2013;45(10). https://doi.org/10.1038/ng.2742.
[90] Tsoi LC, Spain SL, Knight J, et al. Identification of 15 new psoriasis susceptibility loci highlights the role of innate immunity. Nat Genet 2012;44(12). https://doi.org/10.1038/ng.2467.
[91] Nalls MA, Pankratz N, Lill CM, et al. Large-scale meta-analysis of genome-wide association data identifies six new risk loci for Parkinson's disease. Nat Genet 2014; 46(9).
[92] Snyder MW, Adey A, Kitzman JO, et al. Haplotype-resolved genome sequencing: Experimental methods and applications. Nat Rev Genet 2015;16(6). https://doi.org/10.1038/nrg3903.
[93] Tewhey R, Bansal V, Torkamani A, et al. The importance of phase information for human genomics. Nat Rev Genet 2011;12(3). https://doi.org/10.1038/nrg2950.
[94] Goldmann JM, Wong WSW, Pinelli M, et al. Erratum to: Parent-of-origin-specific signatures of de novo mutations. Nat Genet 2016;48(8):935–9, Nature Genetics. 2018;50(11). doi:10.1038/s41588-018-0226-5.
[95] Laver TW, Caswell RC, Moore KA, et al. Pitfalls of haplotype phasing from amplicon-based long-read sequencing. Scientific Rep 2016;6. https://doi.org/10.1038/srep21746.
[96] Wilbe M, Gudmundsson S, Johansson J, et al. A novel approach using long-read sequencing and ddPCR to investigate gonadal mosaicism and estimate recurrence risk in two families with developmental disorders. Prenatal Diagn 2017;37(11). https://doi.org/10.1002/pd.5156.
[97] Zhang S, Liang F, Lei C, et al. Long-read sequencing and haplotype linkage analysis enabled preimplantation genetic testing for patients carrying pathogenic inversions. J Med Genet 2019. https://doi.org/10.1136/jmedgenet-2018-105976.
[98] Gudmundsson S, Wilbe M, Ekvall S, et al. Revertant mosaicism repairs skin lesions in a patient with keratitis-ichthyosis-deafness syndrome by second-site mutations in connexin 26. Hum Mol Genet 2017; 26(6). https://doi.org/10.1093/hmg/ddx017.
[99] Proudfoot N. Pseudogenes *Nat* 1980;286(5776):840–1.
[100] Harrison PM, Gerstein M. Studying Genomes Through the Aeons: Protein Families, Pseudogenes and Proteome Evolution. J Mol Biol 2002;318(5):1155–74.
[101] D'Errico I, Gadaleta G, Saccone C. Pseudogenes in metazoa: Origin and features. Brief Funct Genomics Proteomics 2004;3(2). https://doi.org/10.1093/bfgp/3.2.157.
[102] Pei B, Sisu C, Frankish A, et al. The GENCODE pseudogene resource. Genome Biol 2012;13(9). https://doi.org/10.1186/gb-2012-13-9-r51.
[103] Mandelker D, Schmidt RJ, Ankala A, et al. Navigating highly homologous genes in a molecular diagnostic setting: a resource for clinical next-generation sequencing. Genet Med 2016;18(12):1282–9.
[104] Bardaro T, Falco G, Sparago A, et al. Two cases of misinterpretation of molecular results in incontinentia pigmenti, and a PCR-based method to discriminate NEMO/IKKγ gene deletion. Hum Mutat 2003;21(1). https://doi.org/10.1002/humu.10150.
[105] Claes KBM, de Leeneer K. Dealing with Pseudogenes in Molecular Diagnostics in the Next-Generation Sequencing Era. Methods Mol Biol 2014;303–15.
[106] Ammar R, Paton TA, Torti D, et al. Long read nanopore sequencing for detection of HLA and CYP2D6 variants and haplotypes. F1000Res 2015;4. https://doi.org/10.12688/f1000research.6037.1.
[107] Qiao W, Yang Y, Sebra R, et al. Long-Read Single Molecule Real-Time Full Gene Sequencing of Cytochrome P450-2D6. Hum Mutat 2016;37(3). https://doi.org/10.1002/humu.22936.
[108] Borràs DM, Vossen RHAM, Liem M, et al. Detecting PKD1 variants in polycystic kidney disease patients by single-molecule long-read sequencing. Hum Mutat 2017;38(7): 870–9. https://doi.org/10.1002/humu.23223.
[109] Buermans HPJ, Vossen RHAM, Anvar SY, et al. Flexible and Scalable Full-Length CYP2D6 Long Amplicon PacBio Sequencing. Hum Mutat 2017;38(3):310–6. https://doi.org/10.1002/humu.23166.
[110] Frans G, Meert W, van der Werff Ten Bosch J, et al. Conventional and Single-Molecule Targeted Sequencing Method for Specific Variant Detection in IKBKG while Bypassing the IKBKGP1 Pseudogene. J Mol Diagn 2018;20(2). https://doi.org/10.1016/j.jmoldx.2017.10.005.
[111] Tan AY, Michaeel A, Liu G, et al. Molecular diagnosis of autosomal dominant polycystic kidney disease using next-generation sequencing. J Mol Diagn 2014;16(2). https://doi.org/10.1016/j.jmoldx.2013.10.005.
[112] Stephens Z, Milosevic D, Kipp B, et al. PB-Motif—A Method for Identifying Gene/Pseudogene Rearrangements With Long Reads: An Application to CYP21A2 Genotyping. Front Genet 2021;12. https://doi.org/10.3389/fgene.2021.716586.
[113] Troskie RL, Jafrani Y, Mercer TR, et al. Long-read cDNA sequencing identifies functional pseudogenes in the human transcriptome. Genome Biol 2021;22(1):146. https://doi.org/10.1186/s13059-021-02369-0.
[114] Benson G. Tandem repeats finder: A program to analyze DNA sequences. Nucleic Acids Res 1999;27(2). https://doi.org/10.1093/nar/27.2.573.
[115] Tang H, Kirkness EF, Lippert C, et al. Profiling of Short-Tandem-Repeat Disease Alleles in 12,632 Human Whole Genomes. Am J Hum Genet 2017;101(5). https://doi.org/10.1016/j.ajhg.2017.09.013.

[116] Treangen TJ, Salzberg SL. Repetitive DNA and next-generation sequencing: computational challenges and solutions. Nat Rev Genet 2012;13(1):36–46.

[117] Lee H, Gurtowski J, Yoo S, et al. Third-generation sequencing and the future of genomics. bioRxiv 2016.

[118] Ardui S, Race V, Ravel T de, et al. Detecting AGG interruptions in females with a FMR1 premutation by long-read single-molecule sequencing: A 1 year clinical experience. Front Genet 2018;9. https://doi.org/10.3389/fgene.2018.00150.

[119] Cumming SA, Hamilton MJ, Robb Y, et al. De novo repeat interruptions are associated with reduced somatic instability and mild or absent clinical features in myotonic dystrophy type 1. Eur J Hum Genet 2018;26(11). https://doi.org/10.1038/s41431-018-0156-9.

[120] Höijer I, Tsai YC, Clark TA, et al. Detailed analysis of HTT repeat elements in human blood using targeted amplification-free long-read sequencing. Hum Mutat 2018; 39(9):1262–72. https://doi.org/10.1002/humu.23580.

[121] McFarland KN, Liu J, Landrian I, et al. Paradoxical effects of repeat interruptions on spinocerebellar ataxia type 10 expansions and repeat instability. Eur J Hum Genet 2013;21(11). https://doi.org/10.1038/ejhg.2013.32.

[122] Brook JD, McCurrach ME, Harley HG, et al. Molecular basis of myotonic dystrophy: Expansion of a trinucleotide (CTG) repeat at the 3′ end of a transcript encoding a protein kinase family member. Cell 1992;68(4). https://doi.org/10.1016/0092-8674(92)90154-5.

[123] Ropers HH. Genetics of intellectual disability. Curr Opin Genet Dev 2008;18(3). https://doi.org/10.1016/j.gde.2008.07.008.

[124] Su Y, Fan L, Shi C, et al. Deciphering Neurodegenerative Diseases Using Long-Read Sequencing. Neurology 2021;97(9). https://doi.org/10.1212/WNL.0000000000012466.

[125] Vissers LELM, de Ligt J, Gilissen C, et al. A de novo paradigm for mental retardation. Nat Genet 2010;42(12). https://doi.org/10.1038/ng.712.

[126] Niemi MEK, Martin HC, Rice DL, et al. Common genetic variants contribute to risk of rare severe neurodevelopmental disorders. Nature 2018;562(7726). https://doi.org/10.1038/s41586-018-0566-4.

[127] Mahmoud M, Gobet N, Cruz-Dávalos DI, et al. Structural variant calling: The long and the short of it. Genome Biol 2019;20(1). https://doi.org/10.1186/s13059-019-1828-7.

[128] Hiatt SM, Lawlor JMJ, Handley LH, et al. Long-read genome sequencing for the molecular diagnosis of neurodevelopmental disorders. Hum Genet Genomics Adv 2021;2(2). https://doi.org/10.1016/j.xhgg.2021.100023.

[129] Braat S, Kooy RF. The GABAA Receptor as a Therapeutic Target for Neurodevelopmental Disorders. Neuron 2015;86(5):1119–30.

[130] Huber KM, Klann E, Costa-Mattioli M, et al. Dysregulation of Mammalian Target of Rapamycin Signaling in Mouse Models of Autism. J Neurosci 2015;35(41): 13836–42.

[131] Banerjee A, Ifrim MF, Valdez AN, et al. Aberrant RNA translation in fragile X syndrome: From FMRP mechanisms to emerging therapeutic strategies. Brain Res 2018;1693:24–36.

[132] Sathyanarayana SH, Saunders JA, Slaughter J, et al. Pten heterozygosity restores neuronal morphology in fragile X syndrome mice. Proc Natl Acad Sci U S A 2022; 119(15):e2109448119.

[133] Darnell JC, van Driesche SJ, Zhang C, et al. FMRP Stalls Ribosomal Translocation on mRNAs Linked to Synaptic Function and Autism. Cell 2011;146(2): 247–61.

[134] Bagni C, Tassone F, Neri G, et al. Fragile X syndrome: causes, diagnosis, mechanisms, and therapeutics. J Clin Invest 2012;122(12):4314–22.

[135] Nelson DL, Orr HT, Warren ST. The Unstable Repeats—Three Evolving Faces of Neurological Disease. Neuron 2013;77(5):825–43.

[136] Berry-Kravis EM, Lindemann L, Jønch AE, et al. Drug development for neurodevelopmental disorders: lessons learned from fragile X syndrome. Nat Rev Drug Discov 2018;17(4):280–99.

[137] Yrigollen CM, Durbin-Johnson B, Gane L, et al. AGG interruptions within the maternal FMR1 gene reduce the risk of offspring with fragile X syndrome. Genet Med 2012;14(8). https://doi.org/10.1038/gim.2012.34.

[138] Apessos A, Abou-Sleiman PM, Harper JC, et al. Preimplantation genetic diagnosis of the fragile X syndrome by use of linked polymorphic markers. Prenatal Diagn 2001;21(6). https://doi.org/10.1002/pd.111.

[139] Biancalana V, Glaeser D, McQuaid S, et al. EMQN best practice guidelines for the molecular genetic testing and reporting of fragile X syndrome and other fragile X-associated disorders. Eur J Hum Genet 2015;23(4) https://doi.org/10.1038/ejhg.2014.185.

[140] Zoghbi HY, Orr HT. Glutamine repeats and neurodegeneration. Annu Rev Neurosci 2000;23. https://doi.org/10.1146/annurev.neuro.23.1.217.

[141] Maciel P, Gaspar C, DeStefano AL, et al. Correlation between CAG repeat length and clinical features in Machado- Joseph disease. Am J Hum Genet 1995;57(1).

[142] Matsuura T, Fang P, Pearson CE, et al. Interruptions in the expanded ATTCT repeat of spinocerebellar ataxia type 10: Repeat purity as a disease modifier? Am J Hum Genet 2006;78(1). https://doi.org/10.1086/498654.

[143] Matsuura T, Yamagata T, Burgess DL, et al. Large expansion of the ATTCT pentanucleotide repeat in spinocerebellar ataxia type 10. Nat Genet 2000;26(2). https://doi.org/10.1038/79911.

[144] Schüle B, McFarland KN, Lee K, et al. Parkinson's disease associated with pure ATXN10 repeat expansion. npj Parkinson's Dis 2017;3(1). https://doi.org/10.1038/s41531-017-0029-x.

[145] Wagner LA, Menalled L, Goumeniouk AD, et al. Huntington Disease. In: McArthur RA, Borsini F, editors. Animal and Translational models for CNS drug discovery.

Acedamic Press; 2008. p. 207–66. https://doi.org/10.1016/B978-0-12-373861-5.00018-7.

[146] Huntington T, Macdonald ME, Ambrose CM, et al. A novel gene containing a trinucleotide repeat that is expanded and unstable on Huntington's disease chromosomes. The Huntington's Disease Collaborative Research Group. Cell 1993;72(6). https://doi.org/10.1016/0092-8674(93)90585-E.

[147] Losekoot M, van Belzen MJ, Seneca S, et al. EMQN/CMGS best practice guidelines for the molecular genetic testing of huntington disease. Eur J Hum Genet 2013; 21(5). https://doi.org/10.1038/ejhg.2012.200.

[148] Perfect JR. Fungal diagnosis: how do we do it and can we do better? Curr Med Res Opin 2013;29(sup4):3–11.

[149] Ho CKY, Raghwani J, Koekkoek S, et al. Characterization of Hepatitis C Virus (HCV) Envelope Diversification from Acute to Chronic Infection within a Sexually Transmitted HCV Cluster by Using Single-Molecule, Real-Time Sequencing. J Virol 2017;91(6). https://doi.org/10.1128/jvi.02262-16.

[150] Li Y, zhou HX, hui Li M, et al. Comparison of third-generation sequencing approaches to identify viral pathogens under public health emergency conditions. Virus Genes 2020;56(3). https://doi.org/10.1007/s11262-020-01746-4.

[151] Ko SH, Mokhtari EB, Mudvari P, et al. High-throughput, single-copy sequencing reveals SARS-CoV-2 spike variants coincident with mounting humoral immunity during acute COVID-19. PLoS Pathog 2021;17. https://doi.org/10.1371/journal.ppat.1009431.

[152] Leggett RM, Alcon-Giner C, Heavens D, et al. Rapid MinION profiling of preterm microbiota and antimicrobial-resistant pathogens. Nat Microbiol 2020;5(3):430–42.

[153] Quick J, Loman NJ, Duraffour S, et al. Real-time, portable genome sequencing for Ebola surveillance. Nature 2016;530(7589):228–32.

[154] Yang L, Haidar G, Zia H, et al. Metagenomic identification of severe pneumonia pathogens in mechanically-ventilated patients: a feasibility and clinical validity study. Respir Res 2019;20(1):265.

[155] Charalampous T, Kay GL, Richardson H, et al. Nanopore metagenomics enables rapid clinical diagnosis of bacterial lower respiratory infection. Nat Biotechnol 2019;37(7):783–92.

[156] Moon J, Jang Y, Kim N, et al. Diagnosis of *Haemophilus influenzae* Pneumonia by Nanopore 16S Amplicon Sequencing of Sputum. Emerg Infect Dis 2018;24(10): 1944–6.

[157] Wang K, Li P, Lin Y, et al. Metagenomic Diagnosis for a Culture-Negative Sample From a Patient With Severe Pneumonia by Nanopore and Next-Generation Sequencing. Front Cell Infect Microbiol 2020;10. https://doi.org/10.3389/fcimb.2020.00182.

[158] Hoenen T, Groseth A, Rosenke K, et al. Nanopore sequencing as a rapidly deployable Ebola outbreak tool. Emerg Infect Dis 2016;22(2). https://doi.org/10.3201/eid2202.151796.

[159] Dudas G, Carvalho LM, Bedford T, et al. Virus genomes reveal factors that spread and sustained the Ebola epidemic. Nature 2017;544(7650). https://doi.org/10.1038/nature22040.

[160] Faria NR, Quick J, Claro IM, et al. Establishment and cryptic transmission of Zika virus in Brazil and the Americas. Nature 2017;546(7658). https://doi.org/10.1038/nature22401.

[161] Faria NR, Kraemer MUG, Hill SC, et al. Genomic and epidemiological monitoring of yellow fever virus transmission potential. Science (1979) 2018;(6405):361. https://doi.org/10.1126/science.aat7115.

[162] Kafetzopoulou LE, Efthymiadis K, Lewandowski K, et al. Assessment of metagenomic Nanopore and Illumina sequencing for recovering whole genome sequences of chikungunya and dengue viruses directly from clinical samples. Eurosurveillance 2018;23(50). https://doi.org/10.2807/1560-7917.ES.2018.23.50.1800228.

[163] Greninger AL, Naccache SN, Federman S, et al. Rapid metagenomic identification of viral pathogens in clinical samples by real-time nanopore sequencing analysis. Genome Med 2015;7(1). https://doi.org/10.1186/s13073-015-0220-9.

[164] Lewandowski K, Xu Y, Pullan ST, et al. Metagenomic nanopore sequencing of influenza virus direct from clinical respiratory samples. J Clin Microbiol 2020; 58(1). https://doi.org/10.1128/JCM.00963-19.

[165] Xu Y, Lewandowski K, Jeffery K, et al. Nanopore metagenomic sequencing to investigate nosocomial transmission of human metapneumovirus from a unique genetic group among haematology patients in the United Kingdom. J Infect 2020;80(5). https://doi.org/10.1016/j.jinf.2020.02.003.

[166] Meredith LW, Hamilton WL, Warne B, et al. Rapid implementation of SARS-CoV-2 sequencing to investigate cases of health-care associated COVID-19: a prospective genomic surveillance study. Lancet Infect Dis 2020;20(11). https://doi.org/10.1016/S1473-3099(20)30562-4.

[167] Washington NL, Gangavarapu K, Zeller M, et al. Genomic epidemiology identifies emergence and rapid transmission of SARS-CoV-2 B.1.1.7 in the United States. medRxiv 2021. https://doi.org/10.1101/2021.02.06.21251159.

[168] Wang J. MinION nanopore sequencing of an influenza genome. Front Microbiol 2015;6. https://doi.org/10.3389/fmicb.2015.00766.

[169] Stark R, Grzelak M, Hadfield J. RNA sequencing: the teenage years. Nat Rev Genet 2019;20(11):631–56.

[170] Earl JP, Adappa ND, Krol J, et al. Species-level bacterial community profiling of the healthy sinonasal microbiome using Pacific Biosciences sequencing of full-length 16S rRNA genes 06 Biological Sciences 0604 Genetics 06 Biological Sciences 0605

Microbiology. Microbiome 2018;6(1). https://doi.org/10.1186/s40168-018-0569-2.
[171] Bialasiewicz S, Duarte TPS, Nguyen SH, et al. Rapid diagnosis of *Capnocytophaga canimorsus* septic shock in an immunocompetent individual using real-time Nanopore sequencing: a case report. BMC Infect Dis 2019;19(1). https://doi.org/10.1186/s12879-019-4173-2.
[172] Schmidt K, Mwaigwisya S, Crossman LC, et al. Identification of bacterial pathogens and antimicrobial resistance directly from clinical urines by nanopore-based metagenomic sequencing. J Antimicrob Chemother 2017;72(1). https://doi.org/10.1093/jac/dkw397.
[173] Gargis AS, Cherney B, Conley AB, et al. Rapid Detection of Genetic Engineering, Structural Variation, and Antimicrobial Resistance Markers in Bacterial Biothreat Pathogens by Nanopore Sequencing. Scientific Rep 2019;9(1). https://doi.org/10.1038/s41598-019-49700-1.
[174] Greig DR, Jenkins C, Gharbia S, et al. Comparison of single-nucleotide variants identified by Illumina and Oxford Nanopore technologies in the context of a potential outbreak of Shiga toxin-producing Escherichia coli. Gigascience 2019;8(8). https://doi.org/10.1093/gigascience/giz104.
[175] Sakai J, Tarumoto N, Kodana M, et al. An identification protocol for ESBL-producing gramnegative bacteria bloodstream infections using a MinION nanopore sequencer. J Med Microbiol 2019;68(8). https://doi.org/10.1099/jmm.0.001024.
[176] Taxt AM, Avershina E, Frye SA, et al. Rapid identification of pathogens, antibiotic resistance genes and plasmids in blood cultures by nanopore sequencing. Scientific Rep 2020;10(1). https://doi.org/10.1038/s41598-020-64616-x.
[177] Gu W, Deng X, Lee M, et al. Rapid pathogen detection by metagenomic next-generation sequencing of infected body fluids. Nat Med 2021;27(1). https://doi.org/10.1038/s41591-020-1105-z.
[178] Cuomo CA, Shea T, Yang B, et al. Whole genome sequence of the heterozygous clinical isolate Candida krusei 81-B-5. G3: Genes, Genomes, Genet 2017;7(9). https://doi.org/10.1534/g3.117.043547.
[179] Luo R, Zimin A, Workman R, et al. First draft genome sequence of the pathogenic fungus Lomentospora prolificans (formerly Scedosporium prolificans). G3: Genes, Genomes, Genet 2017;7(11). https://doi.org/10.1534/g3.117.300107.
[180] Vale-Silva L, Beaudoing E, Tran VDT, et al. Comparative genomics of two sequential Candida glabrata clinical isolates. G3: Genes, Genomes, Genet 2017;7(8). https://doi.org/10.1534/g3.117.042887.
[181] Panthee S, Hamamoto H, Ishijima SA, et al. Utilization of hybrid assembly approach to determine the genome of an opportunistic pathogenic fungus, candida albicans timm1768. Genome Biol Evol 2018;10(8). https://doi.org/10.1093/gbe/evy166.
[182] Rhodes J, Abdolrasouli A, Farrer RA, et al. Genomic epidemiology of the UK outbreak of the emerging human fungal pathogen Candida auris article. Emerg Microbes Infect 2018;7(1). https://doi.org/10.1038/s41426-018-0045-x.
[183] Morand SC, Bertignac M, Iltis A, et al. Complete Genome Sequence of Malassezia restricta CBS 7877, an Opportunist Pathogen Involved in Dandruff and Seborrheic Dermatitis. Microbiol Resource Announcements 2019; 8(6). https://doi.org/10.1128/mra.01543-18.
[184] Schultzhaus Z, Cuomo CA, Wang Z. Genome Sequence of the Black Yeast Exophiala lecanii-corni. Microbiol Resource Announcements 2019;8(10). https://doi.org/10.1128/mra.01709-18.
[185] Pchelin IM, Azarov Dv, Churina MA, et al. Whole genome sequence of first Candida auris strain, isolated in Russia. Med Mycol 2020;58(3). https://doi.org/10.1093/mmy/myz078.
[186] Motooka D, Fujimoto K, Tanaka R, et al. Fungal ITS1 deep-sequencing strategies to reconstruct the composition of a 26-species community and evaluation of the gut mycobiota of healthy Japanese individuals. Front Microbiol 2017;8(FEB). https://doi.org/10.3389/fmicb.2017.00238.
[187] Irinyi L, Hu Y, Hoang MTV, et al. Long-read sequencing based clinical metagenomics for the detection and confirmation of Pneumocystis jirovecii directly from clinical specimens: A paradigm shift in mycological diagnostics. Med Mycol 2019;58(5). https://doi.org/10.1093/mmy/myz109.
[188] Sakamoto Y, Sereewattanawoot S, Suzuki A. A new era of long-read sequencing for cancer genomics. J Hum Genet 2020;65(1). https://doi.org/10.1038/s10038-019-0658-5.
[189] Feehan JM, Scheibel KE, Bourras S, et al. Purification of high molecular weight genomic DNA from powdery mildew for long-read sequencing. J Visualized Experiments 2017;2017(121). https://doi.org/10.3791/55463.
[190] Schwessinger B, Rathjen JP. Extraction of high molecular weight DNA from fungal rust spores for long read sequencing. Methods Mol Biol 2017;1659. https://doi.org/10.1007/978-1-4939-7249-4_5.
[191] Inglis PW, Marilia de Castro RP, Resende Lv, et al. Fast and inexpensive protocols for consistent extraction of high quality DNA and RNA from challenging plant and fungal samples for high-throughput SNP genotyping and sequencing applications. PLoS One 2018;13(10). https://doi.org/10.1371/journal.pone.0206085.
[192] Marotz CA, Sanders JG, Zuniga C, et al. Improving saliva shotgun metagenomics by chemical host DNA depletion. Microbiome 2018;6(1). https://doi.org/10.1186/s40168-018-0426-3.
[193] Helmersen K, Aamot HV. DNA extraction of microbial DNA directly from infected tissue: an optimized protocol for use in nanopore sequencing. Sci Rep 2020; 10(1). https://doi.org/10.1038/s41598-020-59957-6.

[194] Heravi FS, Zakrzewski M, Vickery K, et al. Host DNA depletion efficiency of microbiome DNA enrichment methods in infected tissue samples. J Microbiol Methods 2020;170. https://doi.org/10.1016/j.mimet.2020.105856.

[195] Kovaka S, Fan Y, Ni B, et al. Targeted nanopore sequencing by real-time mapping of raw electrical signal with UNCALLED. Nat Biotechnol 2021;39(4). https://doi.org/10.1038/s41587-020-0731-9.

[196] Payne A, Holmes N, Clarke T, et al. Readfish enables targeted nanopore sequencing of gigabase-sized genomes. Nat Biotechnol 2021;39(4). https://doi.org/10.1038/s41587-020-00746-x.

[197] David M, Dursi LJ, Yao D, et al. Nanocall: an open source basecaller for Oxford Nanopore sequencing data. Bioinformatics 2017;33(1):49–55.

[198] Boža V, Brejová B, Vinař T. DeepNano: Deep recurrent neural networks for base calling in MinION nanopore reads. PLoS One 2017;12(6):e0178751.

[199] Teng H, Cao MD, Hall MB, et al. Chiron: translating nanopore raw signal directly into nucleotide sequence using deep learning. Gigascience 2018;7(5). https://doi.org/10.1093/gigascience/giy037.

[200] Koren S, Walenz BP, Berlin K, et al. Canu: scalable and accurate long-read assembly via adaptive *k* -mer weighting and repeat separation. Genome Res 2017;27(5):722–36.

[201] Ruan J, Li H. Fast and accurate long-read assembly with wtdbg2. Nat Methods 2020;17(2):155–8.

[202] Walker BJ, Abeel T, Shea T, et al. Pilon: An Integrated Tool for Comprehensive Microbial Variant Detection and Genome Assembly Improvement. PLoS One 2014;9(11):e112963.

[203] Loman NJ, Quick J, Simpson JT. A complete bacterial genome assembled de novo using only nanopore sequencing data. Nat Methods 2015;12(8):733–5.

[204] Kiełbasa SM, Wan R, Sato K, et al. Adaptive seeds tame genomic sequence comparison. Genome Res 2011;21(3):487–93.

[205] Sović I, Šikić M, Wilm A, et al. Fast and sensitive mapping of nanopore sequencing reads with GraphMap. Nat Commun 2016;7(1):11307.

[206] Jansen HJ, Liem M, Jong-Raadsen SA, et al. Rapid de novo assembly of the European eel genome from nanopore sequencing reads. Scientific Rep 2017;7(1). https://doi.org/10.1038/s41598-017-07650-6.

[207] Shafin K, Pesout T, Lorig-Roach R, et al. Efficient de novo assembly of eleven human genomes using PromethION sequencing and a novel nanopore toolkit. bioRxiv 2019. https://doi.org/10.1101/715722.

[208] Chin CS, Khalak A. Human Genome Assembly in 100 Minutes. bioRxiv 2019.

[209] Kolmogorov M, Yuan J, Lin Y, et al. Assembly of long, error-prone reads using repeat graphs. Nat Biotechnol 2019;37(5). https://doi.org/10.1038/s41587-019-0072-8.

[210] Vaser R, Sikic M. Yet another de novo genome assembler. In: International Symposium on Image and Signal Processing and Analysis, ISPA. Vol 2019-September 23-25th, 2019; Dubrovnik, Croatia. doi:10.1109/ISPA.2019.8868909.

[211] Li H. Minimap2: pairwise alignment for nucleotide sequences. Bioinformatics 2018;34(18):3094–100.

[212] Simpson JT, Workman RE, Zuzarte PC, et al. Detecting DNA cytosine methylation using nanopore sequencing. Nat Methods 2017;14(4). https://doi.org/10.1038/nmeth.4184.

[213] Carson S, Wanunu M. Challenges in DNA motion control and sequence readout using nanopore devices. Nanotechnology 2015;26(7):074004.

[214] Fuller CW, Kumar S, Porel M, et al. Real-time single-molecule electronic DNA sequencing by synthesis using polymer-tagged nucleotides on a nanopore array. Proc Natl Acad Sci 2016;113(19):5233–8.

[215] Pugliese KM, Gul OT, Choi Y, et al. Processive Incorporation of Deoxynucleoside Triphosphate Analogs by Single-Molecule DNA Polymerase I (Klenow Fragment) Nanocircuits. J Am Chem Soc 2015;137(30):9587–94.

[216] Sanders AD, Falconer E, Hills M, et al. Single-cell template strand sequencing by Strand-seq enables the characterization of individual homologs. Nat Protoc 2017;12(6):1151–76.

[217] Ghareghani M, Porubský D, Sanders AD, et al. Strand-seq enables reliable separation of long reads by chromosome via expectation maximization. Bioinformatics 2018;34(13):i115–23.

[218] Lam ET, Hastie A, Lin C, et al. Genome mapping on nanochannel arrays for structural variation analysis and sequence assembly. Nat Biotechnol 2012;30(8):771–6.

[219] Cummings BB, Marshall JL, Tukiainen T, Lek M, Donkervoort S, Foley AR, et al. Improving genetic diagnosis in Mendelian disease with transcriptome sequencing. Sci. Transl. Med 2017;9:eaal5209. https://doi.org/10.1126/scitranslmed.aal5209.

[220] Cretu Stancu M, van Roosmalen MJ, Renkens I, Nieboer MM, Middelkamp S, de Ligt J, et al. Mapping and phasing of structural variation in patient genomes using nanopore sequencing. Nat. Commun 2017;8:1326. https://doi.org/10.1038/s41467-017-01343-4.

Pharmacogenomics

Advances in Molecular Pathology 5 (2022) 109–118
ADVANCES IN MOLECULAR PATHOLOGY

SLCO1B1 Pharmacogenetics in Pediatrics

Laura B. Ramsey, PhD[a,b], Jason A. Sprowl, PhD[c], J. Steven Leeder, PharmD, PhD[d,e], Jonathan B. Wagner, DO[d,e,f,*]

[a]Division of Clinical Pharmacology, Department of Pediatrics, Cincinnati Children's Hospital, University of Cincinnati College of Medicine, Cincinnati, OH, USA; [b]Division of Research in Patient Services, Department of Pediatrics, Cincinnati Children's Hospital, University of Cincinnati College of Medicine, Cincinnati, OH, USA; [c]Department of Pharmaceutical Sciences, School of Pharmacy and Pharmaceutical Sciences, University at Buffalo, State University of New York, Buffalo, NY, USA; [d]Division of Clinical Pharmacology, Toxicology and Therapeutic Innovation, Kansas City, MO, USA; [e]Department of Pediatrics, University of Missouri-Kansas City School of Medicine, Kansas City, MO, USA; [f]Ward Family Heart Center, Children's Mercy, Kansas City, MO, USA

KEYWORDS

• Endogenous biomarkers • Methotrexate • Pediatrics • Pharmacogenetics • Statins • Tyrosine kinase inhibitors

KEY POINTS

- The *SLCO1B1* gene has several common variants that affect function.
- Endogenous biomarkers (bilirubin, CPI, GDCA-3G, and GCDCA-3G) show promise as a tool to individualize drug therapy, but need validation in the pediatric clinical workspace.
- The magnitude of *SLCO1B1* genotype on simvastatin acid systemic exposure in children is greater than observed in adults, but is similar for pravastatin and rosuvastatin.
- Methotrexate pharmacokinetics are impacted by rare and common *SLCO1B1* variants.
- Investigations of inhibitors or substrates, including TKIs, should be a focus for future investigations.

INTRODUCTION

SLCO1B1 Gene

The solute carrier organic anion transporter 1B1 (*SLCO1B1*) gene encodes a major hepatic transporter, which can be called SLCO1B1 or organic polypeptide transporting polypetide 1B1 (OATP1B1). This gene is located on chromosomes 12 and 109 kb in length, including 15 exons. Variants in this gene are combined into alleles, which are cataloged by PharmVar [1], and activity of the allele is determined by expert consensus through the Clinical Pharmacogenetics Implementation Consortium (CPIC) (https://github.com/cpicpgx/cpic-sop/raw/main/CPIC%20Pharmacogene%20Curation%20SOP.pdf). The function of the alleles can be increased, normal, decreased, or no function, depending on the genetic variants [2]. There are some alleles that describe partial or complete deletions of the gene, which have been associated with Rotor Syndrome [3].

SLCO1B1 Genetic Variants and Nomenclature

The most widely studied variant in *SLCO1B1* is rs4149056, which significantly reduces transporter function and is included in several alleles (*5, *15, *40, *46, and *47). The rs4149056 (c.521 T > C) variant has been associated with many pharmacokinetic and adverse event phenotypes due to increased systemic circulation of the substrate. Each of the alleles with this variant is categorized as "no function" alleles for clinical

*Corresponding author. Division of Clinical Pharmacology, Toxicology and Therapeutic Innovation, Kansas City, MO. *E-mail address:* jbwagner@cmh.edu

https://doi.org/10.1016/j.yamp.2022.05.003
2589-4080/22/

purposes but may still have some (albeit little) residual biochemical function. Other alleles categorized as no function by CPIC are: *9, *23, *31, and the full/partial deletion alleles *48 and *49. The only alleles currently categorized as increased function are *14 and *20; their increase in function is likely due to increased expression. A complete list of alleles and their functions is available at CPIC's *SLCO1B1* gene page (https://files.cpicpgx.org/data/report/current/allele_function_reference/SLCO1B1_allele_functionality_reference.xlsx). When combined, a person's alleles make a diplotype that is used to determine the phenotype of the transporter and categorized as increased, normal, decreased, or poor function, whereby decreased means the person has one no function allele, and poor means the person has two no function alleles (Fig. 1) [2]. The phenotype of the transporter is what CPIC uses to make dosing recommendations for statins [4]. The allele and phenotype frequency varies across global populations, and the estimated frequencies of these are also available through CPIC and PharmGKB.

OATP1B1 Protein

The OATP1B1 protein is found almost exclusively in the liver. Other than genetic variants, there are several other factors that can influence the expression and activity of the transporter, including sex, age, and medications.

Ontogeny of OATP1B1

Most discussion of OATP1B1 focuses on its contribution to variability in drug disposition and response in adult patients. In a pediatric context, however, transporters may play important roles in regulating the disposition of endogenous molecules involved in growth and development, as well as defending the developing child against potentially toxic endogenous and exogenous toxicants. Several lines of evidence implicate OATP1B1 in the hepatic uptake of unconjugated bilirubin, the initial step in a process that subsequently involves glucuronidation by UDP glucuronosyltransferase 1 family, polypeptide A1 (UGT1A1) followed by biliary excretion of bilirubin conjugates by Multidrug resistance-associated protein 2 (MRP2) and MRP3 [5]. However, genetic variation in *SLCO1B1* was only associated with neonatal hyperbilirubinemia when accompanied by allelic variants of *UGT1A1* and *G6PD* [6]. Similarly, OATP1B1 substrate concentrations, such as dehydroepiandrosterone-3-sulfate (DHEA-S) [7], increase with increasing postnatal age and play important roles in growth and development [8], implying that developmental regulation of OATP1B1 may have an important physiologic function during childhood.

Although OATP1B1 protein expression seems to be higher and more variable in fetal liver, expression seems to be relatively constant after birth [9,10]. Restricting the analysis to samples with wild-type *SLCO1B1*1 A/*1A* genotypes did reveal higher expression from donors greater than 1 year of age compared with infants less than 1 year of age [10], but the sample size was limited. Similarly, an investigation of *SLCO1B1* messenger RNA (mRNA) expression in pediatric livers explored the potential for age-related changes in alternative splicing as a mechanism for developmental diversity. Several splice variants with age-dependent patterns of expression were identified, but most coded for truncated proteins with limited functional significance [11]. Thus, the available evidence provides little evidence for age-related changes in OATP1B1 protein expression after birth; the potential for developmental changes in transporter *activity* will require studies involving OATP1B1 substrates—drugs or endogenous compounds—as described in more detail later discussion.

Endogenous Substrates as Biomarkers of OATP1B1 Activity

Coproporphyrins

Coproporphyrin I (CPI) is an endogenous biomarker of human hepatic organic anion transporting polypeptide OATP1B activity [12–14]. CPI is a metabolite of porphyrin arising from the heme synthesis pathway. CPI is not enzymatically altered in the hepatocyte and is excreted unchanged in the bile (CPI), making it a potential endogenous biomarker to specifically assess OATP1B activity [15]. Active uptake of CPI by OATP1B1 and 1B3 has been verified in vitro, whereas quantitatively the importance of OATP1B for CPI uptake in vivo has been established using known inhibitors of OATP1B1 and OATP1B3, rifampin and cyclosporin A, where CPI area under the curve (AUC) increased 3-fold and 5-fold, respectively [12]. More recently, the impact of the *SLCO1B1* genotype–phenotype relationship on CPI exposure (ie, AUC) has been established in both adult and pediatric cohorts whereby those with *SLCO1B1* c.521 TC/CC genotype, a genotype known to be associated with impaired hepatic uptake and increased systemic exposure of drug substrates [16–23], have 1.5-fold to 2.5-fold increased AUC relative to those with the reference *SLCO1B1* c.521 TT genotype [24–26]. However, clinically the utility of baseline endogenous biomarkers, such as CPI, to predict drug exposure remains ambiguous. For example, in the

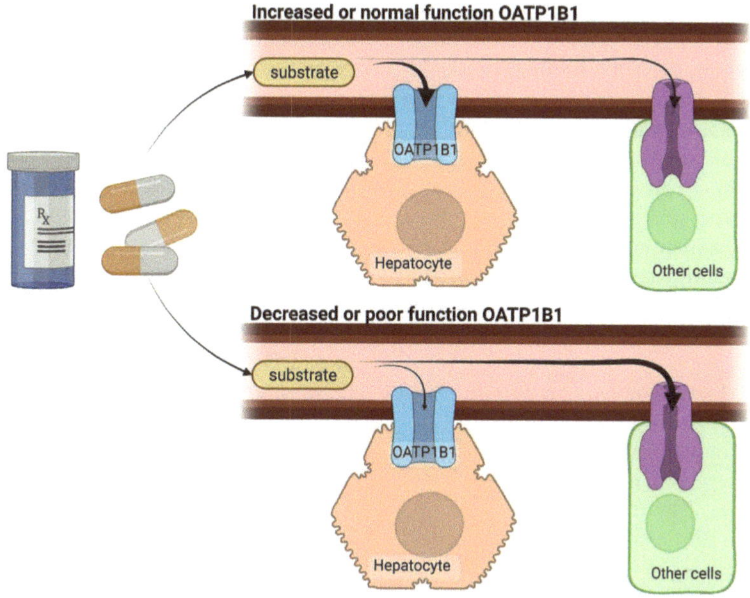

FIG. 1 In people with increased or normal function OATP1B1, the substrate is transported into hepatocytes, leaving less in systemic circulation and available to other cells (illustrated by the width of the *arrow*). In people with decreased or poor function OATP1B1, less of the substrate is transported into the hepatocyte, and more is in systemic circulation and available to other cells, increasing the potential for toxicity. (Created with Biorender.com.)

same aforementioned pediatric cohort enrolled into three separate pharmacogenetic-stratified pharmacokinetic studies involving rosuvstatin, pravastatin, and simvastatin [19,20,22], no consistent relationship between statin exposure and baseline (pre-dose) CPI concentration was observed [27]. The absence of a relationship may reflect the effects of additional factors on systemic stains exposure, namely alternative transporters involved in statin disposition (ie, OATP2B1, MDR-1(P-gp), BCRP). Collectively, this requires further exploration in a larger cohort and in a cohort with other OATP1B1/3 drug substrates.

Glycodeoxycholate 3-O-glucuronide (GDCA-3G) and glycochenodeoxycholate 3-O-glucuronide (GCDCA-3G)

More recently, two bile acid glucuronides, glycodeoxycholate 3-O-glucuronide (GDCA-3G) and glycochenodeoxycholate 3-O-glucuronide (GCDCA-3G), have been identified as OATP1B1 substrates and highly sensitive and specific endogenous biomarkers of OATP1B1 phenotype [28,29]. In fact, GDCA-3G and GCDCA-3G had 6-fold higher OATP1B1-mediated hepatic uptake compared with OATP1B3 and OATP2B1 [28]. In addition, the genotype–phenotype relationship has demonstrated in adults ~6-fold and 9-fold an increase in systemic exposure of GDCA-3G and GCDCA-3G in those with *SLCO1B1* c.521CC genotype relative to *SLCO1B1* c.521 TT genotype can occur. In comparison to CPI, GCDCA-3G demonstrated even higher sensitivity and may become a preferred endogenous biomarker of OATP1B1 [29]. Yet, before GDCA-3G and GCDCA-3G can be used in the assessment of OATP1B1 function in the pediatric cohort, further elucidation is required. Collectively, there is a wide range of endogenous biomarkers associated with OATP1B1 that are used to inform transporter-mediated drug–drug interaction risks in pre-clinical and early phase clinical investigations [30,31]. However, leveraging endogenous biomarkers, as markers of OATP1B1 activity, in the clinical workspace could enhance drug individualization (eg, model-informed decision support tools), and reduce uncertainty nested in the resulting dosage recommendations [32].

Drug Substrates

Pediatric providers are well versed in the impact that development (ontogeny) has on clinical care. Not surprisingly, assimilating pharmacogenomic data into the treatment algorithm for a developing population present challenges given the complexity of patterns of gene expression and, as a result, protein or enzymatic function over a lifespan. In fact, pharmacogenomic-driven pharmacokinetic studies performed in children continue to demonstrate significant variability in systemic exposure, equal to or exceeding variability observed in adults [33]. Thus, simple extrapolation of the genotype–phenotype relationship in adults to a small adult size remains inappropriate. Herein, the authors describe several examples of OATP1B1 drug substrates whereby *SLCO1B1* genotype-informed pediatric data exist.

3-Hydroxy-3-methyl-glutaryl Coenzyme A (HMG-CoA) reductase inhibitors (statins)

Statins, the mainstay for adult and pediatric hypercholesterolemia [34–38], represent one of the largest classes of OATP1B1 substrates. The *SLCO1B1* c.521 T > C variant associated with diminished hepatic uptake and increase systemic exposure [16–23] can lead to clinical adverse events, such as statin-associated musculoskeletal symptoms (SAMS) that have been previously demonstrated in several adult studies [39–41]. However, in children dosed with simvastatin, the magnitude of the *SLCO1B1* c.521 T > C genotype effect on the systemic exposure of the active moiety, simvastatin acid (SVA), was 2-fold greater than that observed in adults [20,21]. It remains unknown if this would lead to an increased risk of SAMS in children relative to adults dosed with simvastatin, but it certainly warrants prospective evaluation in a larger pediatric cohort. An unexpected finding was that SVA systemic exposure was negligible in one-quarter of the children dosed with simvastatin [20] and has not been reported in adults. Although several mechanisms are possible, this phenomenon has not been extensively investigated in adult or pediatric patients.

Although the *SLCO1B1* c.521 T > C genotype–phenotype relationship is similar in adults and children [18,19], an approximately 10-fold range of pravastatin systemic exposure *within genotype* was observed in children indicating that additional factors beyond *SLCO1B1* genotype contribute to the large range of variability among the pediatric cohort. Variability in presystemic conversion to an inactive isomer, 3′ α-iso-pravastatin acid (3αPVA), was one factor contributing to variability in pravastatin systemic exposure, with the effect most pronounced in the c.521 T > C genotype group. Recent in vitro analysis demonstrated that 3αPVA inhibits pravastatin for all genotype groups but was more impactful for those OATP1B1 protein types with c.521 T > C allelic variation [17]. Thus, lower concentrations of 3αPVA alter OATP1B1-mediated pravastatin hepatocellular uptake secondary to lower expression of functional protein in the c.521 T > C expressing cells. In patients with c.521 TT genotypes, a body mass index *Z*-score greater than +2.5 was associated with higher pravastatin systemic exposure [19]. Obesity is a known risk factor contributing to the development of fatty liver disease and, if uncorrected, leading to non-alcoholic steatohepatitis, a pathologic disease state whereby impaired OATP1B1 expression and function is observed [42–44]. Mechanistically, it is hypothesized that these fatty liver disease states lead to impaired N-glycosylation of relevant hepatic uptake transporters (eg, OATP1B1/3, OATP2B1) that result in altered cellular trafficking and expression [45]. Ultimately, this cellular alteration could lead to a state of impaired hepatocellular hepatic uptake of statins, leading to excessive systemic exposure and, thereby, a risk to SAMS. It remains unknown if other forms of lipidation could result in impaired OATP1B1 expression and function that will require further mechanistic investigation. Regardless, the impact of the obese state on hepatocellular transport with a variety of relevant drug substrates needs to be evaluated prospectively in the developing child. Overall, both of these additional variables contributing to interindividual variability in pravastatin systemic exposure must be taken into consideration to accurately inform precision-based dosing of pravastatin.

Similar to pravastatin, the *SLCO1B1* c.521 T > C genotype–phenotype relationship observed with rosuvastatin in adults was also observed in children [22,23]. In this pediatric cohort, 30% of the participants (four c.521 TT, four c.521 TC) were deemed "high outliers" because of excessive rosuvastatin systemic exposure relative to others in the genotype group. Four nonsynonymous sequence variations associated with additional rosuvastatin hepatic uptake (*SLCO1B1* c.767 G > C, *SLC10A1* c.957 G > A) and efflux transporters (*ABCG2* c.34 G > A, *ABCG2* c.421 C > A) were found to be possible additional factors leading to this observation. However, compared with simvastatin and pravastatin, rosuvastatin had the least variability in systemic exposure within genotype groups (~2–5 fold), which could ultimately make rosuvastatin the preferred statin agent for pediatric hypercholesterolemia in the future.

Methotrexate

The influence of *SLCO1B1* on the pharmacokinetics and toxicity induced by methotrexate has been studied in several pediatric populations, including children and adolescents with cancer, juvenile idiopathic arthritis, and inflammatory bowel disease. High-dose methotrexate (>500 mg/m^2) is part of the chemotherapy backbone for kids with cancer, but much lower doses (10–15 mg/m^2) are used in kids with autoimmune disorders. There have been many studies on the influence of *SLCO1B1* on the pharmacokinetics of high-dose methotrexate (*reviewed in* [46]) and several studies on the association with toxicities, including mucositis, hepatotoxicity, gastrointestinal toxicity, and neutropenia [47,48]. One study estimated that genetic variants in *SLCO1B1* explained ~10% of the inter-patient variability in the clearance of high-dose methotrexate, which was more than age, sex, and race combined [49]. In this study, rare variants made a substantial contribution, with effect sizes larger than the common variants. There are few studies of the pharmacokinetics of methotrexate when given at low doses, but *SLCO1B1* variants have been associated with nausea [50–52] and efficacy [53,54]. The decreased function alleles of *SLCO1B1* were associated with more methotrexate-induced nausea, presumably due to higher exposure to methotrexate. In contrast, the increased function allele, *14, was associated with the poorer efficacy of methotrexate.

Tyrosine kinase inhibitors

Tyrosine kinase inhibitors (TKIs), a family of more than 60 approved drugs, are currently used to treat various cancers, rheumatoid arthritis, myelofibrosis, and pulmonary fibrosis and are under investigation for other diseases. TKIs inhibit proteins that catalyze the transfer of phosphates to mediate signal transduction pathways involved in cell proliferation and survival [55]. The activity of these proteins can be altered under diseased states, but TKIs have significantly improved treatment outcome. Unfortunately, several complications can arise, including pharmacokinetic variability and DDIs.

Currently, the prescribing information of 27 TKIs states they are not substrates of OATP1B1; however, many do not report on such information. Meanwhile, some TKIs are reported as potential OATP1B1 substrates, including regorafenib, sorafenib, and lenvatinib (Table 1), although the clinical implications for the most of these observations remain unknown and require further investigation. TKIs have also recently received attention as OATP1B1 inhibitors by the Food and Drug Association and European Medicines Agency, some with confirmation in published reports (see Table 1). Some conflicting data exist, however, involving pazopanib, regorafenib, and sorafenib, indicating there may be a substrate-specific event associated with inhibition [56]. Moreover, the potency of inhibition varies and some may not warrant DDIs risk. For example, fedratinib was shown to have a minimal impact on OATP1B1-mediated pharmacokinetics using a substrate cocktail [57], and EMA prescribing information reports that pexidartinib is expected to have negligible OATP1B1 inhibition properties in hepatocytes, based on physiologic-based pharmacokinetic (PBPK) modeling and simulation.

There are reports of several OATP1B1-mediated DDIs that occur with TKIs. PBPK models have predicted the low potential of dasatinib to inhibit OATP1B1 in vivo [58,59]; however, the *R*-value of dasatinib in hepatocytes is 1.1 [60], and clearance of methotrexate was reduced when patients concurrently received dasatinib [61]. Whether this interaction occurs through OATP1B1 requires further investigation. The use of pazopanib has also been associated with numerous DDIs involving OATP1B1 substrates, including increased rates of rosuvastatin-mediated rhabdomyolysis and increased systemic concentrations of simvastatin and paclitaxel [62,63]. Moreover, coadministration of sorafenib also increased the systemic circulation of docetaxel [64]. Both paclitaxel and docetaxel are recognized as substrates of OATP1B1 based on clinical DDI studies[65].

The mechanism responsible for OATP1B1 inhibition by the most of the above TKIs is unclear. Although inhibition with substrate TKIs such as lenvatinib may be due to competitive inhibition [66], some TKIs demonstrate potent non-competitive properties. For example, nilotinib that is reported to be among the most potent OATP1B1 inhibitors [67–70] is anticipated to suppress the activity of the Src kinase LYN that has been associated with OATP1B1 activity [69]. The mechanism by which LYN mediates OATP1B1 activity and the extent to which TKIs can influence this regulatory pathway, will require in-depth future study.

Clinical Implications

Potential for drug–drug gene interactions

Given the large number of substrates for OATP1B1 (see Table 1), DDIs are common and may be potentiated by no function alleles of *SLCO1B1*. There is potential for drug–drug–gene interactions in pediatric oncology and autoimmune disorders, whereby TKIs are prescribed concomitantly with methotrexate. Some pediatric oncology centers hold TKIs while administering high-dose methotrexate to avoid this DDI.

Infrequency of Statins Prescribed to Children

Admittedly, there exist limited data related to the incidence of adverse events and treatment outcomes in

TABLE 1
OATP1B1 Substrates and Inhibitors

Drug/Endogenous Substrate	Substrate/Inhibitor	Regulatory Recognition	Reference(s)
Atorvastatin	Substrate	FDA and EMA	[16]
Bilirubin	Substrate	N/A	[5]
Bosutinib	Inhibitor	FDA and EMA	[69]
CPI	Substrate	N/A	[12,74]
CPIII	Substrate	N/A	[12,74]
Dabrafenib	Inhibitor	FDA and EMA	[69]
Dasatinib	Inhibitor	None	[68,69]
Encorafenib	Inhibitor	FDA and EMA	[69]
Fedratinib	Inhibitor	FDA and EMA	[69]
GCDCA-3G	Substrate	N/A	[75]
GDCA-3G	Substrate	N/A	[75]
Lapatinib	Inhibitor	FDA and EMA	[69]
Lenvatinib	Inhibitor, Substrate	FDA	[69]
Methotrexate	Substrate	None	
Nilotinib	Inhibitor, Substrate	None	[66–69,76]
Pazopanib	Inhibitor, Substrate	FDA and EMA	[67–70,76]
Pexidartinib	Inhibitor	FDA and EMA	[69]
Pralsetinib	Inhibitor	FDA and EMA	
Pravastatin	Substrate	FDA	[16,17,77,78]
Regorafenib	Inhibitor, Substrate	None	[67–69]
Rosuvastatin	Substrate	FDA and EMA	[79]
Simvastatin	Substrate	FDA and EMA	[16]
Sorafenib	Substrate	None	[76]
Sorafenib (glucuronide metabolite)	Substrate	None	[76,80]

Abbreviations: CPI, Coproporphyrin I; CPIII, Coproporphyrin III; EMA, European Medicines Agency; FDA, United States Food and Drug Administration; GCDCA-3G, glycochenodeoxycholate 3-O-glucuronide; GDCA-3G, glycodeoxycholate 3-O-glucuronide.

the children, especially the obese child prescribed a statin, secondary to the low level of statin use in this population. Reluctance to prescribe statins to children may be due to inadequate information and guidance, especially with respect to toxicity risks [71,72]. Current pediatric dosing recommendations for statins address familial hypercholesterolemia, but a paucity of data surrounding optimal dosing of statins in obese children remains [34]. Thus, prospective evaluation is required as the initiation of statin therapy in this population could provide improved long-term cardiovascular outcomes, even in the obese population with fatty liver disease. However, our previous pharmacokinetic data suggesting higher systemic exposure in obese patient leaves the pediatric provider yet again with trepidation, given the dearth of longitudinal trials elucidating the impact of chronic therapy with sustained supratherapeutic exposures on long-term skeletal muscle function, neurologic maturation, and glucose homeostasis in the developing child. Given that the use of statins may be anticipated to increase with the ongoing childhood obesity epidemic [73], the pediatric community should be proactive in establishing therapeutic guidelines before statins are in widespread use.

SUMMARY

Pediatric data to support clinical pharmacogenetic dosing guidelines are extremely limited, as evidenced by the most recent CPIC guideline for statins [4]. Available evidence indicates that genotype–phenotype relationships for OATP1B1 substrates in adults may not adequately apply to pediatric patients. For example, although each copy of the c.521 T > C variant may be associated with an approximately 2-fold increase in systemic exposure, *within-genotype* variability exceeds *between-genotype* variability, and *SLCO1B1* genotype alone is not sufficient for precision dosing of statins. Similarly, several medications or endogenous compounds may be considered OATP1B1 substrates based on *in vitro* studies, but multiple other pathways are often involved in the disposition of those compounds. Unless OATP1B1 represents the rate-limiting step in the compound's disposition, genotype information may be of limited value for prescribing. Furthermore, pediatric studies characterizing the relationship between systemic exposure of OATP1B1 substrates and clinical response are lacking, and it is recommended that established biomarkers of OATP1B1 activity be included in future exposure-response studies for their potential to inform safer and more effective use of OATP1B1 substrates in pediatrics.

CONFLICTS OF INTEREST

The authors have no conflicts of interest relevant to the topic of this article to disclose.

REFERENCES

[1] Gaedigk A, Whirl-Carrillo M, Pratt VM, et al. PharmVar and the Landscape of Pharmacogenetic Resources. Clin Pharmacol Ther 2020;107(1):43–6.

[2] Caudle KE, Dunnenberger HM, Freimuth RR, et al. Standardizing terms for clinical pharmacogenetic test results: consensus terms from the Clinical Pharmacogenetics Implementation Consortium (CPIC). Genet Med 2017; 19(2):215–23.

[3] van de Steeg E, Stranecky V, Hartmannova H, et al. Complete OATP1B1 and OATP1B3 deficiency causes human Rotor syndrome by interrupting conjugated bilirubin reuptake into the liver. J Clin Invest 2012;122(2):519–28.

[4] Cooper-DeHoff RM, Niemi M, Ramsey LB, et al. The Clinical Pharmacogenetics Implementation Consortium Guideline for SLCO1B1, ABCG2, and CYP2C9 genotypes and Statin-Associated Musculoskeletal Symptoms. Clin Pharmacol Ther 2022. https://doi.org/10.1002/cpt.2557.

[5] Keppler D. The roles of MRP2, MRP3, OATP1B1, and OATP1B3 in conjugated hyperbilirubinemia. Drug Metab Dispos 2014;42(4):561–5.

[6] Watchko JF, Lin Z, Clark RH, et al. Complex multifactorial nature of significant hyperbilirubinemia in neonates. Pediatrics 2009;124(5):e868–77.

[7] Muller F, Sharma A, Konig J, et al. Biomarkers for In Vivo Assessment of Transporter Function. Pharmacol Rev 2018;70(2):246–77.

[8] Remer T, Boye KR, Hartmann MF, et al. Urinary markers of adrenarche: reference values in healthy subjects, aged 3-18 years. J Clin Endocrinol Metab 2005;90(4): 2015–21.

[9] van Groen BD, van de Steeg E, Mooij MG, et al. Proteomics of human liver membrane transporters: a focus on fetuses and newborn infants. Eur J Pharm Sci 2018; 124:217–27.

[10] Prasad B, Gaedigk A, Vrana M, et al. Ontogeny of Hepatic Drug Transporters as Quantified by LC-MS/MS Proteomics. Clin Pharmacol Ther 2016;100(4):362–70.

[11] van Groen BD, Bi C, Gaedigk R, et al. Alternative Splicing of the SLCO1B1 Gene: An Exploratory Analysis of Isoform Diversity in Pediatric Liver. Clin Transl Sci 2020; 13(3):509–19.

[12] Shen H, Dai J, Liu T, et al. Coproporphyrins I and III as Functional Markers of OATP1B Activity: In Vitro and In Vivo Evaluation in Preclinical Species. J Pharmacol Exp Ther 2016;357(2):382–93.

[13] Lai Y, Mandlekar S, Shen H, et al. Coproporphyrins in Plasma and Urine Can Be Appropriate Clinical Biomarkers to Recapitulate Drug-Drug Interactions Mediated by Organic Anion Transporting Polypeptide Inhibition. J Pharmacol Exp Ther 2016;358(3):397–404.

[14] Barnett S, Ogungbenro K, Menochet K, et al. Gaining Mechanistic Insight Into Coproporphyrin I as Endogenous Biomarker for OATP1B-Mediated Drug-Drug Interactions Using Population Pharmacokinetic Modeling and Simulation. Clin Pharmacol Ther 2018;104(3): 564–74.

[15] Kaplowitz N, Javitt N, Kappas A. Coproporphyrin I and 3 excretion in bile and urine. J Clin Invest 1972;51(11): 2895–9.

[16] Kameyama Y, Yamashita K, Kobayashi K, et al. Functional characterization of SLCO1B1 (OATP-C) variants, SLCO1B1*5, SLCO1B1*15 and SLCO1B1*15+C1007G, by using transient expression systems of HeLa and HEK293 cells. Pharmacogenet Genomics 2005;15(7): 513–22.

[17] Wagner JB, Ruggiero M, Leeder JS, et al. Functional Consequences of Pravastatin Isomerization on OATP1B1-Mediated Transport. Drug Metab Dispos 2020;48(11): 1192–8.

[18] Niemi M, Schaeffeler E, Lang T, et al. High plasma pravastatin concentrations are associated with single nucleotide polymorphisms and haplotypes of organic anion transporting polypeptide-C (OATP-C, SLCO1B1). Pharmacogenetics 2004;14(7):429–40.

[19] Wagner JB, Abdel-Rahman S, Gaedigk R, et al. Impact of Genetic Variation on Pravastatin Systemic Exposure in Pediatric Hypercholesterolemia. Clin Pharmacol Ther 2019;105(6):1501–12.

[20] Wagner JB, Abdel-Rahman S, Van Haandel L, et al. Impact of SLCO1B1 Genotype on Pediatric Simvastatin Acid Pharmacokinetics. J Clin Pharmacol 2018. https://doi.org/10.1002/jcph.1080.

[21] Pasanen MK, Neuvonen M, Neuvonen PJ, et al. SLCO1B1 polymorphism markedly affects the pharmacokinetics of simvastatin acid. Pharmacogenet Genomics 2006; 16(12):873–9.

[22] Wagner JB, Abdel-Rahman S, Gaedigk A, et al. Impact of SLCO1B1 genetic variation on rosuvastatin systemic exposure in pediatric hypercholesterolemia. Clin Transl Sci 2020. https://doi.org/10.1111/cts.12749.

[23] Pasanen MK, Fredrikson H, Neuvonen PJ, et al. Different effects of SLCO1B1 polymorphism on the pharmacokinetics of atorvastatin and rosuvastatin. Clin Pharmacol Ther 2007;82(6):726–33.

[24] Yee SW, Giacomini MM, Shen H, et al. Organic Anion Transporter Polypeptide 1B1 Polymorphism Modulates the Extent of Drug-Drug Interaction and Associated Biomarker Levels in Healthy Volunteers. Clin Transl Sci 2019;12(4):388–99.

[25] Mori D, Kashihara Y, Yoshikado T, et al. Effect of OATP1B1 genotypes on plasma concentrations of endogenous OATP1B1 substrates and drugs, and their association in healthy volunteers. Drug Metab Pharmacokinet 2019;34(1):78–86.

[26] Wagner JB, Leeder JS, Ogungbenro K, et al. Effect of SLCO1B1 Genotype on Endogenous Biomarker Coproporhyrin I Baseline in Children and Adolescents. Clin Phamacol Ther 2020;107(SupplS1):S106–7.

[27] Wagner JB, Leeder JS, Ogungbenro K, et al. Utility of Coproprophyrin I to Predict Statin Exposure in Children and Adolescents. Clin Pharmacol Ther 2021;2021(Suppl 1):109. https://doi.org/10.1002/cpt.2167.

[28] Neuvonen M, Hirvensalo P, Tornio A, et al. Identification of Glycochenodeoxycholate 3-O-Glucuronide and Glycodeoxycholate 3-O-Glucuronide as Highly Sensitive and Specific OATP1B1 Biomarkers. Clin Pharmacol Ther 2021;109(3):646–57.

[29] Neuvonen M, Tornio A, Hirvensalo P, et al. Performance of Plasma Coproporphyrin I and III as OATP1B1 Biomarkers in Humans. Clin Pharmacol Ther 2021;110(6): 1622–32.

[30] Yee SW, Giacomini MM, Hsueh CH, et al. Metabolomic and Genome-wide Association Studies Reveal Potential Endogenous Biomarkers for OATP1B1. Clin Pharmacol Ther 2016;100(5):524–36.

[31] Li Y, Talebi Z, Chen X, et al. Endogenous Biomarkers for SLC Transporter-Mediated Drug-Drug Interaction Evaluation. Molecules 2021;26(18). https://doi.org/10.3390/molecules26185500.

[32] Darwich AS, Ogungbenro K, Vinks AA, et al. Why has model-informed precision dosing not yet become common clinical reality? lessons from the past and a roadmap for the future. Clin Pharmacol Ther 2017; 101(5):646–56.

[33] McLaughlin MJ, Wagner J, Shahknovich V, et al. Considerations for Implementing Precision Therapeutics for Children. Clin Transl Sci 2019;12(2):140–50.

[34] Wagner J, Abdel-Rahman SM. Pediatric Statin Administration: Navigating a Frontier with Limited Data. J Pediatr Pharmacol Ther 2016;21(5):380–403.

[35] Baigent C, Keech A, Kearney PM, et al. Efficacy and safety of cholesterol-lowering treatment: prospective meta-analysis of data from 90,056 participants in 14 randomised trials of statins. Lancet 2005;366(9493):1267–78.

[36] Mills EJ, Wu P, Chong G, et al. Efficacy and safety of statin treatment for cardiovascular disease: a network meta-analysis of 170,255 patients from 76 randomized trials. QJM 2011;104(2):109–24.

[37] Tonelli M, Lloyd A, Clement F, et al. Efficacy of statins for primary prevention in people at low cardiovascular risk: a meta-analysis. CMAJ 2011;183(16):E1189–202.

[38] O'Gorman CS, Higgins MF, O'Neill MB. Systematic review and metaanalysis of statins for heterozygous familial hypercholesterolemia in children: evaluation of cholesterol changes and side effects. Pediatr Cardiol 2009;30(4):482–9.

[39] Voora D, Shah SH, Spasojevic I, et al. The SLCO1B1*5 genetic variant is associated with statin-induced side effects. J Am Coll Cardiol 2009;54(17):1609–16.

[40] Group SC, Link E, Parish S, et al. SLCO1B1 variants and statin-induced myopathy–a genomewide study. N Engl J Med 2008;359(8):789–99.

[41] Donnelly LA, Doney AS, Tavendale R, et al. Common nonsynonymous substitutions in SLCO1B1 predispose to statin intolerance in routinely treated individuals with type 2 diabetes: a go-DARTS study. Clin Pharmacol Ther 2011;89(2):210–6.

[42] Fisher CD, Lickteig AJ, Augustine LM, et al. Experimental non-alcoholic fatty liver disease results in decreased hepatic uptake transporter expression and function in rats. Eur J Pharmacol 2009;613(1–3):119–27.

[43] Lake AD, Novak P, Fisher CD, et al. Analysis of global and absorption, distribution, metabolism, and elimination gene expression in the progressive stages of human nonalcoholic fatty liver disease. Drug Metab Dispos 2011;39(10):1954–60.

[44] Clarke JD, Hardwick RN, Lake AD, et al. Experimental nonalcoholic steatohepatitis increases exposure to simvastatin hydroxy acid by decreasing hepatic organic anion transporting polypeptide expression. J Pharmacol Exp Ther 2014;348(3):452–8.

[45] Clarke JD, Novak P, Lake AD, et al. Impaired N-linked glycosylation of uptake and efflux transporters in human non-alcoholic fatty liver disease. Liver Int 2017;37(7): 1074–81.

[46] Taylor ZL, Vang J, Lopez-Lopez E, et al. Systematic Review of Pharmacogenetic Factors That Influence High-Dose Methotrexate Pharmacokinetics in Pediatric

Malignancies. Cancers (Basel) 2021;13(11). https://doi.org/10.3390/cancers13112837.
[47] Trevino LR, Shimasaki N, Yang W, et al. Germline genetic variation in an organic anion transporter polypeptide associated with methotrexate pharmacokinetics and clinical effects. J Clin Oncol 2009;27(35):5972–8.
[48] Cheng Y, Chen MH, Zhuang Q, et al. Genetic factors involved in delayed methotrexate elimination in children with acute lymphoblastic leukemia. Pediatr Blood Cancer 2021;68(5):e28858.
[49] Ramsey LB, Bruun GH, Yang W, et al. Rare versus common variants in pharmacogenetics: SLCO1B1 variation and methotrexate disposition. Genome Res 2012;22(1):1–8.
[50] Mehta RS, Taylor ZL, Martin LJ, et al. SLCO1B1 *15 allele is associated with methotrexate-induced nausea in pediatric patients with inflammatory bowel disease. Clin Transl Sci 2022;15(1):63–9.
[51] Kyvsgaard N, Mikkelsen TS, Als TD, et al. Single nucleotide polymorphisms associated with methotrexate-induced nausea in juvenile idiopathic arthritis. Pediatr Rheumatol Online J 2021;19(1):51.
[52] Roszkiewicz J, Michalek D, Ryk A, et al. SLCO1B1 variants as predictors of methotrexate-related toxicity in children with juvenile idiopathic arthritis. Scand J Rheumatol 2021;50(3):213–7.
[53] Ramsey LB, Moncrieffe H, Smith CN, et al. Association of SLCO1B1 *14 Allele with Poor Response to Methotrexate in Juvenile Idiopathic Arthritis Patients. ACR Open Rheumatol 2019;1(1):58–62.
[54] Takahashi K, Nakamura H, Watanabe A, et al. Polymorphism in Organic Anion-Transporting Polypeptide Gene Related to Methotrexate Response in Rheumatoid Arthritis Treatment. J Nippon Med Sch 2019;86(3):149–58.
[55] Arora A, Scholar EM. Role of tyrosine kinase inhibitors in cancer therapy. J Pharmacol Exp Ther 2005;315(3):971–9.
[56] Sato T, Ito H, Hirata A, et al. Interactions of crizotinib and gefitinib with organic anion-transporting polypeptides (OATP)1B1, OATP1B3 and OATP2B1: gefitinib shows contradictory interaction with OATP1B3. Xenobiotica 2018;48(1):73–8.
[57] Ogasawara K, Wood-Horrall RN, Thomas M, et al. Impact of fedratinib on the pharmacokinetics of transporter probe substrates using a cocktail approach. Cancer Chemother Pharmacol 2021;88(6):941–52.
[58] Chang M, Bathena S, Christopher LJ, et al. Prediction of drug-drug interaction potential mediated by transporters between dasatinib and metformin, pravastatin, and rosuvastatin using physiologically based pharmacokinetic modeling. Cancer Chemother Pharmacol 2022;89(3):383–92.
[59] Pahwa S, Alam K, Crowe A, et al. Pretreatment With Rifampicin and Tyrosine Kinase Inhibitor Dasatinib Potentiates the Inhibitory Effects Toward OATP1B1- and OATP1B3-Mediated Transport. J Pharm Sci 2017;106(8):2123–35.
[60] Farasyn T, Pahwa S, Xu C, et al. Pre-incubation with OATP1B1 and OATP1B3 inhibitors potentiates inhibitory effects in physiologically relevant sandwich-cultured primary human hepatocytes. Eur J Pharm Sci 2021;165:105951.
[61] Ramsey LB, Mizuno T, Vinks AA, et al. Delayed methotrexate clearance in patients with acute lymphoblastic leukemia concurrently receiving dasatinib. Pediatr Blood Cancer 2019;66(5):e27618.
[62] Logue JM, Kiani B, Bitting RL. Pazopanib and Statin-Induced Rhabdomyolysis. Case Rep Oncol 2017;10(3):954–7.
[63] Kendra KL, Plummer R, Salgia R, et al. A multicenter phase I study of pazopanib in combination with paclitaxel in first-line treatment of patients with advanced solid tumors. Mol Cancer Ther 2015;14(2):461–9.
[64] Awada A, Hendlisz A, Christensen O, et al. Phase I trial to investigate the safety, pharmacokinetics and efficacy of sorafenib combined with docetaxel in patients with advanced refractory solid tumours. Eur J Cancer 2012;48(4):465–74.
[65] https://www.fda.gov/drugs/drug-interactions-labeling/drug-development-and-drug-interactions-table-substrates-inhibitors-and-inducers. (Accessed April 20, 2022).
[66] Koide H, Tsujimoto M, Takeuchi A, et al. Substrate-dependent effects of molecular-targeted anticancer agents on activity of organic anion transporting polypeptide 1B1. Xenobiotica 2018;48(10):1059–71.
[67] Hu S, Mathijssen RH, de Bruijn P, et al. Inhibition of OATP1B1 by tyrosine kinase inhibitors: in vitro-in vivo correlations. Br J Cancer 2014;110(4):894–8.
[68] Leblanc AF, Sprowl JA, Alberti P, et al. OATP1B2 deficiency protects against paclitaxel-induced neurotoxicity. J Clin Invest 2018;128(2):816–25.
[69] Hayden ER, Chen M, Pasquariello KZ, et al. Regulation of OATP1B1 Function by Tyrosine Kinase-mediated Phosphorylation. Clin Cancer Res 2021;27(15):4301–10.
[70] Khurana V, Minocha M, Pal D, et al. Inhibition of OATP-1B1 and OATP-1B3 by tyrosine kinase inhibitors. Drug Metabol Drug Interact 2014;29(4):249–59.
[71] de Ferranti SD, Rodday AM, Parsons SK, et al. Cholesterol Screening and Treatment Practices and Preferences: A Survey of United States Pediatricians. J Pediatr 2017;185:99–105 e2.
[72] Dixon DB, Kornblum AP, Steffen LM, et al. Implementation of lipid screening guidelines in children by primary pediatric providers. J Pediatr 2014;164(3):572–6.
[73] McCrindle BW, Tyrrell PN, Kavey RE. Will obesity increase the proportion of children and adolescents recommended for a statin? Circulation 2013;128(19):2162–5.
[74] Bednarczyk D, Boiselle C. Organic anion transporting polypeptide (OATP)-mediated transport of coproporphyrins I and III. Xenobiotica 2016;46(5):457–66.
[75] Mori D, Kimoto E, Rago B, et al. Dose-Dependent Inhibition of OATP1B by Rifampicin in Healthy Volunteers:

Comprehensive Evaluation of Candidate Biomarkers and OATP1B Probe Drugs. Clin Pharmacol Ther 2020; 107(4):1004–13.
[76] Zimmerman EI, Hu S, Roberts JL, et al. Contribution of OATP1B1 and OATP1B3 to the disposition of sorafenib and sorafenib-glucuronide. Clin Cancer Res 2013; 19(6):1458–66.
[77] Hsiang B, Zhu Y, Wang Z, et al. A novel human hepatic organic anion transporting polypeptide (OATP2). Identification of a liver-specific human organic anion transporting polypeptide and identification of rat and human hydroxymethylglutaryl-CoA reductase inhibitor transporters. J Biol Chem 1999;274(52):37161–8.
[78] Nakai D, Nakagomi R, Furuta Y, et al. Human liver-specific organic anion transporter, LST-1, mediates uptake of pravastatin by human hepatocytes. J Pharmacol Exp Ther 2001;297(3):861–7.
[79] Ho RH, Tirona RG, Leake BF, et al. Drug and bile acid transporters in rosuvastatin hepatic uptake: function, expression, and pharmacogenetics. Gastroenterology 2006;130(6):1793–806.
[80] Bins S, van Doorn L, Phelps MA, et al. Influence of OATP1B1 Function on the Disposition of Sorafenib-beta-D-Glucuronide. Clin Transl Sci 2017;10(4):271–9.

Advances in Molecular Pathology 5 (2022) 119–129

ADVANCES IN MOLECULAR PATHOLOGY

Implementation of a Clinical Pharmacogenomics Service in a Large Freestanding Pediatric Health System

Courtney Paetznick, PharmD[a], David Gregornik, PharmD[a,*], Lane Miller, MD, MS[b], Damon Olson, MD[c], Jacob Brown, PharmD, MS[d]

[a]Pharmacogenomics Program, Children's Minnesota, 2545 Chicago Avenue South Suite 700, Minneapolis, MN 55404, USA; [b]Center for Cancer and Blood Disorders, Children's Minnesota, 2530 Chicago Avenue South Suite 175, Minneapolis, MN 55404, USA; [c]Molecular Pathology Program, Children's Minnesota, 2525 Chicago Avenue South Suite 32-B600, Minneapolis, MN 55404, USA; [d]University of Minnesota College of Pharmacy, Duluth Department of Pharmacy Practice and Pharmaceutical Sciences, 232 Life Science, 1110 Kirby Drive, Duluth, MN 55812, USA

KEYWORDS

• Pediatrics • Pharmacogenetics • Pharmacogenomics • Implementation

KEY POINTS

- Pharmacogenomics (PGx) implementation in a pediatric health system has unique considerations compared with adult health systems.
- System-wide implementation of PGx requires several team members.
- Children's Minnesota is currently in its sixth year of PGx implementation across the health system, with the most application occurring in oncology and behavioral health programs.
- Children's Minnesota has customized the electronic health record to host genotype results for 13 pharmacogenes and has created more than 260 customized rules to drive electronic clinical decision support for 40 medications with drug/gene interactions.
- Deciding to do PGx testing in-house versus send-outs is complex and depends on capacity and interest.

INTRODUCTION

Implementation of pharmacogenomics (PGx) into health systems has notably increased in recent years, though in varied capacity [1]. Although some institutions have implemented pre-emptive PGx testing, others have imparted the responsibility to clinicians as to when and for whom these tests should be ordered. Due to the various types of institutional settings with unique variations of electronic health records (EHRs) and stages of PGx utilization, different approaches are and will be necessary.

PGx testing in pediatric health systems has seen considerable progress and, in many ways, has provided a blueprint for large-scale implementation. Implementation practices in pediatric institutions range from minimum uptake to full-scale clinical services [2]. Of note, the drug/gene pairs of interest may differ between pediatric and adult institutions. A recent survey through the Children's Hospital Association showed the most common drug/gene pairs tested for at high use centers were codeine/opioids and cytochrome P450 2D6 (*CYP2D6*), selective serotonin reuptake inhibitors

*Corresponding author, *E-mail address:* david.gregornik@childrensmn.org

https://doi.org/10.1016/j.yamp.2022.05.004
2589-4080/22/

(SSRIs) and *CYP2D6*/cytochrome P450 2C19 (*CYP2C19*), thiopurines and thiopurine S-methyltransferase (*TPMT*) ± nudix hydrolase 15 (*NUDT15*), and voriconazole and *CYP2C19* [3]. The PGx evidence for these drug/gene pairs in children has been further characterized in a recent review [4]. The Clinical Pharmacogenetics Implementation Consortium (CPIC) guidelines typically also comment on the use of these within children and even have separate pediatric and adult recommendations for atomoxetine and *CYP2D6* [5], and voriconazole and *CYP2C19* [6].

While some challenges to PGx implementation apply to both children and adults (eg, clinician familiarity with PGx testing, storage of PGx results in the medical record, cost concerns), others are intrinsically unique to children [2]. Central among these include ontogeny and the developmental changes children undergo from birth onward, especially in premature infants, and the evolving effects these changes have on pharmacokinetics and pharmacodynamics [7]. Additionally, when pediatric data is lacking, dosing guidance has been extrapolated from adult data, which is not always appropriate [8]. Although these challenges result in an additional layer of complexity, children may also be among the most likely to benefit from PGx testing, as this information will ideally be available to them as they progress into adulthood. The preemptive use of PGx testing has improved clinical and safety outcomes [9].

Children's Minnesota implemented a Clinical PGx service in 2016. The primary objective of this review is to provide a comprehensive overview of a broadly implemented PGx service at a large freestanding pediatric health system.

HISTORY OF CHILDREN'S MINNESOTA PHARMACOGENOMICS PROGRAM

Children's Minnesota is the seventh-largest independent, nonprofit pediatric health system in the United States. The system includes two hospitals, nine primary care clinics, seven rehabilitation, and nine specialty care sites. The Medical Genetics and Genomics Program at Children's Minnesota provides care for patients prenatally through early adulthood, including most neonates born in Minnesota with an abnormal genetics screen. With the hiring of a new medical director for the Medical Genetics and Genomics Program, a new strategy and business plan were developed that included the eventual creation of an interdisciplinary precision therapeutics program. The first stage of that program implemented a clinical PGx service, with the medical director identifying members of the professional staff from the oncology and behavioral health programs who were interested in promoting PGx within their practices. This team participated in early program planning and hired a clinical pharmacist with PGx implementation experience to lead the service.

The implementation of any new service within a health system requires multiple long-term projects that must take place in parallel. The clinical PGx pharmacist joined Children's Minnesota in August 2016 and, working with the medical director, continued PGx service planning. Fig. 1 describes an implementation framework adapted from a guide to starting a new Comprehensive Medication Management (CMM) service and was used to systematically implement the Children's Minnesota PGx service [10]. The first steps (Getting Started) included an assessment of the current use of PGx testing and an evaluation of medications used health system-wide with PGx recommendations in Food and Drug Administration (FDA) labeling, CPIC, and Dutch Pharmacogenetic Working Group (DPWG) guidelines. In addition, policies and standard operating procedures needed to be developed for the service, and a professional staff survey was developed to capture an understanding of PGx utility in clinical care.

At the time of inception, the utilization of PGx testing could not be determined due to PGx tests being ordered under a generic, nondescript test code within the health system. The PGx pharmacist and the medical director of Genetics and Genomics met with current medical staff who had requested genetic consults specifically for PGx evaluation or had expressed interest in PGx testing. This interview process determined that the hematology/oncology and behavioral/mental health services regularly ordered some form of PGx tests, either through single-gene or multi-gene panels. Primary care, immunology, and pain and palliative care services also expressed interest in exploring clinical PGx utility within their services.

To evaluate Children's Minnesota's use of medications with PGx implications, order information was extracted from the EHR. This information demonstrated regular use of medications with evidence-based PGx implications for selection and dosing, including antiepileptic agents, oncology supportive care medications, pain management, SSRIs, tricyclic antidepressants, and thiopurines (Table 1).

With the information gathered during the Get Started activities, the PGx pharmacist began the Build Your Team phase, with the medical director initially recruiting a genetic counselor to partner with the PGx

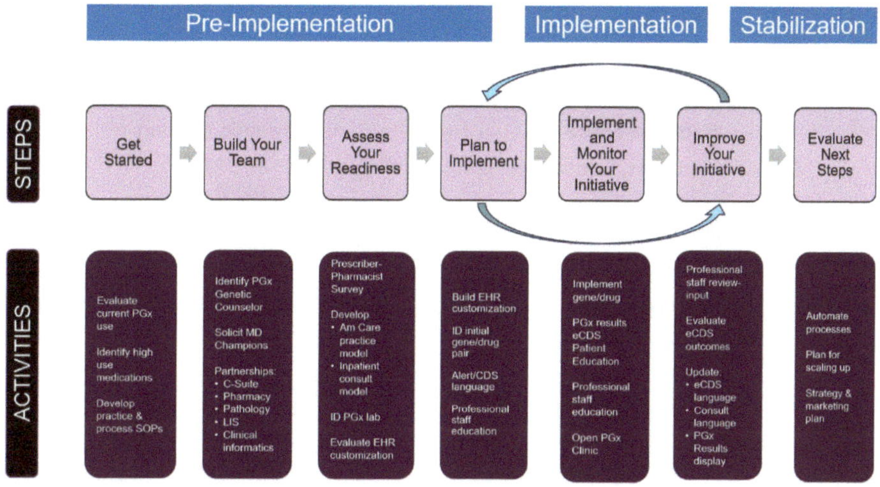

FIG. 1 Implementation framework for Children's Minnesota PGx Program.

pharmacist. Additionally, a new clinical informatics position was specifically created to support the PGx EHR implementation. Around the time the PGx program was starting, the Children's Minnesota EHR, a Cerner product, scanned PDFs of PGx test reports into an external document database and did not support hosting genetic results as discrete data. Discrete data is necessary to obtain the full benefits of PGx testing with electronic clinical decision support (eCDS). This newly formed team discussed how PGx data would be used in a clinical setting, how it should appear in the EHR, and how prescribers would be expected to interpret and use these results. This group worked to facilitate the customization of the Children's EHR to support the PGx service, and a process of integrating PGx results and eCDS was designed to describe the work needed to customize the EHR (Fig. 2). In conjunction with this work, a multidisciplinary PGx oversight committee (POC) composed of internal and external engaged Children's Minnesota stakeholders was established. The POC was incorporated into the health system reporting structure as a sub-committee of the Pharmacy and Therapeutics committee and began the review and approval process of the implementation steps, the clinical interpretation results, and the related eCDS.

For the initial implementation, a manual process using a Cerner PowerForm allowed the posting of discrete PGx results for display on a custom-designed Cerner MPage. Fig. 3 is an example of the current "landing page" for PGx results. This MPage can pull information throughout the EHR to display PGx genotypes paired with an interpretive consult (see red box in the figure) and current inpatient and home medications. In this example, passive eCDS is demonstrated by the drug mercaptopurine, which is bolded and highlighted in red, indicating a significate drug/gene interaction with *TPMT*. Once a genotype result is posted in the EHR it can be used for further eCDS, such as point-of-care interruptive alerts (Supplemental Fig. 1) or passive display of relevant genotypes during the medication ordering process (Supplemental Fig. 2). Lastly, as a continuous improvement process, the authors regularly evaluate the practice and make changes to the customization to enhance the utility of PGx implementation for the end-users, prescribers, and pharmacists.

To date, Children's Minnesota has customized the EHR to host genotype results for 13 pharmacogenes and has created more than 260 customized rules to drive eCDS for 40 medications with drug/gene interactions. This process is ongoing as new CPIC guidelines are published, older guidelines are updated, and our own experience is driving continuous improvement in the clinical utility of PGx for our patients.

PHARMACOGENOMICS CLINIC WORKFLOW AND PATIENT CARE PROCESS

Referral Patients to Pharmacogenomics Clinic

The Children's Minnesota PGx Program is currently a referral-based service using a two-appointment model (Fig. 4). Patients and families meet with a PGx pharmacist and a genetic counselor during the initial visit. The PGx pharmacist begins the appointment by performing

TABLE 1
Medications with Pharmacogenomics Implications Used Regularly at Children's Minnesota from January 2014 Through July 2016

Medication	Medical Service	Genetic Biomarker	Clinical Guideline
Amitriptyline	Psychiatry, Concussion clinic, Oncology	*CYP2C19* *CYP2D6*	CPIC Guideline
Abacavir	Infectious disease	*HLA-B*	CPIC Guideline
Allopurinol	Oncology	*HLA-B*	CPIC Guideline
Aripiprazole	Psychiatry	*CYP2D6*	FDA Labeling
Azathioprine	Gastrointestinal	*TPMT* *NUDT15*	CPIC Guideline
Carbamazepine	Neuroscience, Psychiatry	*HLA-A* *HLA-B*	CPIC Guideline
Citalopram/escitalopram	Primary care, Psychiatry	*CYP2C19*	CPIC Guideline
Clobazam	Neuroscience	*CYP2C19*	FDA Labeling
Clomipramine	Psychiatry	*CYP2C19* *CYP2D6*	CPIC Guideline
Doxepin	Psychiatry, Sleep clinic	*CYP2C19* *CYP2D6*	CPIC Guideline
Fluvoxamine	Psychiatry	*CYP2D6*	CPIC Guideline
Ondansetron	Oncology, Emergency department, Primary care, Surgery	*CYP2D6*	CPIC Guideline
Paroxetine	Primary care	*CYP2D6*	CPIC Guideline
Phenytoin	Neuroscience	*CYP2C9* *HLA-B*	CPIC Guideline
Sertraline	Primary care, Psychiatry	*CYP2C19*	CPIC Guideline
Tacrolimus	Transplant	*CYP3A5*	CPIC Guideline
Tramadol	Primary care, Emergency department, Ears-Nose-Throat	*CYP2D6*	CPIC Guideline
Venlafaxine	Psychiatry	*CYP2D6*	DPWG Guideline
Voriconazole	Infectious disease, Oncology	*CYP2D19*	CPIC Guideline
Warfarin	Cardiology, Hematology	*CYP2C9* *VKORC1* *CYP4F2*	CPIC Guideline

a CMM assessment, which includes evaluating the patient's conditions and medication therapy, medication allergy review, immunization assessment, and a review of systems. Throughout the appointment, the PGx pharmacist makes note of the medication(s) that were not effective in treating a patient's condition and/or an adverse drug event(s) from current or previousmedication(s). At the end of the visit, the PGx pharmacist discusses the evaluation based on our clinical criteria for testing (Box 1) and provides a recommendation as to whether PGx testing may help address the primary concern(s). When PGx testing is recommended and pursued, the patient and family meet with a genetic counselor during the visit to discuss the benefits and limitations of PGx testing and walk through several examples of how the information is applied in clinical practice. The genetic counselor also discusses the potential for incidental genetic findings (eg, UDP-glucuronosyltransferase 1A1 (*UGT1A1*) and Gilbert's syndrome) and obtains laboratory consent. Currently, PGx testing

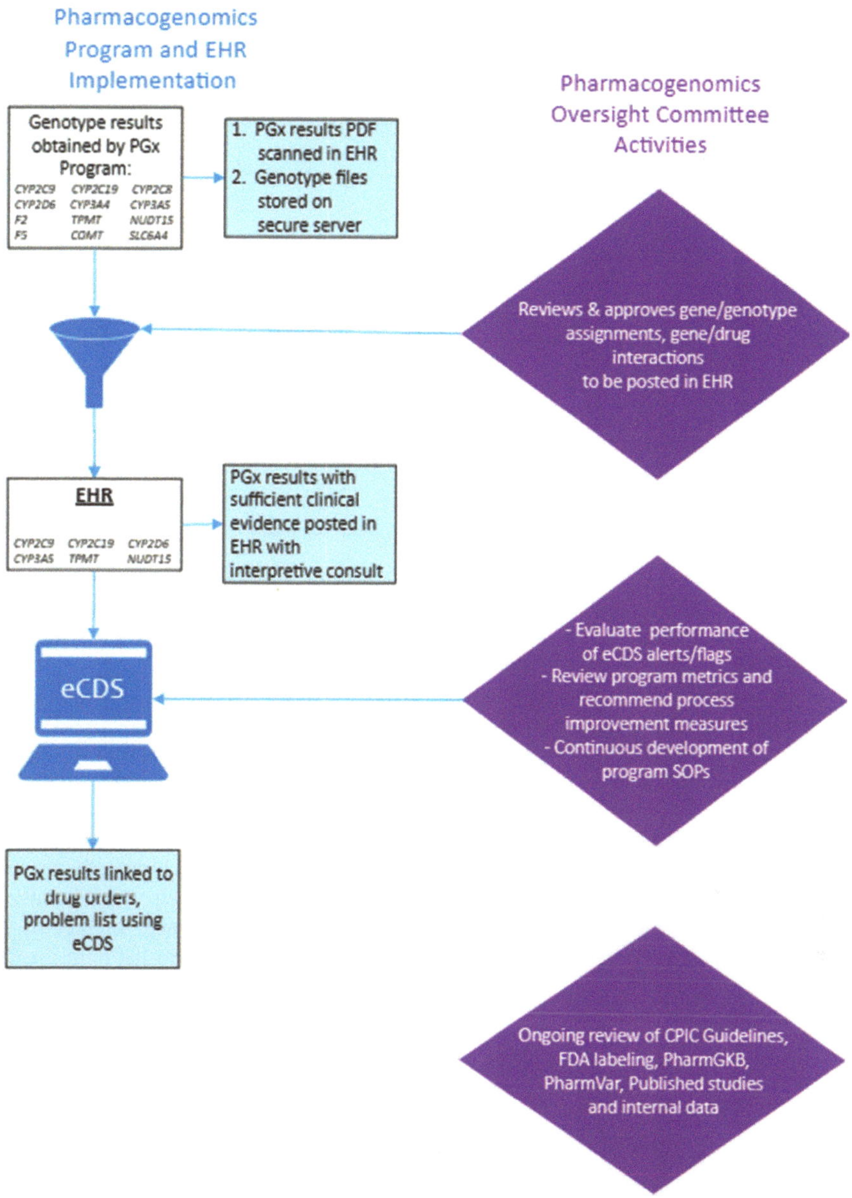

FIG. 2 Overview of integrating genotype results and eCDS into EHR. CPIC, clinical pharmacogenetics implementation consortium; eCDS, electronic clinical decision support; EHR, electronic health record; SOP, standard of practice.

is completed by external laboratories. A return of results visit is then scheduled with the family in 4 to 6 weeks from the initial visit. This timeframe allows the laboratory to run the DNA sample, and the Children's Minnesota PGx team to enter the actionable genes into the EHR and create a patient report based on CPIC guidelines, DPWG guidelines, and FDA labeling. At Children's Minnesota, clinical decision support based on proprietary, "black box" algorithms provided by laboratory companies are not used due to limited evidence for improved outcomes in pediatrics [11]. At the follow-up visits, the patients and families receive education about the common terminology used in PGx that is displayed on the report (eg, allele, genotype, phenotype).

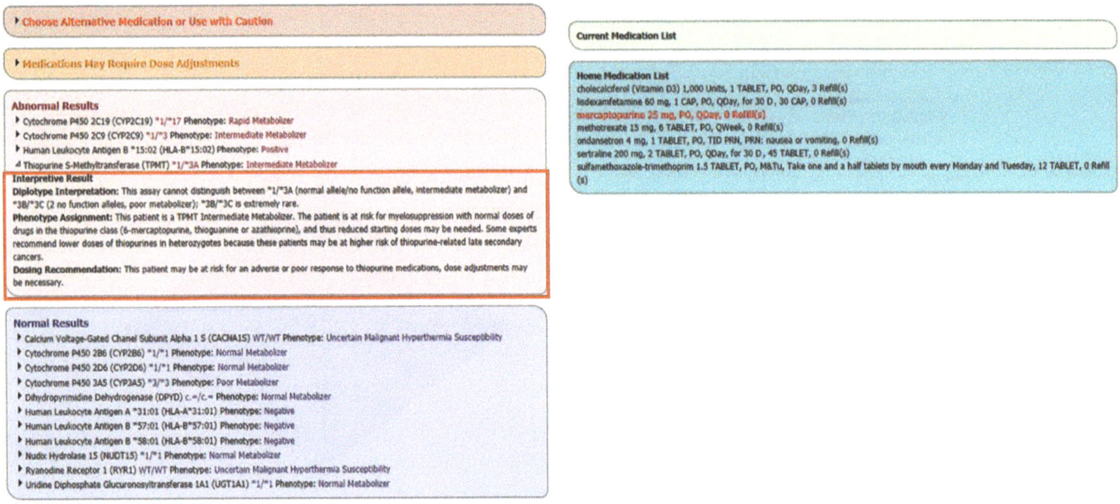

FIG. 3 EHR landing page for PGx.

This is followed by a discussion of the patient's specific PGx results and their relationships with past, current, and potential future medications that may be pertinent throughout the patient's life. Patients who receive PGx testing as part of a research study follow a similar clinic workflow, except the two appointments are combined into one hybrid appointment (see Fig. 4). The genetic counselor provides a review of the background education, and the PGx pharmacist discusses the patient's PGx results in the same appointment. If any incidental findings are noted, the patient and family meet with a genetic counselor to discuss the results and any implications. Patients and families are encouraged to share the results with any clinician they see outside of Children's Minnesota. It is recommended that patients/families follow up with the PGx clinic annually to receive updated information about new drug/gene interactions or modifications.

Transitions of Care

As a pediatric health system providing lifelong PGx results, the authors face unique challenges of transitions of care (see Fig. 4). This is especially challenging with the limited operability of health-system EHRs to share laboratory results, including PGx results. One way the authors currently help with transitions of care is through the EHR design of priority genotype results. Upon entry, a problem list item displaying the phenotype (eg, CYP2D6 poor metabolizer) is automatically placed in the EHR. The PGx team also monitors that a

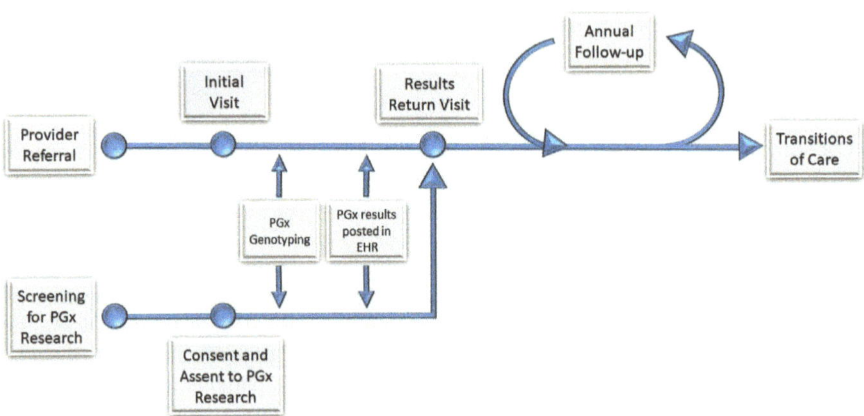

FIG. 4 PGx patient care process at Children's Minnesota.

BOX 1
Clinical Criteria for Pharmacogenomic Testing at Children's Minnesota

- Patient has experienced an adverse reaction to one or more medications
- One or more medications has failed to treat the medical indication the patient is experiencing
- Patient has a family history of significant adverse drug reactions
- Patient is anticipated to begin therapy on a medication with a narrow therapeutic window that is known to be metabolized by a polymorphic enzyme for which a genotype test is clinically available
- Patient is experiencing polypharmacy with three or more maintenance medications and is at risk for drug-drug interactions and potential drug-gene interactions
- Pending allogeneic stem cell or liver transplant
- Patient is unable to communicate side effects or ineffective treatment either due to immaturity or nonverbal/inability to speak
- Patient has been placed into foster care or adopted; limited or no family history is available

phenotype from a patient's problem list is not accidently removed via weekly reports. Future plans include continuing to improve transitions of care by developing a report that will alert the PGx team when patients with PGx results are about to turn 18 years of age. This will allow the PGx team to contact the families to ensure they have the most current PGx information to date before the patient transitions to an adult health system. Although this may reduce the risk of unnecessary retesting in the future, new variants of significance, new genes, or even identification of rare variants with sequencing may indicate additional testing based on advances in technology and standards of care.

PROVIDER PERSPECTIVE OF PHARMACOGENOMICS IMPLEMENTATION FROM A PEDIATRIC HEMATOLOGY/ ONCOLOGY PHYSICIAN

In selective ways, pediatric oncology centers have become increasingly comfortable assessing and utilizing PGx results for specific patient care scenarios, the most evident being *TPMT* and *NUDT15* genotyping and dosing of 6-mercaptopurine (6-MP) and 6-thioguanine (6-TG). In fact, the Children's Oncology Group (COG) has provided guidance on 6-MP and 6-TG dosing based on TPMT status within its acute lymphoblastic leukemia (ALL) protocols since 2002 and has been assessing the effects of TPMT genetic variation on treatment [12]. Moreover, St Jude Children's Research Hospital has assimilated TPMT status into thiopurine dosing since the 1990s [13]. The hematology/ oncology department has used PGx in clinical practice for several years, predominantly following medication intolerance or ineffectiveness and post hoc suspicions for gene\drug interactions. Still, common PGx barriers limited utilization, most notably due to cost restraints of the test itself, unfamiliarity within the EHR PGx framework, and reduced provider comfort in general with the interpretation and implementation of results [14]. Regardless, our current system of consenting families to PGx testing, coordinating the paper and electronic orders needed to send PGx testing from the inpatient and outpatient settings, receiving distilled results and relevant alerts through the EHR, and translating applicable results into medication adjustments was not entirely unfamiliar to our providers and was readily welcomed into practice in the context of a pre-emptive PGx research study.

Children's Minnesota Institutional Review Board approved the pre-emptive PGx protocol to evaluate the clinical utility of incorporating early PGx testing in patients undergoing cancer treatment, a hematopoietic stem cell, or heart transplant. The current process used by the hematology/oncology service to identify patient eligibility and experience using PGx in clinical practice is described herein. During a patient's initial hospitalization with a new cancer diagnosis, our inpatient rounding service has used a daily safety checklist that includes enrollment status on the pre-emptive PGx research protocol, serving as a prompt to the pharmacy and clinician teams. The inpatient pharmacist then performs daily drug/gene interaction assessments on all applicable inpatients as a component of the same safety checklist. Alternatively, in the outpatient setting, the PGx team circulates a regularly amended list of eligible outpatients who have not yet been approached to consent to the PGx protocol to the appropriate clinical personnel. Following permission/assent and once the specimen has been collected and sent, the return of results typically takes 3 to 4 weeks. At this time a structured display of these results is made available in the

"Pharmacogenomics" tab under the EHR workflow, readily accessible to any practitioner. This includes medications that may require dose adjustments, explains the variant gene involved, details the risk of standard dosing, provides evidence-based suggestions on adjusting starting or subsequent dosing decisions, and explains normal results. Concurrently, drug/gene alerts will prompt ordering providers when applicable (ie, suggesting 6-MP dose reduction in a TPMT poor metabolizer for whom 6-MP is being ordered).

PHARMACOGENOMICS RESEARCH

Clinical trials and research in PGx are essential to support the use of genotype-guided therapy in optimizing outcomes in patient care [15]. Evidence has shown that PGx results can guide treatment selection and dose, improving efficacy and reducing adverse events [16]. As a clinical PGx program in pediatrics, the authors are often challenged by the lack of drug/gene evaluations in pediatric patients. With a clinical PGx service in place, this has created a unique opportunity to harness this information and provide novel insights into drug/gene pairs in children. To date, Children's Minnesota has performed chart reviews for three drug/gene pairs of interest, including *CYP2D6* and atomoxetine , *CYP2D6*/*CYP2C9* and fluoxetine, and *CYP2C19* and sertraline [17].

Atomoxetine and CYP2D6

Atomoxetine is a non-stimulant medication used to treat attention deficit hyperactivity disorder in children and is predominantly metabolized by CYP2D6. A records review of 62 patients with *CYP2D6* genotypes and prescribed atomoxetine at Children's Minnesota were examined to compare clinical outcomes with the CYP2D6 phenotype group. This review showed a trend that children who were normal/ultrarapid metabolizers of CYP2D6 were more likely to discontinue atomoxetine due to a lack of efficacy as compared with those who were poor/intermediate metabolizers (HR: 2.4, $P = .068$). Furthermore, children with higher CYP2D6 activity scores were more likely to discontinue atomoxetine because of a lack of efficacy ($P = .04$) (unpublished data).

Fluoxetine and CYP2D6/CYP2C9

Fluoxetine is a first-line antidepressant used to treat depression in children and is metabolized by CYP2D6 and CYP2C9. To date, limited data is available on fluoxetine use in children as it relates to their *CYP2D6* and *CYP2C9* genotypes. Thus, a retrospective review was conducted of children prescribed fluoxetine at Children's Minnesota with documented *CYP2D6* and *CYP2C9* genotypes. In all, 177 patients were identified with a *CYP2D6* and *CYP2C9* genotype on file, of which 63 were eligible for study inclusion. Data analysis will primarily examine the response to fluoxetine based on genotype and phenoconversion predicted CYP2D6 and CYP2C9 activity scores, in addition to associations with adverse effects, time to medication discontinuation, and dosing requirements.

Sertraline and CYP2C19

Sertraline is metabolized in part by CYP2C19 and is commonly prescribed in children to treat generalized anxiety disorder. A records review of 90 patients prescribed sertraline with *CYP2C19* genotypes was assessed, displaying unique prescribing characteristics. In all children, rapid/ultrarapid metabolizers had a trend for higher dosing at the second dose titration as compared with normal metabolizers ($P = .067$). Additional comparisons were made when excluding individuals with *CYP2C19* genotypes before starting sertraline, which showed significantly higher doses in intermediate/poor metabolizers at the first dose titration as compared with normal metabolizers ($P = .03$). When looking only at individuals with *CYP2C19* genotypes before starting sertraline, a trend showed intermediate/poor metabolizers received lower dosing at the first titration as compared with normal metabolizers ($P = .064$). Although it was difficult to assess health outcomes with this study, it is notable that prescribing trends differed across CYP2C19 phenotypes in children prescribed sertraline, particularly when CYP2C19 phenotypes were known at the start of sertraline as compared with those without [17].

DEVELOPING A PHARMACOGENOMICS GENOTYPING ASSAY

An important consideration for a PGx program is how and whereby testing will be performed. Traditionally, most PGx testing has been approached on a gene-by-gene, single nucleotide polymorphism (SNP) or variant (SNV) and copy number variant (CNV) basis with genotyping assays. These types of assays identify the nucleotides, ie, the "genotype," at specific locations within the genome. When the nucleotide at that location matches the reference genome nucleotide, it is referred to as a "wild type," and any other variation is then referred to as a "variant." By interrogating several sites within a gene, a collection of genotypes can be determined, leading to a description of the sample's haplotype, of which essentially shorthand descriptions make up the star allele nomenclature. Similarly, focused approaches to determining CNV (ie, deletions or duplications) have traditionally been used via various techniques, such as real-time polymerase chain reaction (PCR) and multiplex ligation probe amplification assays.

In the present state, many reference laboratories offer PGx testing with a variety of gene panels and techniques available that are predominantly genotyping assays, but there has been a more recent shift over the last few years towards sequencing technologies. Sequencing, whether via classic Sanger sequencing or next-generation sequencing, is more comprehensive than genotyping approaches since the entire nucleotide sequence within a genomic region of interest is ascertained. Next-generation sequencing (also known as massively parallel sequencing) generally allows interrogation of many genes and is becoming a preferred approach in reference laboratories over genotyping or Sanger sequencing [18]. Further discussion regarding sequencing approaches in this article refers to next-generation sequencing.

Genotyping or sequencing approaches each have advantages and disadvantages, and a brief discussion is provided here while a more detailed review of the approaches can be found elsewhere [18]. Genotyping is historically well established, and there are many different commercially available products for this approach. Depending on the technology, there is generally flexibility in batch sizes, the overall cost is low, and the turnaround times are faster relative to sequencing. If a laboratory is looking to develop testing in-house, implementation of genotyping assays is relatively straightforward, especially if using an FDA-approved/cleared assay. In contrast, genotyping assays may not identify relevant or rare variants because they are based on SNPs occurring in specific, well-researched populations and commercially available assays are largely limited to this existing knowledge. This may lead to false-negative results, particularly for patient populations who have not been well-studied and whose potentially relevant minor allele variants have not been characterized and codified [19,20].

Sequencing approaches are attractive because of the ability to interrogate many different genes and identify all or most potential variants within the interrogated regions. For example, a typical PGx panel may include anywhere from less than 10 to a few dozen genes. Although some larger genotyping microarray-based chips have just as many genes or even more, they are again limited to only the specific SNPs or loci. In addition to sequencing allowing identification of nearly all variants in the interrogated region, it may also help determine the allelic configuration (ie, cis or trans) of any identified variants if they occur within the same next-generation sequencing read. This is in contrast to genotyping assays, where this knowledge is often inferred via known variant linkage disequilibrium but still may not always be known or correct. However, with the identification of more variants comes the unique challenge of interpreting the clinical significance of any new or poorly characterized variants, requiring additional interpretive expertise and resource consumption. Related to this challenge is the potential for discovering incidental findings, such as identifying a tumor predisposition variant or other pathogenic germline variants if those genes are part of the panel. PGx programs receiving sequencing results need to have a policy for handling incidental findings. For laboratories looking to develop in-house sequencing assays, these are much more challenging and resource-intensive than genotyping assays. Next-generation sequencers are generally much more expensive than genotyping systems and have complex and prolonged workflows, including extensive bioinformatics processes and reporting formats. Reagents and chips are more expensive, often forcing laboratories to batch samples for extended periods and resulting in longer turnaround times.

The decision of how and where a PGx program might pursue clinical testing is complex. There are practical factors to consider, such as the preferred turnaround time, cost of testing to ensure access to a broad patient population, ability to incorporate new variant evidence and guidelines, how many and what variants need interrogation for clinical utility [21,22], and how results will be integrated into the EHR and interact with clinical decision support tools [19,23]. If considering in-house development, the capabilities and resources of the local laboratory, technological approaches, and alignment with organizational goals are essential as well [23]. More programmatic questions to consider include the characteristics of the target patient populations that may require specialized testing or inclusion of rare variants, degree of desired control over assay development and operations, and concurrent research objectives.

Our PGx program was initially built on and currently remains based on external reference laboratory testing, using genotyping assays mainly but with a more recent introduction of sequencing technologies. However, we have also elected to move forward with the development of an in-house assay based on the Agena

Bioscience's MassARRAY platform using several commercially available, "off-the-shelf" assays in combination with a custom panel. This platform is a genotyping-based approach using Matrix-Assisted Laser Desorption Ionization-Time of Flight technology. Briefly, genomic regions of interest in extracted genomic DNA from patient samples are amplified via PCR via an initial set of primers. The amplicons are then purified via shrimp alkaline phosphatase to remove excess nucleotides and subjected to a second set of primers with chain-terminating dideoxy nucleotides. This results in a single-base extension overlying single nucleotides of interest and imparting a known molecular mass to the amplicon molecule. The MassARRAY instrument then pulses laser light onto the samples, inducing charge and acceleration through a vacuum tube to a detector at the end. Each molecule is then identified by its molecular weight, allowing detection of the genotype for each targeted region with a multiplexing capability on average of approximately 10 markers per well for our assay.

With the intention to provide this in-house PGx panel as a clinical test, the assay will be fully validated per the Clinical Laboratory Improvements Act of 1988 and its Amendments utilizing commercially available reference samples and previously characterized patient samples to ensure test accuracy as has been described elsewhere [19,23]. Genotypes will be provided from the assay with subsequent software analysis providing the most likely haplotypes and subsequent star allele designations. After initial intralaboratory quality checks and reviews, results will automatically transfer into the EHR to drive eCDS. The interpretive analysis and predicted phenotypes will be provided by pharmacists with specialized PGx training.

SUMMARY

As a large, freestanding pediatric health system, Children's Minnesota is faced with unique challenges and opportunities with PGx implementation compared with adult health systems. The PGx program was initially developed to meet a growing desire to incorporate PGx information into clinical decision making, particularly in hematology/oncology and behavioral health, and to lead the clinical PGx implementation. Since the launch of the PGx program, new possibilities have emerged with contributions to PGx research and the development of an in-house genotyping assay as ways to better serve our diverse pediatric population.

DISCLOSURE

C. Paetznick, D. Gregornik and L. Miller have received financial and research support from the Children's Minnesota Foundation for the Pre-emptive PGx Protocol.

SUPPLEMENTARY DATA

Supplementary data related to this article can be found online at https://doi.org/10.1016/j.yamp.2022.05.004.

REFERENCES

[1] Luczak T, Brown SJ, Armbruster D, et al. Strategies and settings of clinical pharmacogenetic implementation: a scoping review of pharmacogenetics programs. Pharmacogenomics 2021;22(6):345–64.
[2] Gregornik D, Salyakina D, Brown M, et al. Pediatric pharmacogenomics: challenges and opportunities: on behalf of the Sanford Children's Genomic Medicine Consortium. Pharmacogenomics J 2021;21(1):8–19.
[3] Brown JT, Ramsey LB, Van Driest SL, et al. Characterizing Pharmacogenetic Testing Among Children's Hospitals. Clin Transl Sci 2021;14(2):692–701.
[4] Ramsey LB, Brown JT, Vear SI, et al. Gene-Based Dose Optimization in Children. Annu Rev Pharmacol Toxicol 2020;60:311–31.
[5] Brown JT, Bishop JR, Sangkuhl K, et al. Clinical Pharmacogenetics Implementation Consortium Guideline for Cytochrome P450 (CYP)2D6 Genotype and Atomoxetine Therapy. Clin Pharmacol Ther 2019;106(1):94–102.
[6] Moriyama B, Obeng AO, Barbarino J, et al. Clinical Pharmacogenetics Implementation Consortium (CPIC) Guidelines for CYP2C19 and Voriconazole Therapy. Clin Pharmacol Ther 2017;102(1):45–51.
[7] Funk RS, Brown JT, Abdel-Rahman SM. Pediatric pharmacokinetics: human development and drug disposition. Pediatr Clin North Am 2012;59(5):1001–16.
[8] Green DJ, Mummaneni P, Kim IW, et al. Pharmacogenomic information in FDA-approved drug labels: Application to pediatric patients. Clin Pharmacol Ther 2016;99(6):622–32.
[9] Roden DM, Van Driest SL, Mosley JD, et al. Benefit of Preemptive Pharmacogenetic Information on Clinical Outcome. Clin Pharmacol Ther 2018;103(5):787–94.
[10] Blanchard C, Livet M, Ward C, et al. The Active Implementation Frameworks: A roadmap for advancing implementation of Comprehensive Medication Management in Primary care. Res Social Adm Pharm 2017;13(5):922–9.
[11] Vande Voort JL, Orth SS, Shekunov J, et al. A Randomized Controlled Trial of Combinatorial Pharmacogenetics Testing in Adolescent Depression. J Am Acad Child Adolesc Psychiatry 2022;61(1):46–55.

[12] Sepe DM, McWilliams T, Chen J, et al. Germline genetic variation and treatment response on CCG-1891. Pediatr Blood Cancer 2012;58(5):695–700.

[13] Relling MV, Pui CH, Cheng C, et al. Thiopurine methyltransferase in acute lymphoblastic leukemia. Blood 2006;107(2):843–4.

[14] Moyer AM, Caraballo PJ. The challenges of implementing pharmacogenomic testing in the clinic. Expert Rev Pharmacoecon Outcomes Res 2017;17(6):567–77.

[15] Roden DM, McLeod HL, Relling MV, et al. Pharmacogenomics. Lancet 2019;394(10197):521–32.

[16] Luzum JA, Pakyz RE, Elsey AR, et al. The Pharmacogenomics Research Network Translational Pharmacogenetics Program: Outcomes and Metrics of Pharmacogenetic Implementations Across Diverse Healthcare Systems. Clin Pharmacol Ther 2017;102(3): 502–10.

[17] Brown JT, Gregornik DB, Jorgenson A, et al. Sertraline dosing trends in children and adolescents stratified by CYP2C19 genotype. Pharmacogenomics 2022;23(4): 247–53.

[18] Hippman C, Nislow C. Pharmacogenomic Testing: Clinical Evidence and Implementation Challenges. J Pers Med 2019;9(3):E40.

[19] Scott SA, Scott ER, Seki Y, et al. Development and Analytical Validation of a 29 Gene Clinical Pharmacogenetic Genotyping Panel: Multi-Ethnic Allele and Copy Number Variant Detection. Clin Transl Sci 2021;14(1): 204–13.

[20] Zhou Y, Ingelman-Sundberg M, Lauschke VM. Worldwide Distribution of Cytochrome P450 Alleles: A Meta-analysis of Population-scale Sequencing Projects. Clin Pharmacol Ther 2017;102(4):688–700.

[21] Pratt VM, Turner A, Broeckel U, et al. Characterization of Reference Materials with an Association for Molecular Pathology Pharmacogenetics Working Group Tier 2 Status: CYP2C9, CYP2C19, VKORC1, CYP2C Cluster Variant, and GGCX: A GeT-RM Collaborative Project. J Mol Diagn 2021;23(8):952–8.

[22] Pratt VM, Cavallari LH, Del Tredici AL, et al. Recommendations for Clinical CYP2D6 Genotyping Allele Selection: A Joint Consensus Recommendation of the Association for Molecular Pathology, College of American Pathologists, Dutch Pharmacogenetics Working Group of the Royal Dutch Pharmacists Association, and the European Society for Pharmacogenomics and Personalized Therapy. J Mol Diagn 2021;23(9):1047–64.

[23] Mroz P, Michel S, Allen JD, et al. Development and Implementation of In-House Pharmacogenomic Testing Program at a Major Academic Health System. Front Genet 2021;12:712602.

Advances in Molecular Pathology 5 (2022) 131–139
ADVANCES IN MOLECULAR PATHOLOGY

Artificial Intelligence/Machine Learning and Mechanistic Modeling Approaches as Translational Tools to Advance Personalized Medicine Decisions

George A. Mystridis, MSc, MBA[a,b], Fani Chatzopoulou, MSc, PhD[b], George P. Patrinos, PhD[c,*], Ioannis S. Vizirianakis, PhD[a,*]

[a]Laboratory of Pharmacology, School of Pharmacy, Aristotle University of Thessaloniki, Thessaloniki 54124, Greece; [b]Laboratory of Microbiology, School of Medicine, Aristotle University of Thessaloniki, Thessaloniki 54124, Greece; [c]Laboratory of Pharmacogenomics and Individualized Therapy, Department of Pharmacy, School of Health Sciences, University of Patras, GR-26504, Greece

KEYWORDS

• Personalized medicine • Individualized therapy • Machine learning • Artificial intelligence • Pharmacogenomics • Mechanistic modeling

KEY POINTS

- Artificial intelligence/machine learning (ML) and mechanistic modeling offer the required simulation capacity of biological and physiologic processes in order to enhance translational research efforts and advance personalized medicine decisions and patient care.
- ML predictive models are adjustable and account for the molecular heterogeneity of biological systems in real-time, allowing for accuracy and reproducibility in the clinical setting.
- The power in computerized systems allows the clinical implementation of data-driven ML platforms to guide treatment decisions.
- Data-driven ML platforms may be used to affordably implement the information extracted from the biological systems and increase innovation and productivity in the pharmaceutical and health-care sectors.
- Computerized platforms and algorithms allow analysis of vast amounts of health-related biological data beneficial to the advancement of pharmacogenomics and precision medicine interventions and therapeutics.

INTRODUCTION

Every scientific biomedical sector is now witnessing rapidly increasing computing power capacity, thus allowing the simulation and modeling of complex biological processes. Machine learning (ML) and mechanistic modeling consist of different but complementary approaches of mathematical and computational modeling. They now offer the required computational capacity for the simulation of biological and physiologic processes for research efforts that may be translated to therapeutics and the clinical setting. ML algorithms integrate and analyze big data sets, aiming to identify and visualize patterns, trends, and correlations in the data to unveil which biological processes contribute to biological outcomes. Mechanistic models that are based on physiology allow the generation of

*Corresponding authors. *E-mail addresses:* gpatrinos@upatras.gr; ivizir@pharm.auth.gr

https://doi.org/10.1016/j.yamp.2022.06.003
2589-4080/22/

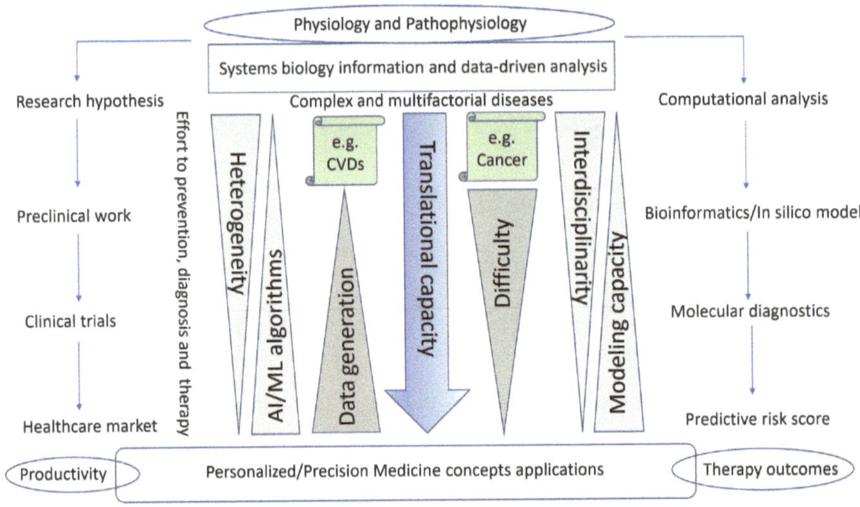

FIG. 1 Impact of AI/ML algorithms implementation and mechanistic modeling on personalized (precision) medicine interventions in health care. The massive information flow and the data derived from systems biology methodologies that are related to physiology and pathophysiology present a challenge in translational research efforts. The application of AI/ML algorithms and the development of predictive simulation models along with mechanistic modeling provide the tools to overcome the issues of complexity, heterogeneity, and multifactorial nature of diseases, such as cancer and CVDs. In this way, both research and the clinical setting are favored in efforts aiming to increase the productivity in health-care research and to improve the therapy outcomes, respectively.

hypotheses, thus contributing new insights on how biological processes cause/produce biological outcomes. Together, between inputs and outputs, mechanistic modeling works toward establishing a mechanistic relationship, whereas ML seeks to create statistical relationships and correlations [1].

The recent increases in power in computerized systems support the implementation of data-driven ML platforms in health care to guide therapeutic decisions, as well as strengthen translational research efforts that aim to affordably implement information extracted from the biological systems in the clinical setting [2]. Artificial intelligence (AI) methodologies and mathematical algorithms drive innovation in the pharmaceutical and health-care sectors by creating a fertile ground for the analysis of vast amounts of health-related biological data beneficial to the advancement of pharmacologic, pharmacogenomic, and personalized (precision) medicine interventions and therapeutics. In fact, for multifactorial diseases, such as cardiovascular disorders (CVDs) and cancer, this approach can be used for the development of effective predictive, diagnostic, and treatment options. Indeed, AI approaches can be used to create practical tools with clinical utility for complex classification, clustering, and predictive modeling tasks in research and the clinical environment. For example, patient management and monitoring have greatly benefited from such AI-based algorithms and practices that use imaging and other clinical markers and have been applied to CVDs [3–6]. These efforts are happening in the current health-care environment where the creation of a framework for CVD risk-stratification using ML data-driven models contributes to noninvasive and more accurate prediction of illnesses, such as severity of coronary artery disease (CAD) [4]. By being able to include pharmacogenomics-related information in these models, personalized therapy management could be achieved for patients [7]. It is also noteworthy that the use of ML platforms and the continuous development of relevant algorithms applied to predictive modeling can facilitate practice improvement for individual practitioners and advance the progression of precision medicine. The impact of AI/ML algorithms and mechanistic modeling when implemented to deliver personalized (precision) medicine interventions in health care is shown diagrammatically in Fig. 1.

Nowadays, the advances in "omics" disciplines, and in nanotechnology provide new clinical and therapeutic directions in the health-care environment. The concept of personalized (precision) medicine is based on the exploitation of molecular knowledge in clinical practice to allow health-care practitioners to more precisely diagnose illnesses and evaluate prognosis, as well as to deliver therapeutics. By working toward the establishment of precision medicine, however, scientists and clinicians face challenging issues in health care. Efforts to achieve practical clinical utility by exploiting a diverse source of information, knowledge, and methodologies are underway to address challenges in implementing precision medicine. Moreover, demonstration of the added value gained by translation of the generated molecular knowledge into the clinical setting to guide personalized therapeutic decisions for patient populations, and/or individual patients is still challenging [2,8–10]. Factors that limit the utilization of molecular knowledge to guide personalized therapeutic decisions for patient populations and/or individual patients are related to the large volume of unstructured data, velocity of data generation, and variability, as well as the lack of clinical validation and inability of some models to accurately predict the associated outcome [6,8,11–13].

Existing heterogeneity within clinical phenotypes contributes to differential pharmacologic response profiles observed in patient populations and limits outcomes and also poses significant societal and economic burdens on the health-care system. This interindividual variability represents the intrinsic capacity of an organism to respond to various environmental stimuli and how biological systems, that are dynamic in nature, behave at the molecular level by adapting and regulating their functions. In fact, by trying to translate the molecular knowledge and to exploit it therapeutically, the experimental approaches used must efficiently address this heterogeneity [2]. This can be done by establishing machine-learning predictive models that are adjustable and account for the molecular heterogeneity of biological systems in real-time. To be implemented, these models must be accurate and reproducible in the clinical setting as well as achieve broad clinical utility, and be compliant with regulatory guidelines worldwide [14].

ARTIFICIAL INTELLIGENCE-BASED AND MACHINE LEARNING-BASED APPROACHES FOR PERSONALIZED CARDIOVASCULAR MEDICINE

The enormous volume of molecular data generated by research efforts requires suitable statistical analysis and proper algorithm development. Additionally, the use of AI and ML approaches in health care must fulfill the ethical considerations that the World Health Organization has recently published to guide their design, development, and clinical implementation [15]. This is particularly necessary in CVDs due to the heterogenous nature of the data that must be correlated to allow the practical utility of clinically relevant information, because the data used in these algorithms are derived from various repositories, for example, chemical, pharmacologic, molecular, clinical, and epidemiologic. In recent years, the exponential increase in computational power has allowed for big data analytical platforms to be applied to diverse dataset collections to generate pattern associations and create predictive models of prognostic, diagnostic and therapeutic value [2,8,14,16]. Incorporation of molecular-level biomarker, or multiomics information, in CVDs coincides with the development of predictive models that may be clinically validated to accurately predict the associated outcome in patient populations and/or individuals [6,12,17,18]. By developing machine-learning platforms as hands-on approaches to precisely predict disease risk in real-time, robust personalized medicine decisions for specific populations, or individual patients, may be reliably made in the clinical setting. Several studies have evaluated the application of predictive machine-learning models to CVDs as compared with traditional predictors, and demonstrated utility of ML approaches in the care of patients suffering from acute coronary syndrome [19] and non-ST–segment elevation myocardial infarction [20]. This approach provided practitioners with a 1-year risk prediction of ischemic and major bleeding events in these patients. Such an application of a ML risk-stratification model has resulted in the improvement of the quality of care of these patients by guiding personalized clinical decision-making [21,22].

In the current health-care environment, the power in computerized systems has allowed the clinical implementation of data-driven ML platforms to guide therapy decisions in the clinical setting. To this end, the management of CVD patients has tremendously benefited from such AI-based algorithms and practices [3,5]. Importantly, the use of ML frameworks requires automated connection of information coming through interfaces from various sources, which also facilitates data availability for practitioners to improve outcomes in their practice. Consequently, the continuous development and application of ML algorithms clearly contributes to the progression of precision cardiovascular medicine. As far as CAD is concerned, ML algorithm approaches have been implemented in the clinical setting to (a) predict the occurrence of obstructive CAD by evaluating multiple clinical variables and the coronary artery calcium score [23]; (b) improve the detection of functionally obstructive CAD [24], as well as to detect lesion-specific ischemia [25] by using computational fluid dynamics algorithms; (c) estimate the pretest probability of CAD [26]; and (d) evaluate the automatic prediction of obstructive CAD from myocardial perfusion imaging [27,28]. To this end, an ML risk-stratification framework was recently published to predict the severity of CAD, as assessed by the SYNTAX score [4]. The SYNTAX score combines anatomic and clinical prognostic variables to predict outcomes in CAD patients and guide the choice between percutaneous coronary intervention and coronary artery bypass graft surgery. Higher scores are associated with more complex or severe disease [29]. In this model, the combination of both classification and regression ML techniques into a unified risk-score assessment process was used to build a 2-stage modeling approach: (1) the zero/nonzero SYNTAX score and (2) the strictly positive SYNTAX score distribution. Using that data-driven ML approach, the model demonstrated that hypertension, diabetes mellitus, and atherogenic index of plasma levels are considered important risk factors for discriminating patients into zero SYNTAX and nonzero SYNTAX score groups. Body mass index, peripheral vascular disease, and diastolic and systolic arterial blood pressure were the significant risk factors for providing an accurate estimation of the expected SYNTAX score and were identified in the second stage. Although this ML model needs further clinical validation, it may contribute to a more personalized approach in the clinical setting by stratifying patients with CVDs to guide therapy via the implementation of automated noninvasive systems that are based on data-driven analytics algorithms [4]. Future studies incorporating genetic and other multiomic data may further add to the existing models that are based primarily on imaging and clinical biomarkers. They may lead to advances in efficacy and safety outcomes through improved selection of medication therapy as well as procedural interventions.

ARTIFICIAL INTELLIGENCE-BASED AND MACHINE LEARNING-BASED APPROACHES FOR PERSONALIZED CANCER MEDICINE

Tumor cell heterogeneity represents a challenge in both research and clinical settings and is considered a major factor in preventing cancer therapeutics from achieving maximum clinical outcomes [2]. It is a well-known established notion that intratumor cell and genome heterogeneity limits the efficacy and safety profiles of therapeutics and is a key contributor to mortality [30]. During therapeutic development, ideally the pharmacologic and translational experimental methodologies would successfully tackle this heterogeneity when identifying phenotype–genotype associations. However, this remains a challenge. Nowadays, patient data are ever increasingly digitized. At the same time, the medical imaging archives/records are growing and the Omics databases are getting bigger. However, the application of powerful approaches to exploit genomics information in large-scale therapeutics-oriented studies, such as genome-wide association studies, have questionable usefulness in predicting clinical phenotypes, although they have been successful in population-based disease-gene discovery correlations [31]. It must be emphasized that big data analytical platforms and the applied computational methodologies (eg, data mining and ML algorithms) allow the manipulation and processing of large and diverse data sets. Their capacity to generate predictive models of pattern associations with prognostic, diagnostic, and therapeutic value has led to high expectations in society for these tools to improve health-care practices worldwide [32,33].

An urgent need for efforts focusing on innovative therapeutic approaches while considering the tumor heterogeneity stands in the frontline of cancer research globally [34]. Recent developments in generating and studying in vitro tumor models that mimic the tumor structure and behavior of cancer cells have enriched our understanding of cell composition, biochemical, and biophysical characteristics of human tumors [35]. This experimental approach allows tumor microenvironment heterogeneity to be pharmacologically investigated and targeted, a fact that empowers therapeutics development. Importantly, ML and mechanistic modeling approaches can further contribute to the prediction of individual tumor growth capacity, thus further advancing personalized cancer therapy decisions. Recently, the combined use of ML and mechanistic modeling has led to accurate predictions of clinical outcomes in human patients with cancer such as gliomas, chronic lymphoblastic leukemia, and ovarian cancer [36]. Moreover, the predictive capacity of the synergistic application of ML and mechanistic modeling has been shown for metastatic relapse in patients with early-stage breast cancer [37]. Moreover, ML methodologies are successfully applied to predict the presence of residual cancer in patients with gynecologic malignancies following hysterectomy [38]. Overall, the implementation of ML and mechanistic modeling in cancer therapy reinforces the use of these tools for the development of individualized treatment care options in patients along with the identification of potential cancer molecular signatures for the development of new and more diverse targeted therapies. The application of ML to such data can provide many different types of clinically relevant information, ranging from the automatic detection of lesions from medical images to their diagnosis and characterization, their grading and staging, as well as a prognosis for the patient and a prediction of the therapeutic response [39,40]. At the same time, mathematical or mechanistic models are constantly being developed to predict the progression and evolution of cancer [41,42]. Such methodologies can now be combined with the predictive capacity of AI and ML in image processing to better understand and predict cancer progression [43].

TACKLING MOLECULAR PATHOLOGY HETEROGENEITY WITH PHYSIOLOGICALLY BASED PHARMACOKINETIC MODELS TO ADVANCE TRANSLATIONAL RESEARCH EFFORTS AND PERSONALIZED MEDICINE DECISIONS

The constant progress made in recent years in quantitative systems pharmacology (QSP) has led to the development and validation of advanced patient-specific predictive simulation models. Physiologically based pharmacokinetic (PBPK) modeling and simulation is an approach that incorporates multiple variables, such as blood flow and tissue composition, to predict the absorption, distribution, metabolism, and excretion of medications and substances. PBPK models have come a long way toward accurately predicting the pharmacokinetic (PK) profiles of many drugs using in vitro in-vivo extrapolation methodologies [44]. Striving to be as mechanistic in nature as possible, they are based on the underlying anatomic, physiologic, and biochemical characteristics of an organism [45] comprised of many physiologically relevant compartments connected through a system of differential equations describing different procedures such as blood flow, and so forth [46]. Over time, these models have integrated more and more physiologically relevant parameters, including but not limited to physiologic, molecular, and genetic information as they have become available. Thus, they can be valuable tools to identify the sources of PK variability and allow extrapolation to different populations, as well as investigating the effects of changing other variables.

A lot of progress has been made in the pharmacodynamic (PD) models as well. PD modeling methodologies can adapt to incorporate many different response systems. Besides the classic receptor-binding action [47], PD models can also predict more complex medication responses such as those from the usage of therapeutic antibodies [48] to the effects of antibiotics on killing bacteria at the site of action/infection [49] to the prediction and management of the immunogenicity of therapeutics [50]. The latter can be useful both for trying to lower the immunogenicity of therapeutic proteins or for maximizing the immunogenicity for vaccines. Coupling PBPK with PD models can be very useful in predicting the pharmacologic response for each individual patient. Such capabilities can be used in different areas ranging from new drug development to drug repurposing, and from stratifying patients by identifying crucial differences in pharmacogenomics (PGx) to personalized dosage selection, realizing the promises of precision medicine. Of note, these models demonstrated their power as drugs were identified to be repurposed as coronavirus disease drugs [51].

Such an approach could be considered as the individual patient "pan-simulation" hands-on approach to precisely predict in real-time the PK/PD behavior of therapeutics in the body [2]. By building a combined PBPK/bioinformatic model, this simulation-based analysis will include key biomarkers, signaling pathways and convergence in the crossroads of molecular knowledge within the patient network.

The datasets to create the individual patient "pan-simulation" avatar model will be based on the: (a) Omics data, (b) PK/PD drug parameters, (c) clinical and laboratory test measurements, and (d) information on environmental and drug interactions. The tremendously increasing power in computing capacity suggests that the generation of a dual PBPK/bioinformatic "pan-simulation" avatar model for individual patients could be achieved in the years to come, provided strategies are developed to maximize both safety and efficacy and that the regulatory environment is developed to account for this type of information. Of note, PBPK modeling along with other QSP approaches was proposed as a way for clinical trials to continue despite the pandemic, which further supports the future possibility of this approach [52].

Linking PBPK with PD models can be used in predicting the impact that many different parameters (eg, genotypic variability, differences in formulation, differences in binding capacity) can have in the response of a drug and its variability among individuals [47]. In fact, massive amounts of data could be generated using such approaches and then be analyzed by ML in order to identify the most crucial factors that affect the observed response, thus enabling changes in prescribing or development of new drugs to increase of the efficacy while minimizing the adverse effects at the same time (Fig. 2).

MACHINE LEARNING-BASED TRANSLATIONAL PHARMACOGENOMICS TOOLS TO ADVANCE PERSONALIZED MEDICINE

Pharmacogenomics focuses on how an individual's genome affects drug efficacy and/or toxicity, aiming to guide drug treatment individualization both in terms of drug regimen and dose, so that it maximizes the clinical benefits and minimizes the risks for the patients. The recent technological advancements in genome sequencing approaches, combined with the development of improved computational methods for the efficient analysis of the vast amount of generated data, have allowed the fast and cost-effective sequencing of a patient's genome, hence expediting its incorporation into routine clinical practice. This approach has catalyzed the development of web-based tools that are used to translate pharmacogenomic variants into a clinically meaningful format [53,54]. However, only a handful of these tools exploit AI/ML to interpret the functional impact of sequence variants, including single nucleotide variants, within genes involved in drug metabolism and transport. In particular, these tools use well-characterized pharmacogenomic variants to train a classifier that would categorize novel variants according to their expected effect on the enzyme functionality. This categorization is based on the available in silico prediction and/or conservation scores, which are selected with the use of a recursive feature elimination process.

We have recently developed such a tool that exploits AI/ML to translate pharmacogenomic information into a clinically meaningful format that uses 4 ML algorithms, namely AdaBoost, XGBoost, Multinomial logistic regression, and Random Forest, of which the performance was assessed through 5-fold cross-validation [55]. In this case, all models achieved similar performance toward making informed conclusions. Importantly, when applied on real-world whole-genome sequencing data from a patient, the tool determined that 2 missense variants were expected to lead to an enzyme of decreased function and 1 variant to enzyme of increased function. Moreover, when data derived from targeted pharmacogene resequencing were used, the tool indicated that 71 variants would lead to enzyme of decrease function, 41 variants of no function, and 1 variant as increased function. For a subset of these variants, the predictions were supported by data available in PharmGKB. This novel tool, as well as other tools using improved prediction algorithms that will be developed in the future, holds promise to lead to extremely efficient variant prioritization and to improve variant classification with significant clinical implications for integrating pharmacogenomics and personalized medicine into routine clinical care.

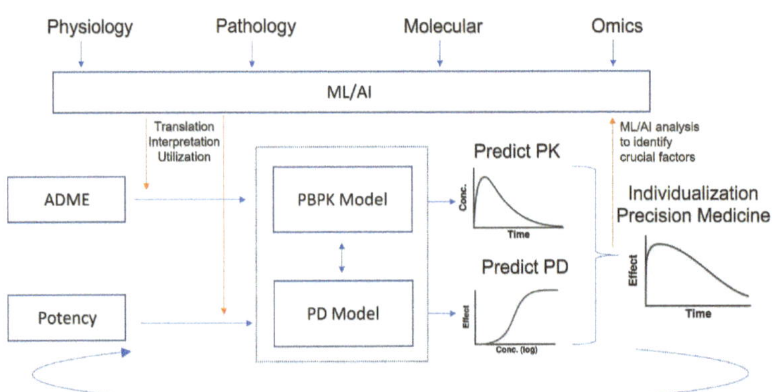

FIG. 2 Interaction between AI/ML algorithms and PBPK/PD modeling. Big data can be analyzed to provide informed input for mechanistic PBPK and PD models. At the same time, big data produced from such models can be analyzed using AI/ML to identify key factors for successful treatment (eg, favorable PK properties).

NEW DRUG DEVELOPMENT AND DRUG REPURPOSING THROUGH THE APPLICATION OF ARTIFICIAL INTELLIGENCE AND MACHINE LEARNING APPROACHES IN DRUG DEVELOPMENT

For a new drug to be a successful candidate, it needs to deliver a therapeutic benefit with minimal adverse effects and be administered at a practical schedule. At the early stages of drug discovery, the PK parameters that would lead to such favorable behavior are not usually known because they depend on many factors. Many of the required physicochemical properties to predict the PK of the drug can be calculated in silico, whereas the quantitative structure-activity relationship approaches can predict the biological effect/outcome. Thus, it is possible to predict the pharmacologic effect of a molecule only by its structure by predicting its PK profile and then using the predicted concentrations over time to predict its effect on the biological system (PD).

This approach can be used in conjunction with ML techniques in a "reverse translation" approach. By generating thousands of such predictions using the aforementioned methodologies a huge amount of data will be produced. Using ML, the data can be analyzed to identify the crucial parameters to obtain the desired effect. This novel approach can be particularly helpful in new drug development, saving a lot of time and money in lead optimization and selection. Such an approach, termed model-based target pharmacology assessment, is used by GlaxoSmithKline [56]. The recent case of the severe acute respiratory syndrome coronavirus 2 (SARS-CoV-2) pandemic has vividly demonstrated the usefulness and need for drug repurposing [57]. The advantages of PBPK modeling are clearly demonstrated in this case, as many simulations have been performed for the repurposing of drugs for SARS-CoV-2 as well as for the study of different aspects of their PKs [58–60].

SUMMARY

Nowadays, the obstacles holding back wider adoption of AI/ML and mechanistic modeling in drug discovery and development as well as in the clinical setting are systematically being dismissed, thus helping scientists to provide solutions faster and with more accuracy and success. In the CVD space, models mostly based on imaging and clinical parameters have demonstrated clinical utility. It is our responsibility to proceed toward improving the implementation processes of these and future models for which the accuracy, reproducibility, and clinical validity have been established in order to facilitate application of AI/ML approaches to the health-care environment and market. These efforts will increase the development and translation of tools to advance personalized medicine and to benefit patient care globally in the years to come.

CLINICS CARE POINTS

- AI/ML approaches provide to the point of care predictive models for disease prognosis, diagnosis, and therapy.
- The mechanistic PBPK modeling increases in the point of care accuracy in drug dosage schemes for specific patient populations.
- AL/ML and mechanistic modeling in the point of care facilitate medical practitioners to achieve improved patient therapy outcomes.
- The adoption of AI/ML methodologies in the point of care helps clinicians to interpret laboratory results better clinically with molecular and genetic information for their patients.
- AI/ML methodologies contribute to the epidemiological analysis to minimize the burden of illnesses and improve the patient quality of life for heterogenous diseases, e.g., CVDs and cancer.
- The adoption of AL/ML techniques and mechanistic modeling in the point of care permit practitioners to achieve quicker multi-specialty clinical decisions as well as handling their patients at real-time with safety and better efficacy.

DISCLOSURE

The authors declare no conflict of interest.

REFERENCES

[1] Baker RE, Pena JM, Jayamohan J, et al. Mechanistic models versus machine learning, a fight worth fighting for the biological community? Biol Lett 2018;14(5). https://doi.org/10.1098/rsbl.2017.0660.

[2] Vizirianakis IS, Miliotou AN, Mystridis GA, et al. Tackling pharmacological response heterogeneity by PBPK modeling to advance precision medicine productivity of nanotechnology and genomics therapeutics. Expert Rev Precision Med Drug Development 2019;4(3): 139–51.

[3] Judd RM. Machine learning in medical imaging: all journeys begin with a single step. JACC Cardiovasc Imaging 2020;13(3):696–8.
[4] Mittas N, Chatzopoulou F, Kyritsis KA, et al. A risk-stratification machine learning framework for the prediction of coronary artery disease severity: insights from the GESS trial. Front Cardiovasc Med 2021;8:812182.
[5] Seetharam K, Brito D, Farjo PD, et al. The role of artificial intelligence in cardiovascular imaging: state of the art review. Front Cardiovasc Med 2020;7:618849.
[6] Silverio A, Cavallo P, De Rosa R, et al. Big health data and cardiovascular diseases: a challenge for research, an opportunity for clinical care. Front Med (Lausanne) 2019;6:36.
[7] Chatzopoulou F, Kyritsis KA, Papagiannopoulos CI, et al. Dissecting miRNA-gene networks to map clinical utility roads of pharmacogenomics-guided therapeutic decisions in cardiovascular precision medicine. Cells 2022; 11(4):607.
[8] Hulsen T, Jamuar SS, Moody AR, et al. From Big Data to Precision Medicine. Front Med (Lausanne) 2019;6:34.
[9] Vizirianakis IS. Nanomedicine and personalized medicine toward the application of pharmacotyping in clinical practice to improve drug-delivery outcomes. Nanomedicine 2011;7(1):11–7.
[10] Vizirianakis IS, Fatouros DG. Personalized nanomedicine: paving the way to the practical clinical utility of genomics and nanotechnology advancements. Adv Drug Deliv Rev 2012;64(13):1359–62.
[11] Bhatt DK, Mehrotra A, Gaedigk A, et al. Age- and Genotype-Dependent Variability in the Protein Abundance and Activity of Six Major Uridine Diphosphate-Glucuronosyltransferases in Human Liver. Clin Pharmacol Ther 2019;105(1):131–41.
[12] Lau E, Wu JC. Omics, big data, and precision medicine in cardiovascular sciences. Circ Res 2018;122(9):1165–8.
[13] Olivera P, Danese S, Jay N, et al. Big data in IBD: a look into the future. Nat Rev Gastroenterol Hepatol 2019; 16(5):312–21.
[14] Ngiam KY, Khor IW. Big data and machine learning algorithms for health-care delivery. Lancet Oncol 2019;20(5): e262–73.
[15] World Health Organization. Ethics and governance of artificial intelligence for health: WHO guidance. World Health Organization; 2021. Available at: https://apps.who.int/iris/handle/10665/341996. Accessed 2021.
[16] Krittanawong C, Johnson KW, Rosenson RS, et al. Deep learning for cardiovascular medicine: a practical primer. Eur Heart J 2019;40(25):2058–73.
[17] Krittanawong C, Zhang H, Wang Z, et al. Artificial intelligence in precision cardiovascular medicine. J Am Coll Cardiol 2017;69(21):2657–64.
[18] Ranka S, Reddy M, Noheria A. Artificial intelligence in cardiovascular medicine. Curr Opin Cardiol 2021; 36(1):26–35.
[19] Gibson WJ, Nafee T, Travis R, et al. Machine learning versus traditional risk stratification methods in acute coronary syndrome: a pooled randomized clinical trial analysis. J Thromb Thrombolysis 2020;49(1):1–9.
[20] Lee W, Lee J, Woo SI, et al. Machine learning enhances the performance of short and long-term mortality prediction model in non-ST-segment elevation myocardial infarction. Sci Rep 2021;11(1):12886.
[21] Fernandez-Ruiz I. Machine learning predicts risk in. ACS *Nat Rev Cardiol* 2021;18(4):230.
[22] D'Ascenzo F, De Filippo O, Gallone G, et al. Machine learning-based prediction of adverse events following an acute coronary syndrome (PRAISE): a modelling study of pooled datasets. Lancet 2021;397(10270): 199–207.
[23] Al'Aref SJ, Maliakal G, Singh G, et al. Machine learning of clinical variables and coronary artery calcium scoring for the prediction of obstructive coronary artery disease on coronary computed tomography angiography: analysis from the CONFIRM registry. Eur Heart J 2020;41(3): 359–67.
[24] Coenen A, Kim YH, Kruk M, et al. Diagnostic accuracy of a machine-learning approach to coronary computed tomographic angiography-based fractional flow reserve: result From the MACHINE consortium. Circ Cardiovasc Imaging 2018;11(6):e007217.
[25] Tang CX, Liu CY, Lu MJ, et al. CT FFR for ischemia-specific CAD with a new computational fluid dynamics algorithm: a chinese multicenter study. JACC Cardiovasc Imaging 2020;13(4):980–90.
[26] Hou ZH, Lu B, Li ZN, et al. Machine learning for pretest probability of obstructive coronary stenosis in symptomatic patients. JACC Cardiovasc Imaging 2019;12(12): 2584–6.
[27] Betancur J, Commandeur F, Motlagh M, et al. Deep learning for prediction of obstructive disease from fast myocardial perfusion SPECT: a multicenter study. JACC Cardiovasc Imaging 2018;11(11):1654–63.
[28] Betancur J, Hu LH, Commandeur F, et al. Deep learning analysis of upright-supine high-efficiency SPECT myocardial perfusion imaging for prediction of obstructive coronary artery disease: a multicenter study. J Nucl Med 2019;60(5):664–70.
[29] Vizirianakis IS, Chatzopoulou F, Papazoglou AS, et al. The GEnetic Syntax Score: a genetic risk assessment implementation tool grading the complexity of coronary artery disease-rationale and design of the GESS study. BMC Cardiovasc Disord 2021;21(1):284.
[30] McGranahan N, Swanton C. Clonal heterogeneity and tumor evolution: past, present, and the future. *Cell.* 2017;168(4):613–28.
[31] Marigorta UM, Rodriguez JA, Gibson G, et al. Replicability and prediction: lessons and challenges from GWAS. Trends Genet 2018;34(7):504–17.
[32] Doudican NA, Kumar A, Singh NK, et al. Personalization of cancer treatment using predictive simulation. J Translational Med 2015;13:43.
[33] Gal J, Milano G, Ferrero JM, et al. Optimizing drug development in oncology by clinical trial simulation:

Why and how? Brief Bioinformatics 2018;19(6): 1203–17.
[34] Mo H, Breitling R, Francavilla C, et al. Data integration and mechanistic modelling for breast cancer biology: Current state and future directions. Curr Opin Endocr Metab Res 2022;24:100350.
[35] Fong ELS, Iyer NG. Next generation in vitro tumor models guiding cancer therapy. Adv Drug Deliv Rev 2021;179:114047.
[36] Mascheroni P, Savvopoulos S, Alfonso JCL, et al. Improving personalized tumor growth predictions using a Bayesian combination of mechanistic modeling and machine learning. Commun Med 2021;1(1):19.
[37] Nicolo C, Perier C, Prague M, et al. Machine learning and mechanistic modeling for prediction of metastatic relapse in early-stage breast cancer. JCO Clin Cancer Inform 2020;4(4):259–74.
[38] Ganguli R, Franklin J, Yu X, et al. Machine learning methods to predict presence of residual cancer following hysterectomy. Sci Rep 2022;12(1):2738.
[39] Cuocolo R, Caruso M, Perillo T, et al. Machine learning in oncology: a clinical appraisal. Cancer Lett 2020;481: 55–62.
[40] Benzekry S. Artificial intelligence and mechanistic modeling for clinical decision making in oncology. Clin Pharmacol Ther 2020;108(3):471–86.
[41] Thomas RM, Van Dyke T, Merlino G, et al. Concepts in cancer modeling: a brief history. Cancer Res 2016; 76(20):5921–5.
[42] Tabassum S, Rosli NB, Binti Mazalan MSA. Mathematical modeling of cancer growth process: a review. J Phys Conf Ser 2019;1366(1):012018.
[43] Zangooei MH, Margolis R, Hoyt K. Multiscale computational modeling of cancer growth using features derived from microCT images. Sci Rep 2021;11(1):18524.
[44] Rostami-Hodjegan A. Reverse translation in PBPK and QSP: going backwards in order to go forward with confidence. Clin Pharmacol Ther 2018;103(2):224–32.
[45] Jones H, Rowland-Yeo K. Basic concepts in physiologically based pharmacokinetic modeling in drug discovery and development. CPT Pharmacometrics Syst Pharmacol 2013;2:e63.
[46] Rowland M, Peck C, Tucker G. Physiologically-based pharmacokinetics in drug development and regulatory science. Annu Rev Pharmacol Toxicol 2011;51(1):45–73.
[47] Chetty M, Rose RH, Abduljalil K, et al. Applications of linking PBPK and PD models to predict the impact of genotypic variability, formulation differences, differences in target binding capacity and target site drug concentrations on drug responses and variability. Front Pharmacol 2014;5:258. https://doi.org/10.3389/fphar.2014.00258.
[48] Tang Y, Cao Y. Modeling pharmacokinetics and pharmacodynamics of therapeutic antibodies: progress, challenges, and future directions. Pharmaceutics 2021; 13(3):422.
[49] Sadiq MW, Nielsen EI, Khachman D, et al. A whole-body physiologically based pharmacokinetic (WB-PBPK) model of ciprofloxacin: a step towards predicting bacterial killing at sites of infection. J Pharmacokinet Pharmacodyn 2017;44(2):69–79.
[50] Kierzek AM, Hickling TP, Figueroa I, et al. A quantitative systems pharmacology consortium approach to managing immunogenicity of therapeutic proteins. CPT Pharmacometrics Syst Pharmacol 2019;8(11):773–6.
[51] Pilla Reddy V, El-Khateeb E, Jo H, et al. Pharmacokinetics under the COVID-19 storm. Br J Clin Pharmacol 2020; 23:14668.
[52] Geerts H, van der Graaf P. A modeling informed quantitative approach to salvage clinical trials interrupted due to COVID-19. Alzheimers Dement (N Y) 2020;6(1): e12053.
[53] Piriyapongsa J, Sukritha C, Kaewprommal P, et al. PharmVIP: A Web-Based Tool for Pharmacogenomic Variant Analysis and Interpretation. J Pers Med 2021; 11(11). https://doi.org/10.3390/jpm11111230.
[54] Bousman CA, Wu P, Aitchison KJ, et al. Sequence2Script: a web-based tool for translation of pharmacogenetic data into evidence-based prescribing recommendations. Front Pharmacol 2021;12. https://doi.org/10.3389/fphar.2021.636650.
[55] Pandi MT, Koromina M, Tsafaridis I, et al. A novel machine learning-based approach for the computational functional assessment of pharmacogenomic variants. Hum Genomics 2021;15(1):51.
[56] Chen EP, Bondi RW, Michalski PJ. Model-based target pharmacology assessment (mTPA): an approach using PBPK/PD modeling and machine learning to design medicinal chemistry and DMPK strategies in early drug discovery. J Med Chem 2021;64(6):3185–96.
[57] Chakraborty C, Sharma AR, Bhattacharya M, et al. The drug repurposing for COVID-19 clinical trials provide very effective therapeutic combinations: lessons learned from major clinical studies. Front Pharmacol 2021;12: 704205.
[58] Cui C, Zhang M, Yao X, et al. Dose selection of chloroquine phosphate for treatment of COVID-19 based on a physiologically based pharmacokinetic model. Acta Pharm Sin B 2020;10(7):1216–27.
[59] Verscheijden LFM, van der Zanden TM, van Bussel LPM, et al. Chloroquine dosing recommendations for pediatric covid-19 supported by modeling and simulation. Clin Pharmacol Ther 2020;108(2):248–52.
[60] Zhang M, Yao X, Hou Z, et al. Development of a physiologically based pharmacokinetic model for hydroxychloroquine and its application in dose optimization in specific COVID-19 patients. Front Pharmacol 2020; 11:585021.

Solid Tumors

Advances in Molecular Pathology 5 (2022) 141–148
ADVANCES IN MOLECULAR PATHOLOGY

Advances in Cell-Free DNA

Elizabeth S. Barrie, PhD*, Andrea Ferreira-Gonzalez, PhD
Department of Pathology, Virginia Commonwealth University Health System, 403 North 13th Street, Room 247, Richmond, VA 23298, USA

KEYWORDS
• Liquid biopsy • Non-invasive cancer monitoring • Non-invasive cancer screening • Solid tumor • Cell-free DNA • Exosomes

KEY POINTS

- Cell-free DNA can aid in detecting and monitoring solid tumors with improved patient safety, turnaround time, and the ability to sample more frequently over time.
- Preanalytic factors significantly impact result quality, and proper sample collection is essential to ensure the best testing outcomes.
- There are several Food and Drug Administration-cleared/approved assays for liquid biopsy of solid tumors across different tumor types and technology.
- Further work is needed to increase the sensitivity of these assays, which could be achieved with the analysis of additional analytes such as exosomes.

SIGNIFICANCE

Biological Basis

Liquid biopsy is a broad term that encompasses analyses involving circulating cell-free DNA (cfDNA), circulating cell-free RNA (cfRNA), circulating tumor cells, and/or exosomes. Following the discovery of cfDNA in 1948 by Mandel and Metais [1], it was understood that this material could be informative in the context of autoimmune disease [2], cancer [3], and pregnancy [4]. After cellular apoptosis, necrosis, or another cellular turnover, DNA is released and can be detected in bodily fluids such as blood, urine, saliva, stool, pleural fluid, cerebrospinal fluid (CSF), or peritoneal fluid. This double-stranded genetic material is generally referred to as circulating cfDNA. While cfDNA is released from both normal and tumor cells, there are typically increased levels of cfDNA in individuals with cancer due to higher cell turnover [5]. cfDNA is fragmented, with a modal size of 167 basepairs [6]. The fragment size is typically smaller in individuals with cancer than in healthy individuals. The cfDNA derived from the tumor is then more specifically referred to as circulating tumor DNA (ctDNA). Of note, the fragment size can also vary by tumor type. Efforts have successfully sorted profiles of the tumor by origin based on the size of the fragments [6,7], albeit with overlap between the categories.

Preanalytic Factors

Proper sample collection is essential to ensure the best testing outcomes. Variability in preanalytic factors can lead to variability in test sensitivity due to sample degradation. A large gauge needle is needed for collection to avoid DNA fragmentation. It is recommended by some that the blood be collected in a tube that stabilizes the fragments. However, these tubes are more expensive and typically made of glass, which poses an increased risk of breakage and sample loss, leading to a need for re-collection. Interestingly, recent studies regarding the short-term processing of liquid biopsies have shown that there might not be significant advantages to using leukocyte lysis-preventive tubes compared with

*Corresponding author, *E-mail address:* Elizabeth.barrie@vcuhealth.org

https://doi.org/10.1016/j.yamp.2022.08.002
2589-4080/22/

Ethylenediaminetetraacetic acid (EDTA) tubes. This is true as long as the storage and transport of the samples are carried out at low temperatures and do not exceed 48 hours [8–11]. While others suggest that if an EDTA tube is used, the specimen should be processed within 6 hours of collection [12], which may be challenging to implement for many centers. Adequate sample volume, which provides sufficient DNA yield, is vital for optimal sensitivity. A higher volume may be required for minimal residual disease monitoring.

The extraction, purification, and enrichment methods need to be tailored to the clinical setting. A recent review asserts that the preferred specimen for ctDNA testing is plasma from a cell stabilization tube kept at room temperature and cfDNA extracted with a bead-based method [12]. Although more DNA is present in the serum, there is a higher proportion of ctDNA in the plasma; therefore, this is the preferred fraction [12]. Due to fragment size variation between specimens from healthy individuals and those with cancer, enrichment for a target fragment size with higher levels of mutant ctDNA could improve sensitivity. One study, specific to double stranded DNA (dsDNA) extracted from plasma specimens across multiple tumor types, found enriching for 2 cell populations, fragments 90 to 150 bp as well as 250 to 320 bp, yielded maximum enrichment of ctDNA [6].

Test Metrics/Characteristics

When evaluating the utility and application for this test, liquid biopsy will have different performance metrics (sensitivity, specificity, positive predictive value [PPV], negative predictive value[NPV]) when compared to standard sequencing of a tissue biopsy specimen. Liquid biopsy has the advantage of being less invasive and more convenient; however, there is a trade-off for decreased sensitivity when using standard techniques. Conversely, liquid biopsy allows more frequent sampling and decreased testing intervals. Of note, there are challenges in establishing a set value for the sensitivity of an assay as this will vary significantly depending on the tumor burden in each patient, as well as the type of primary tumor, as both these factors influence the total amount of ctDNA present in each specimen.

There may be different requirements/standards for a diagnostic specimen compared to monitoring for residual disease. During initial diagnosis, distinguishing tumor signal from white blood cell signal is vital. Clonal hematopoiesis of indeterminate potential (CHIP) describes genetic changes in the blood due to aging but are not typically associated with neoplasm. Since myeloid-derived variants are detected in liquid biopsy and account for most variants detected in patients with cancer, separating these patterns is important to ensure only signal from tumor cells is encompassed in the signature for monitoring [13]. One mechanism to adjust for this is the sequencing of white blood cells using a paired whole-blood control, including additional sequencing data beyond that derived solely from plasma aids in interpreting variants detected in the liquid biopsy. Mutations seemingly derived from the tumor may be CHIP-associated changes and, without paired testing, could be reported as false positives.

Laboratory Techniques

A variety of approaches are available, with different molecular techniques available to answer these questions. For example, one can monitor single, more common mutations (such as in the epidermal growth factor receptor gene *EGFR* in lung), create a personalized profile, or use an agnostic whole-exome approach. To create a personalized profile, submission of a diagnostic, treatment-naive specimen from both the tumor and a blood specimen is most informative. Having a known profile of mutations detectable in the diagnostic specimen(s) is beneficial for monitoring and decreases false negatives. A negative result in a follow-up specimen has different implications depending on diagnostic testing results. For example, if the diagnostic specimen had no observed mutations, this would not be a beneficial test to use for monitoring.

Conversely, suppose the mutations initially detected in the diagnostic specimen are no longer detectable. In that case, this suggests that the treatment is effective at decreasing the tumor burden, at least below the limit of detection of the assay. When using a personalized profile and a targeted approach for monitoring, it is possible that not every mutation is identified; however, if at least one can be tracked, this can be informative.

Liquid biopsy can be applied to 2 main groups of assays: NGS and targeted polymerase chain reaction (PCR). The advantage of targeted PCR is increased sensitivity. However, these assays can only detect known, previously detected mutations, and prior knowledge is required. Conversely, NGS can provide important phasing data that may not be evident from PCR. For example, EGFR resistance mutations p.T790M and p.C797S are close enough that NGS reads can determine if multiple EGFR resistance mutations are in *cis* (together on the same read/chromosome) or in *trans* (on the other copy of the gene). Their orientation will inform therapy options and efficacy [14]. This is not possible with targeted PCR for single mutations.

There is a high concordance between mutational profiles from cfDNA sequencing and tumor sequencing when analyzing metastatic tumors [15]; however, tumor shedding of ctDNA is different among different tumor types, as discussed in the next section.

Clinical applications

Randomized clinical trials are needed to demonstrate the clinical utility of this testing for many tumor types and guide how liquid biopsy results should be used and interpreted to inform clinical practice. Several studies are currently underway. Feasibility studies such as that of Lennon and colleagues [16] have shown promise, leading to a clinical trial (NCT04213326) which has completed enrollment, but the data have not been published at the time of writing of this chapter.

Across tumor types, an advantage of liquid biopsy is improved detection of mutations independent of tumor heterogeneity compared to a traditional tumor biopsy. In 2020, companion diagnostics were approved for use in non-small-cell lung cancer (NSCLC), prostate, ovarian, and breast cancer using real-time PCR and NGS methods (Table 1).

Bladder Cancer

Until recently, most monitoring techniques in bladder cancer (BC) have focused on urine-based biomarkers to reduce or even avoid the complications and the discomfort related to multiple cystoscopies and, simultaneously, provide a safe, readily available diagnostic method in the detection and surveillance of BC. However, the urine is a dynamic body fluid; therefore, the concentrations of potential biomarkers could vary with hydration status, renal pathologies, and the effect of medications. As a result, a high degree of variability is still possible. The limitations of urine-based biomarkers related to sensitivity and specificity are highlighted in the case of lower clinical stages (0a, 0is, and 1), thus partially limiting the use of urinary biomarkers in recurrence detection.

A unique advantage of blood-based biomarkers in patients with BC is they can be used after cystectomy since urinary biomarkers could not be used [17]. A recent systematic evidence review reported some genes as common targets tested across multiple studies; however, these were a combination of somatic sequence changes and methylation differences. They also suggest changes in microRNA (miRNA) may be a useful biomarker, which is more abundant in the serum [18]. For future tests, methylation and miRNA studies on serum may be beneficial in patients with BC. In the current National Comprehensive Cancer Network (NCCN) guidelines (v1.2022), there is no specific mention or direction regarding liquid biopsy in BC [19]. Several clinical trials are currently underway to evaluate the clinical utility of ctDNA in the management of advanced BC (eg, NCT02053662, NCT00962052, NCT02546661, NCT03563443, NCT01198808, NCT02177695; Clinical Trials.gov). One recent study addressing biomarker-guided treatment selection in patients with metastatic BC found similar mutational profiles between tissue and paired ctDNA, indicating that ctDNA could be used to guide patient treatment selection in patients that lack tissue specimens for genomic characterization [20].

Brain Tumors

The detection rate of ctDNA for gliomas and medulloblastomas is low, and the quantity of mutant fragments present in samples from these patients is significantly lower than that in other tumors [7]. This makes brain tumors challenging to detect using standard liquid biopsy methods [8]. Due to the interference of the blood-brain barrier in ctDNA crossing to the blood, CSF is a potential alternative in these cases [21,22]. The use of CSF decreases the background signal in the blood due to the reduced number of other cell types present in this fluid [23] although the levels of ctDNA present in the CSF vary by tumor location and may be affected by tumor heterogeneity [24]. Still, the diagnosis would need to be established (no screening method available), and this specimen type validated separately.

Breast Cancer

Most genetic tests for tumor prognosis in breast cancer focus on *HER2* (*ERBB2*). Due to the availability of targeted therapy, more recently, *PIK3CA* mutations have also become an important biomarker. The Food and Drug Administration (FDA) recently approved the therascreen PIK3CA RGQ PCR companion diagnostic test to detect PIK3CA mutations in both tissue and liquid biopsies to identify patients eligible for targeted therapies. The current NCCN guidelines for breast cancer (v2.2022) suggest that HR-positive/HER-2-negative metastatic breast cancers be assessed for *PIK3CA* mutations [25]. It also states explicitly that this may be done using either tumor tissue or liquid biopsy (ctDNA from peripheral blood). However, if the liquid biopsy is negative, reflex testing of the tumor tissue is recommended. Of note, this is specifically for diagnostic testing for advanced breast cancer that has failed hormonal therapy and not for monitoring residual disease. Liquid biopsies in breast cancer have yielded cautiously promising results thus far, and the outlook remains encouraging. With time and prospective clinical trials, liquid

TABLE 1
FDA clearance/approvals for cancer liquid biopsy of solid tumors

FDA-Approved/Cleared Assays	Indications
CELLSEARCH	Circulating tumor cell (CTC) test with prognosis indication for colon, prostate, and breast. 2007
Epi proColon	cfDNA Plasma test identifies epigenetic markers used for colorectal cancer screening. 2016
cobas EGFR mutation test v2. qPCR	cfDNA Plasma companion diagnostic test to aid in treatment selection for targeted therapies in NSCLC patients. 2016
therascreen PIK3CA RGQ qPCR	cfDNA Plasma companion diagnostic test to identify advanced breast cancer patients who may be eligible for treatment with targeted therapy. 2019
Guardant 360 CDx NGS	cfDNA Plasma companion diagnostic test for identifying NSCLC patients eligible for targeted therapies, those with EGFR mutations for treatment with osimertinib, and those with KRAS G12 C mutations for treatment with sotorasib. 2020
FoundationOne Liquid CDx NGS	cfDNA Plasma companion diagnostic test to identify eligible patients for treatment with targeted therapies in NSCLC, prostate, ovarian, and breast cancer. 2020

biopsy could play an even more significant role in the breast cancer clinic.

Colon Cancer

In colon cancer's pathology and molecular workup process, the current NCCN guidelines (v1.2022) now include both blood and formalin-fixed paraffin-embedded (FFPE) tissue as acceptable sample types for diagnosis and prognosis. However, FFPE, if available, is still preferred [26]. They also state that NGS is beneficial in detecting rare mutations which may be actionable. Studies have shown that analysis of ctDNA has a prognostic impact on colon cancer after surgery and chemotherapy as well as response to molecularly targeted drugs [27–29]. Some of these assays require diagnostic sequencing of the primary tumor tissue to develop a patient-specific mutation profile that can then be used for monitoring residual or metastatic disease with liquid biopsy, also referred to as a tumor-informed approach. A recent National Cancer Institute (NCI) consensus statement provides detailed recommendations on integrating ctDNA into care for patients with colorectal cancer [30]. A systematic evidence review determined that most publications assessed found that the presence of ctDNA detected by liquid biopsy was associated with decreased survival in patients with colorectal cancer. However, like with other tumor types, the authors caution that laboratory standardization, especially with preanalytical variables, is vital [31]. Multiple ongoing trials will provide additional insights regarding the application and utility of this testing, especially for minimal residual disease (MRD) monitoring [32].

Liquid biopsy is gaining momentum as a way to screen for certain tumors at very early stages. Multiple commercial assays are available to aid with colon cancer screening and/or detection. Epi proColon (Polymedco, Cortlandt Manor, NY) was given FDA approval for colon cancer screening in those at the average risk age of 50 years or above and for those "unwilling or unable to be screened by recommended methods." The Epi proColon works by detecting methylated SEPT9. This assay has also overcome billing and reimbursement challenges, as the Centers for Medicare and Medicaid Services recognize CPT code 81,327 [33]. They do note the following caveats: Positive results are not diagnostic and need to be followed with colonoscopy, and false positive results increase with age.

GIST

Gastrointestinal stromal tumors (GISTs) are tumors of mesenchymal origin arising in the gastrointestinal tract and constituting the most common subtype of sarcomas. Genetic changes often involve *KIT* and/or *PDGFRA*, which are essential drivers of GIST progression throughout all stages of the disease. Significantly, *KIT/PDGFRA* genotype predicts response to imatinib. Despite the high initial activity of imatinib as a first-line agent, most patients will eventually progress in 20 to 24 months since treatment initiation. GISTs have low DNA shedding, which can be challenging for the detection of localized disease, leading to lower assay sensitivity, but they can be advantageous when positive. In contrast, metastatic and particularly imatinib-resistant GISTs have increased ctDNA shedding with higher mutated allele fractions, which has been associated with tumor burden and improved ctDNA detection [34–36]. The use of liquid biopsy as a diagnostic tool for GISTs remains challenging, especially considering the wide variety of *KIT* primary mutations. These limitations also apply to using ctDNA as a biomarker for early detection of tumor relapse after GIST surgery and/or adjuvant imatinib. Based on GIST clinical behavior and biology, the major promise for this tumor type would be implementing ctDNA-based therapeutic decisions in imatinib-resistant disease through serial monitoring of clonal evolution.

Lung Cancer

There are multiple FDA-approved tests for liquid biopsy applications in patients with advanced NSCLC. EGFR sensitizing mutations detected using PCR on the companion diagnostic Roche cobas assay are eligible to be treated with Tarceva (erlotinib) (see Table 1). Next, approval was given to use a liquid biopsy test to detect the EGFR T790M resistance mutation on the Roche cobas for treatment with osimertinib or Tagrisso, when a tumor biopsy could not be obtained. Two commercially available plasma-based NGS assays have recently received FDA approval to assess solid tumors, including NSCLC for molecularly targeted drugs (see Table 1). There is a growing number of guideline-recommended biomarkers to be evaluated in advanced NSCLC, which poses significant challenges in tumor tissue adequacy for complete tissue genotyping, making plasma ctDNA testing with a clinically validated NGS platform highly desirable in treatment-naïve patients and those with multiple mechanisms of acquired resistance. The choice of tumor tissue genotyping or liquid biopsy, either sequentially or concurrently, should be individualized based on patient disease characteristics and expected results. An emerging body of literature supports both approaches simultaneously to increase identification rates of relevant targetable biomarkers. The concurrent approach seems practical and a reasonable option with small tumor biopsies or fine-needle-aspiration specimens with uncertain adequacy for tumor genotyping despite the not negligible caveat of high cost of this approach. At the time of acquired resistance after tyrosine kinase inhibitor therapy, ctDNA can be used to evaluate the resistance mechanism. Providers should consider retesting with a tissue biopsy in the case of a negative result. Given the ease of serial sampling, ctDNA is also emerging as a preferred method for real-time monitoring of response to treatment.

The following validation and methodology questions are to be answered by the individual testing laboratory:

- What are the required specimen types and storage conditions? Will one be indicated as preferred and others still accepted? Additional validation needed for exceptions (longer transit time, different tube type) and additional disclaimers (such as decreased sensitivity)?
- Will specimens need to be transported by a local courier or shipped across the country?
- Initial processing to use serum or plasma?
- Is there another more informative specimen type other than blood (such as CSF)?
- Will analysis be restricted to sequence changes in the DNA, or will methylation signatures and/or cfRNA be analyzed?
- Will additional size selection be performed to increase the proportion of tumor DNA in the sample? Will a size selection be performed using bioinformatics methods?
- Will a paired whole blood sample also be sequenced as a control to aid interpretation?
- Will single common mutations be tested, or will a personalized profile be created for each patient? For NGS, which error-correction method will be used? Will NGS or targeted PCR be used?
- Which tumor types are validated? How many of each need to be tested?
- Can this only be used for initial diagnosis in symptomatic patients or appropriate as screening? For disease monitoring, when should tumor biopsy be used?

Factors to improve sensitivity include standardization of storage and collection conditions that minimize fragmentation and degradation, deeper sequencing, use of error correction (in silico and/or experimentally), testing of advanced-stage tumors, testing of tumor types with increased shedding, and inclusion of additional analytes (discussed in the next section).

Present Relevance and Future Avenues to Consider

Surgical tissue biopsies are still considered the gold standard for diagnosing and treating solid tumors. Still, molecular profiling testing has increased because of its clinical utility in guiding treatment decisions and outcome-based predictions. Furthermore, this approach does not consider tumor heterogeneity, critical for evaluating therapeutic options based on the patient's tumor biomarker profiling. It is well accepted that various tumor parts can present a related but different genetic profile. Moreover, the tumor's molecular makeup can evolve dynamically because of clonal selection under treatment pressure and microenvironmental stimuli, rendering future therapeutic decisions based on historical tissue biopsy suboptimal. Another major caveat is that tissue is not always available for molecular testing. Surgical biopsy procedures may be limited by accessibility, repeatability, clinical status, age, cost, and potential to cause clinical complications. These constraints of tissue biopsy and the paradigm shift to include molecular analysis have begun a transition to molecular profiling of biofluids. Measuring biofluids offers a significant advantage as it is less invasive and can provide a real-time state of tumor status. The ease of use of liquid biopsies can benefit patients over time, even at a lower sensitivity than the gold standard tissue test.

Most efforts to develop liquid biopsy tests have focused on circulating tumor cells and ctDNA. Despite the progress, 1 limitation of this approach is that it relies on a single type of analyte, ctDNA, to be present in sufficient quantities for analysis. Some studies indicate that detecting ctDNA-derived mutations requires impractically large input volumes of plasma to allow for adequate numbers of ctDNA-derived mutations. It is imperative to increase the sensitivity of these assays, which could be achieved by analyzing additional analytes such as exosomes.

Exosomes and other extracellular vesicular particles present an exciting complement to ctDNA and could improve traditional liquid biopsies for better diagnostic performance. Exosomes are released continuously by all living cells, providing a broad range of content as they contain DNA, RNA, and protein. The difference in how ctDNA and exosomes are released from cells suggests that exosomes provide information about living tumor cells. One could envision that it could lead to early lesion detection. Detection of mutations in RNA present in exosomes can be added to the findings from ctDNA to increase the sensitivity of mutation detection. Furthermore, a multianalyte approach could improve sensitivity for these assays [37]. Studies have shown that combining cfDNA with exosomal RNA is advantageous over cfDNA analysis alone [38,39]. The unique composition of the exosome compartment makes these vesicles particularly amenable for multianalyte analysis. They carry many informative cancer molecules such as DNA, RNA, protein, lipids, oligosaccharides, and metabolites with the ability to be evaluated simultaneously. Improvements in technology for analyzing tumor-derived exosomes should bring robust and content-rich cancer diagnostics to the forefront.

A recent novel approach is monitoring cancer and potential infection through liquid biopsy. Using plasma DNA sequencing, a proof-of-principle study was able to monitor acute lymphoblastic leukemia relapse and detect microbes that could become problematic in these patients with suppressed immune systems [40].

SUMMARY

Cell-free ctDNA presents an opportunity to expand our tools to detect and monitor solid tumors that significantly benefit patients. Studies have confirmed the promising roles of liquid biopsy in solid tumors. In the past decade, various biomarkers detected in liquid biopsies in cancers have been useful in multiple areas, including diagnosis, prognosis prediction, monitoring of therapy, and even early cancer detection. However, this testing presents additional complexities. Preanalytic factors must be monitored and controlled for best results. While there are several FDA-approved assays, further studies are needed across tumor types. The practical clinical applications of these biomarkers have limitations. One of the reasons for this challenge is that most of the studies on the potential application of these biomarkers have had a relatively small number of patients. Therefore, there is a need for larger, multicenter, and, more importantly, prospective clinical validation trials to understand the clinical implications of clinical decision-making. To improve the sensitivity of these assays, advancing technology needs to be applied. Decreasing sequencing costs may allow for deeper sequencing. Also, new error-correction algorithms may be developed to improve sensitivity. The inclusion of exosomes in the analysis is another possible approach.

CLINICS CARE POINTS

- Cell-free ctDNA presents an opportunity to expand our tools to detect and monitor solid tumors with significant benefit to patients. Various biomarkers detected in liquid biopsies have been helpful in multiple areas, including diagnosis, prognosis, monitoring, and even early cancer detection.
- NCCN guidelines now include blood and formalin-fixed paraffin-embedded (FFPE) tissue as acceptable sample types for a subset of tumor types. However, FFPE, if available, is still preferred.

- There are multiple FDA-approved tests for liquid biopsy applications in patients with different types of advanced cancer.
- Some of the challenges in applying liquid biopsy have been due to limited data in previous studies. Therefore, there is a need for large, multicenter, prospective clinical trials to understand the advantages and limitations of this testing and what the best applications are moving forward

DISCLOSURE

The authors have nothing to disclose.

REFERENCES

[1] Mandel P, Metais P. Les acides nucléiques du plasma sanguin chez l'homme [Nuclear Acids In Human Blood Plasma]. C R Seances Soc Biol Fil 1948;142(3–4):241–3, PMID: 18875018.

[2] Tan EM, Schur PH, Carr RI, et al. Deoxyribonucleic acid (DNA) and antibodies to DNA in the serum of patients with systemic lupus erythematosus. J Clin Invest 1966;45:1732–40, PMID: 4959277.

[3] Leon SA, Shapiro B, Sklaroff DM, et al. Free DNA in the serum of cancer patients and the effect of therapy. Cancer Res 1977;37:646–50, PMID: 837366.

[4] Lo YM, Corbetta N, Chamberlain PF, et al. Presence of fetal DNA in maternal plasma and serum. Lancet 1997;350:485–7.

[5] Fiorentino F, Bono S, Pizzuti F, et al. The importance of determining the limit of detection of non-invasive prenatal testing methods. Prenat Diagn 2016;36(4):304–11, Epub 2016 Feb 21. PMID: 26815144.

[6] Mouliere F, Chandrananda D, Piskorz AM, et al. Enhanced detection of circulating tumor DNA by fragment size analysis. Sci Transl Med 2018;10(466):eaat4921, PMID: 30404863.

[7] Bettegowda C, Sausen M, Leary RJ, et al. Detection of circulating tumor DNA in early- and late-stage human malignancies. Sci Transl Med 2014;6(224):224ra24, PMID: 24553385.

[8] Gerber T, Taschner-Mandl S, Saloberger-Sindhöringer L, et al. Assessment of pre-analytical sample handling conditions for comprehensive liquid biopsy analysis. J Mol Diagn 2020;22(8):1070–86, Epub 2020 Jun 1. PMID: 32497717.

[9] Johansson G, Andersson D, Filges S, et al. Considerations and quality controls when analyzing cell-free tumor DNA. Biomol Detect Quantif 2019;17:100078, PMID: 30906693.

[10] Markus H, Contente-Cuomo T, Farooq M, et al. Evaluation of pre-analytical factors affecting plasma DNA analysis. Sci Rep 2018;8(1):7375.

[11] Nikolaev S, Lemmens L, Koessler T, et al. Circulating tumoral DNA: preanalytical validation and quality control in a diagnostic laboratory. Circulating tumoral DNA: Preanalytical validation and quality control in a diagnostic laboratory. Anal Biochem 2018;542:34–9, Epub 2017 Nov 11. PMID: 29137972.

[12] Merker JD, Oxnard GR, Compton C, et al. Circulating Tumor DNA Analysis in Patients With Cancer: American Society of Clinical Oncology and College of American Pathologists Joint Review. J Clin Oncol 2018;36(16):1631–41, Epub 2018 Mar 5. PMID: 29504847.

[13] Razavi P, Li BT, Brown DN, et al. High-intensity sequencing reveals the sources of plasma circulating cell-free DNA variants. Nat Med 2019;25(12):1928–37, PMID: 31768066.

[14] Leonetti A, Sharma S, Minari R, et al. Resistance mechanisms to osimertinib in EGFR-mutated non-small cell lung cancer. Br J Cancer 2019;121(9):725–37, Epub 2019 Sep 30. PMID: 31564718.

[15] Adalsteinsson VA, Ha G, Freeman SS, et al. Scalable whole-exome sequencing of cell-free DNA reveals high concordance with metastatic tumors. Nat Commun 2017;8(1):1324, PMID: 29109393.

[16] Lennon AM, Buchanan AH, Kinde I, et al. Feasibility of blood testing combined with PET-CT to screen for cancer and guide intervention. Science 2020;369(6499):eabb9601, Epub 2020 Apr 28. PMID: 32345712.

[17] Ellinger J, El Kassem N, Heukamp LC, et al. Hypermethylation of cell-free serum DNA indicates worse outcome in patients with bladder cancer. J Urol 2008;179:346–52, PMID: 18006010.

[18] Khetrapal P, Lee MWL, Tan WS, et al. The role of circulating tumour cells and nucleic acids in blood for the detection of bladder cancer: A systematic review. Cancer Treat Rev 2018;66:56–63, Epub 2018 Apr 17. PMID: 29684744.

[19] National Comprehensive Cancer Network. Bladder Cancer (Version 1.2022). https://www.nccn.org/professionals/physician_gls/pdf/bladder.pdf. [Accessed 3 May 2022].

[20] Agarwal N, Pal SK, Hahn AW, et al. Characterization of metastatic urothelial carcinoma via comprehensive genomic profiling of circulating tumor DNA. Cancer 2018;124:2115–24, Epub 2018 Mar 8. PMID: 29517810.

[21] Mouliere F, Mair R, Chandrananda D, et al. Detection of cell-free DNA fragmentation and copy number alterations in cerebrospinal fluid from glioma patients. EMBO Mol Med 2018;10(12):e9323.

[22] Miller AM, Shah RH, Pentsova EI, et al. Tracking tumour evolution in glioma through liquid biopsies of cerebrospinal fluid. Nature 2019;565(7741):654–8, Epub 2019 Jan 23. PMID: 30675060.

[23] Pentsova EI, Shah RH, Tang J, et al. Evaluating cancer of the central nervous system through next-generation sequencing of cerebrospinal fluid. J Clin Oncol 2016;34:2404–15, PMID: 27161972.

[24] Wang Y, Springer S, Zhang M, et al. Detection of tumor-derived DNA in cerebrospinal fluid of patients with primary tumors of the brain and spinal cord. Proc Natl Acad Sci 2015;112(31):9704–9, Epub 2015 Jul 20. PMID: 26195750.

[25] National Comprehensive Cancer Network. Breast Cancer (Version 2.2022). https://www.nccn.org/professionals/physician_gls/pdf/breast.pdf. [Accessed 3 May 2022].

[26] National Comprehensive Cancer Network. Colon Cancer (Version 1.2022). https://www.nccn.org/professionals/physician_gls/pdf/colon.pdf. [Accessed 3 May 2022].

[27] Tie J, Cohen JD, Wang Y, et al. Circulating Tumor DNA Analyses as Markers of Recurrence Risk and Benefit of Adjuvant Therapy for Stage III Colon Cancer. JAMA Oncol 2019;5(12):1710–7.

[28] Reinert T, Henriksen TV, Christensen E, et al. Analysis of Plasma Cell-Free DNA by Ultradeep Sequencing in Patients With Stages I to III Colorectal Cancer. JAMA Oncol 2019;5(8):1124–31.

[29] Henriksen TV, Tarazona N, Frydendahl A, et al. Circulating Tumor DNA in Stage III Colorectal Cancer, beyond Minimal Residual Disease Detection, toward Assessment of Adjuvant Therapy Efficacy and Clinical Behavior of Recurrences. Clin Cancer Res 2022;28(3):507–17, Epub 2021 Oct 8. PMID: 34625408.

[30] Dasari A, Morris VK, Allegra CJ, et al. ctDNA applications and integration in colorectal cancer: an NCI Colon and Rectal-Anal Task Forces whitepaper. Nat Rev Clin Oncol 2020;17(12):757–70, Epub 2020 Jul 6. PMID: 32632268.

[31] Vymetalkova V, Cervena K, Bartu L, et al. Circulating Cell-Free DNA and Colorectal Cancer: A Systematic Review. Int J Mol Sci 2018;19(11):3356.

[32] Bent A, Raghavan S, Dasari A, et al. The Future of ctDNA-Defined Minimal Residual Disease: Personalizing Adjuvant Therapy in Colorectal Cancer. Clin Colorectal Cancer 2022;21(2):89–95, Online ahead of print. PMID: 35450837.

[33] Epi proColon. https://www.epiprocolon.com/us/laboratories/coding-and-reimbursement. [Accessed 3 May 2022].

[34] Serrano C, Vivancos A, López-Pousa A, et al. Clinical value of next generation sequencing of plasma cell-free DNA in gastrointestinal stromal tumors. BMC Cancer 2020;20(1):99, PMID: 32024476.

[35] Namløs HM, Boye K, Mishkin SJ, et al. Non-invasive Detection of ctDNA Reveals Intratumor Heterogeneity and Is Associated with Tumor Burden in Gastrointestinal Stromal Tumor. Mol Cancer Ther 2018;17(11):2473–80, Epub 2018 Aug 10. PMID: 30097488.

[36] Ravegnini G, Sammarini G, Serrano C, et al. Clinical relevance of circulating molecules in cancer: focus on gastrointestinal stromal tumors. Ther Adv Med Oncol 2019;11: 1758835919831902.

[37] Cohen JD, Li L, Wang Y, et al. Detection and localization of surgically resectable cancers with a multianalyte blood test. Science 2018;359(6378):926–30, Epub 2018 Jan 18. PMID: 29348365.

[38] Krug AK, Enderle D, Karlovich C, et al. Improved EGFR mutation detection using combined exosomal RNA and circulating tumor DNA in NSCLC patient plasma. Ann Oncol 2018;29(10):2143.

[39] Castellanos-Rizaldos E, Grimm DG, Tadiglota V, et al. Exosomes-based detection of EGFR T790M in plasma from non-small cell lung cancer patients. Clin Cancer Res 2018; 24(12):2944–50, Epub 2018 Mar 13. PMID: 29535126.

[40] Barsan V, Xia Y, Klein D, et al. Simultaneous monitoring of disease and microbe dynamics through plasma DNA sequencing in pediatric patients with acute lymphoblastic leukemia. Sci Adv 2022;8(16):eabj1360, Epub 2022 Apr 20. PMID: 35442732.